BIOSIGNAL PROCESSING

PRINCIPLES AND PRACTICES

BIOSIGNAL PROCESSING
PRINCIPLES AND PRACTICES

Edited by
Hualou Liang
Joseph D. Bronzino
Donald R. Peterson

CRC Press
Taylor & Francis Group
Boca Raton London New York

CRC Press is an imprint of the
Taylor & Francis Group, an **informa** business

First published 2013 by CRC Press

Published 2019 by CRC Press
Taylor & Francis Group
6000 Broken Sound Parkway NW, Suite 300
Boca Raton, FL 33487-2742

Version Date: 20120608

ISBN-13: 978-1-4398-7143-0 (hbk)

Library of Congress Cataloging-in-Publication Data

Biosignal processing : principles and practices / edited by Hualou Liang, Joseph D. Bronzino, and Donald R. Peterson.
p. ; cm.
Includes bibliographical references and index.
ISBN 978-1-4398-7143-0 (hardcover : alk. paper)
I. Liang, Hualou II. Bronzino, Joseph D., 1937- III. Peterson, Donald R.
[DNLM: 1. Brain Mapping. 2. Brain--physiology. 3. Brain Waves--physiology. 4. Electrodiagnosis--methods. 5. Nervous System Physiological Phenomena. 6. Signal Processing, Computer-Assisted. WL 335]

612.8'2--dc23 2012022198

Visit the Taylor & Francis Web site at
http://www.taylorandfrancis.com

and the CRC Press Web site at
http://www.crcpress.com

Contents

Preface

Biosignal processing has been around for decades, but it still seems to be growing in popularity. With the rise of advanced computerized data collection systems, monitoring devices, and instrumentation technologies, large and complex datasets simply accrue as an inevitable part of biomedical enterprise. The availability of large quantities of biomedical data not only offers unprecedented opportunities to advance our understanding of the underlying biological and physiologic functions, structures, and dynamics but also drives tremendous progress toward innovative methods in biosignal processing. As such, this field has advanced to a conspicuous stage that biosignal processing has become an integral part in all phases of biomedical research and development.

The purpose of this book is to provide state-of-the-art coverage of contemporary methods in biosignal processing with an emphasis on brain signal analysis. The first two chapters in this book present fundamental aspects of biomedical signal processing, which should be accessible to the general audience. Chapter 1 provides a general overview of basic concepts in biomedical signal acquisition and processing, whereas Chapter 2 deals with the nonstationary and transient nature of signals by introducing time–frequency analysis and discusses its applications to signal analysis and detection problems in bioengineering.

The next four chapters address emerging methods for brain signal processing, each focusing on specific noninvasive imaging techniques such as electroencephalography (EEG), magnetoencephalography (MEG), magnetic resonance imaging (MRI), and functional near-infrared spectroscopy (fNIR). Chapter 3 covers a multivariate spectral analysis of EEG data using power, coherence, and second-order blind identification. Chapter 4 introduces a general linear modeling approach for the analysis of induced and evoked responses in MEG. Chapter 5 presents the progress in groupwise registration algorithms for effective MRI medical image analysis. Chapter 6 describes the basis of optical imaging, fNIR instrumentation, and signal analysis in various cognitive studies.

Chapter 7 reviews recent advances of causal influence measures such as the Granger causality for analyzing multivariate neural data. For basic applications, the emphasis is on the typical analysis of spike trains, EEG, and fMRI BOLD data, each representing a major recording modality used in neuroscience research. For clinical applications, epileptogenic seizure localization is selected as a direct demonstration.

The topics covered in this book reflect an ongoing evolution in biosignal processing. As biomedical datasets grow larger and more complicated, emerging signal processing methods that analyze and interpret these data have gained in importance. We hope that this book will aid the process for biosignal analysis and stimulate new ideas and opportunities for developing cutting-edge computational methods for biosignal processing, which will in turn accelerate laboratory discoveries into treatments for patients. All the contributors of this book share this vision and herein are gratefully recognized for donating their talent and time so that the promise of biosignal processing will be fulfilled.

Hualou Liang
Philadelphia, Pennsylvania

Editors

Hualou Liang is a professor at Drexel University, School of Biomedical Engineering. Dr. Liang received his PhD in physics from the Chinese Academy of Sciences, Beijing, China. He studied signal processing at Dalian University of Technology, Dalian, China. Dr. Liang has been a postdoctoral researcher in Tel-Aviv University, Israel, Max Planck Institute for Biological Cybernetics, Germany, and the Center for Complex Systems and Brain Sciences, Florida Atlantic University, USA.

Professor Liang focuses his research study on neuroengineering, neuroinformatics, functional brain imaging, cognitive and computational neuroscience, and biomedical signal processing. Dr. Liang's team explores neural mechanisms of visual perception during various cognitive tasks using computational approaches. His recent work deals with (1) development of software package (www.brain-smart.org) for analyzing brain circuits, (2) neuronal oscillations and attentional control, (3) development of advanced signal processing methods for the analysis of nonstationary, multivariate neurobiological data (spikes, field potentials, EEG/MEG, fMRI, etc.), and (4) algorithm development for brain–computer interface or brain–machine interface.

Joseph D. Bronzino earned a BSEE from Worcester Polytechnic Institute, Worcester, Massachusetts, in 1959, an MSEE from the Naval Postgraduate School, Monterey, California, in 1961, and a PhD in electrical engineering from Worcester Polytechnic Institute in 1968. He is presently the Vernon Roosa Professor of Applied Science, an endowed chair at Trinity College, Hartford, Connecticut, and president of the Biomedical Engineering Alliance and Consortium (BEACON), a nonprofit organization consisting of academic and medical institutions as well as corporations dedicated to the development and commercialization of new medical technologies (www.beaconalliance.org).

Dr. Bronzino is the author of over 200 articles and 11 books, including *Technology for Patient Care* (C.V. Mosby, 1977), *Computer Applications for Patient Care* (Addison-Wesley, 1982), *Biomedical Engineering: Basic Concepts and Instrumentation* (PWS Publishing Co., 1986), *Expert Systems: Basic Concepts* (Research Foundation of State University of New York, 1989), *Medical Technology and Society: An Interdisciplinary Perspective* (MIT Press and McGraw-Hill, 1990), *Management of Medical Technology* (Butterworth/Heinemann, 1992), *The Biomedical Engineering Handbook* (CRC Press, 1st Ed., 1995; 2nd Ed., 2000; 3rd Ed., 2005), and *Introduction to Biomedical Engineering* (Academic Press 1st Ed., 1999; 2nd Ed., 2005),

Dr. Bronzino is a fellow of IEEE and the American Institute of Medical and Biological Engineering (AIMBE), an honorary member of the Italian Society of Experimental Biology, past chairman of the Biomedical Engineering Division of the American Society for Engineering Education (ASEE), a charter member and former vice president of the Connecticut Academy of Science and Engineering (CASE), and a charter member of the American College of Clinical Engineering (ACCE), the Association for the Advancement of Medical Instrumentation (AAMI), past president of the IEEE-Engineering in Medicine and Biology Society (EMBS), past chairman of the IEEE Health Care Engineering Policy Committee

(HCEPC), past chairman of the IEEE Technical Policy Council in Washington, DC, and presently editor-in-chief of Elsevier's BME Book Series and CRC Press's *The Biomedical Engineering Handbook*.

Dr. Bronzino received the Millennium Award from IEEE/EMBS in 2000 and the Goddard Award from Worcester Polytechnic Institute for Professional Achievement in June 2004.

Donald R. Peterson is an associate professor of medicine and the director of the biodynamics laboratory in the School of Medicine at the University of Connecticut (UConn). He serves jointly as the director of the biomedical engineering undergraduate program in the School of Engineering and recently served as the director of the graduate program and as the BME Program chair. He earned a PhD in biomedical engineering and an MS in mechanical engineering at UConn and a BS in aerospace engineering and a BS in biomechanical engineering from Worcester Polytechnic Institute. Dr. Peterson has 16 years of experience in biomedical engineering education and offers graduate-level and undergraduate-level courses in BME in the areas of biomechanics, biodynamics, biofluid mechanics, and ergonomics, and he teaches in medicine in the subjects of gross anatomy, occupational biomechanics, and occupational exposure and response. Dr. Peterson's scholarly activities include over 50 published journal articles, 3 textbook chapters, and 12 textbooks, including his new appointment as co-editor-in-chief for *The Biomedical Engineering Handbook* by CRC Press.

Dr. Peterson has over 21 years of experience in biomedical engineering research and has been recently focused on measuring and modeling human, organ, and/or cell performance, including exposures to various physical stimuli and the subsequent biological responses. This work also involves the investigation of human–device interaction and has led to applications on the design and development of tools and various medical devices. Dr. Peterson is faculty within the occupational and environmental medicine group at the UConn Health Center, where his work has been directed toward the objective analysis of the anatomic and physiological processes involved in the onset of musculoskeletal and neuromuscular diseases, including strategies of disease mitigation. Recent applications of his research include human interactions with existing and developmental devices such as powered and non-powered tools, spacesuits and space tools for NASA, surgical and dental instruments, musical instruments, sports equipment, and computer-input devices. Other overlapping research initiatives focus on cell mechanics and cellular responses to fluid shear stress, the acoustics of hearing protection and communication, human exposure and response to vibration, and the development of computational models of biomechanical performance.

Dr. Peterson is also the co-executive director of the Biomedical Engineering Alliance and Consortium (BEACON; www.beaconalliance.org), which is a nonprofit entity dedicated to the promotion of collaborative research, translation, and partnership among academic, medical, and industry people in the field of biomedical engineering to develop new medical technologies and devices.

Contributors

Anna M. Bianchi
Department of Biomedical Engineering
Politecnico di Milano
Milan, Italy

G. Faye Boudreaux-Bartels
Department of Electrical Computer and Biomedical Engineering
University of Rhode Island
Kingston, Rhode Island

Sergio Cerutti
Department of Biomedical Engineering
Politecnico di Milano
Milan, Italy

Siyi Deng
Department of Cognitive Science
and
Department of Biomedical Engineering
University of California, Irvine
Irvine, California

Meltem Izzetoglu
School of Biomedical Engineering, Science and Health Systems
Drexel University
Philadelphia, Pennsylvania

Hongjun Jia
Department of Radiology and BRIC
University of North Carolina
Chapel Hill, North Carolina

Maciej Kamiński
Department of Biomedical Physics
University of Warsaw
Warsaw, Poland

Richard M. Leahy
Signal and Image Processing Institute
University of Southern California
Los Angeles, California

Hualou Liang
School of Biomedical Engineering, Science and Health Systems
Drexel University
Philadelphia, Pennsylvania

Luca T. Mainardi
Department of Biomedical Engineering
Politecnico di Milano
Milan, Italy

Robin Murray
Department of Electrical Computer and Biomedical Engineering
University of Rhode Island
Kingston, Rhode Island

and

Environmental and Target Physics
Naval Undersea Warfare Center
Newport, Rhode Island

Dimitrios Pantazis
Signal and Image Processing Institute
University of Southern California
Los Angeles, California

Dinggang Shen
Department of Radiology and BRIC
University of North Carolina
Chapel Hill, North Carolina

Feng Shi
Department of Radiology and BRIC
University of North Carolina
Chapel Hill, North Carolina

Juan Luis Poletti Soto
Signal and Image Processing Institute
University of Southern California
Los Angeles, California

Ramesh Srinivasan
Department of Cognitive Science
and
Department of Biomedical Engineering
University of California, Irvine
Irvine, California

Qian Wang
Department of Radiology and BRIC
and
Department of Computer Science
University of North Carolina
Chapel Hill, North Carolina

Guorong Wu
Department of Radiology and BRIC
University of North Carolina
Chapel Hill, North Carolina

Pew-Thian Yap
Department of Radiology and BRIC
University of North Carolina
Chapel Hill, North Carolina

1

Digital Biomedical Signal Acquisition and Processing

Luca T. Mainardi
Politecnico di Milano

Anna M. Bianchi
Politecnico di Milano

Sergio Cerutti
Politecnico di Milano

Biologic signals carry information that is useful for the comprehension of the complex pathophysiologic mechanisms underlying the behavior of living systems. Nevertheless, such information cannot be available directly from the raw recorded signals; it can be masked by other biologic signals contemporaneously detected (endogenous effects) or buried in some additive noise (exogenous effects). For such reasons, some additional processing is usually required to enhance the relevant information and to extract from it parameters that quantify the behavior of the system under study, mainly for physiologic studies, or that define the degree of pathology for routine clinical procedures (diagnosis, therapy, or rehabilitation).

Several processing techniques can be used for such purposes (they are also called preprocessing techniques): time- or frequency-domain methods, including filtering, *averaging*, spectral estimation, and others. Even if it is possible to deal with continuous time waveforms, it is usually convenient to convert them into a numerical form before processing. The recent progress of digital technology, in terms of both hardware and software, makes digital rather than analog processing more efficient and flexible. Digital techniques have several advantages: their performance is generally powerful, being able to easily implement even complex algorithms, and accuracy depends only on the truncation and round-off errors, whose effects can be predicted and controlled by the designer and are largely unaffected by other unpredictable variables such as component aging and temperature, which can degrade the performances of analog devices. Moreover, design parameters can be more easily changed because they involve software rather than hardware modifications.

A few basic elements of signal acquisition and processing will be presented in the following; our aim is to stress mainly the aspects connected with acquisition and analysis of biologic signals, leaving to the cited literature a deeper insight into the various subjects for both the fundamentals of digital signal processing and the applications.

1.1 Acquisition

A schematic representation of a general acquisition system is shown in Figure 1.1. Several physical magnitudes are usually measured from biologic systems. They include electromagnetic quantities (currents, potential differences, field strengths, etc.), as well as mechanical, chemical, or generally

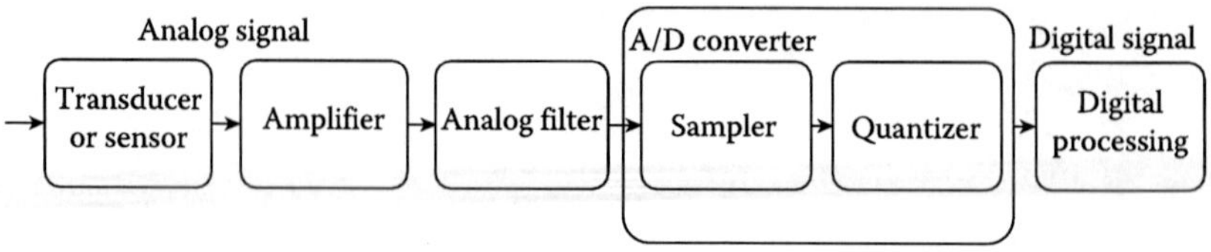

FIGURE 1.1 General block diagram of the acquisition procedure of a digital signal.

nonelectrical variables (pressure, temperature, movements, etc.). Electric signals are detected by sensors (mainly electrodes), while nonelectric magnitudes are first converted by transducers into electric signals that can be easily treated, transmitted, and stored. Several books of biomedical instrumentation give detailed descriptions of the various transducers and the hardware requirements associated with the acquisition of the different biologic signals (Tompkins and Webster, 1981; Cobbold, 1988; Webster, 2009).

An analog preprocessing block is usually required to amplify and filter the signal (in order to make it satisfy the requirements of the hardware such as the dynamic of the analog-to-digital converter), to compensate for some unwanted sensor characteristics, or to reduce the portion of undesired noise. Moreover, the continuous-time signal should be bandlimited before analog-to-digital (A/D) conversion. Such operation is needed to reduce the effect of *aliasing* induced by sampling, as will be described in the next section. Here it is important to remember that the acquisition procedure should preserve the information contained in the original signal waveform. This is a crucial point when recording biologic signals, whose characteristics may often be considered by physicians as indices of some underlying pathologies (i.e., the ST-segment displacement on an ECG signal can be considered a marker of ischemia, the peak-and-wave pattern on an EEG tracing can be a sign of epilepsy, and so on). Thus, the acquisition system should not introduce any form of distortion that can be misleading or can destroy real pathologic alterations. For this reason, the analog prefiltering block should be designed with constant modulus and linear phase (or zero-phase) *frequency response*, at least in the passband, over the frequencies of interest. Such requirements make the signal arrive undistorted up to the A/D converter.

The analog waveform is then A/D converted into a digital signal, that is, it is transformed into a series of numbers, discretized both in time and in amplitude, that can be easily managed by digital processors. The A/D conversion ideally can be divided into two steps, as shown in Figure 1.1: the sampling process, which converts the continuous signal in a discrete-time series and whose elements are named samples, and a quantization procedure, which assigns the amplitude value of each sample within a set of determined discrete values. Both processes modify the characteristics of the signal, and their effects will be discussed in the following sections.

1.1.1 Sampling Theorem

The advantages of processing a digital series instead of an analog signal have been reported previously. Furthermore, the basic property when using a sampled series instead of its continuous waveform lies in the fact that the former, under certain hypotheses, is completely representative of the latter. When this happens, the continuous waveform can be perfectly reconstructed just from the series of sampled values. This is known as the sampling theorem (or Shannon theorem) (Shannon, 1949). It states that a continuous-time signal can be completely recovered from its samples if, and only if, the sampling rate is greater than twice the signal bandwidth.

In order to understand the assumptions of the theorem, let us consider a continuous bandlimited signal $x(t)$ (up to f_b) whose Fourier transform $X(f)$ is shown in Figure 1.2a and let us suppose to uniformly sample it. The sampling procedure can be modeled by the multiplication of $x(t)$ with an impulse train:

$$i(t) = \sum_{k=-\infty,\infty} \delta(t - kT_s) \tag{1.1}$$

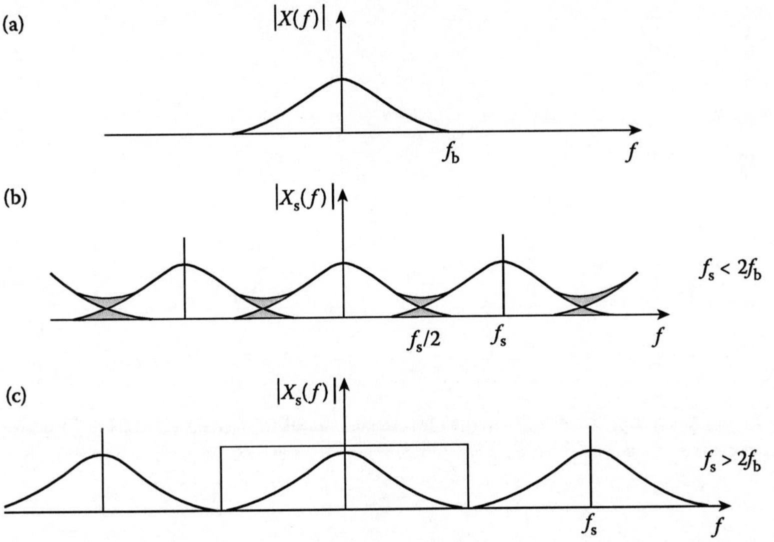

FIGURE 1.2 Effect of sampling frequency (f_s) on a bandlimited signal (up to frequency f_b). Fourier transform of the original time signal (a), of the sampled signal when $f_s < 2f_b$ (b), and when $f_s > 2f_b$ (c). The dark areas in part (b) indicate the frequency range affected by aliasing.

where $\delta(t)$ is the delta (Dirac) function, k is an integer, and T_s is the sampling interval. The sampled signal becomes

$$x_s(t) = x(t) \cdot i(t) = \sum_{k=-\infty,\infty} x(t) \cdot \delta(t - kT_s) \tag{1.2}$$

Taking into account that convolution in time domain implies multiplication in frequency domain, we obtain

$$X_s(f) = X(f) \cdot I(f) = X(f) \cdot \frac{1}{T_s} \sum_{k=-\infty,\infty} \delta(f - kf_s) = \frac{1}{T_s} \sum_{k=-\infty,\infty} X(f - kf_s) \tag{1.3}$$

where $f_s = 1/T_s$ is the sampling frequency.

Thus, $X_s(f)$, that is, the Fourier transform of the sampled signal, is periodic and consists of a series of identical repeats of $X(f)$ centered around multiples of the sampling frequency, as depicted in Figure 1.2b and c. It is worth noting in Figure 1.2b that the frequency components of $X(f)$ placed above $f_s/2$ appears, when $f_s < 2f_b$, as folded back, summing up to the lower-frequency components. This phenomenon is known as aliasing (higher component look "alias" lower components). When aliasing occurs, the original information (Figure 1.2a) cannot be recovered because the frequency components of the original signal are irreversibly corrupted by the overlaps of the shifted versions of $X(f)$.

A visual inspection of Figure 1.2 allows one to observe that such frequency contamination can be avoided when the original signal is bandlimited ($X(f) = 0$, for $f > f_b$) and sampled at a frequency $f_s > 2f_b$. In this case, as shown in Figure 1.2c, no overlaps exist between adjacent reply of $X(f)$, and the original waveform can be retrieved by low-pass filtering the sampled signal (Oppenheim and Schafer, 1975). Such observations are the basis of the sampling theorem previously reported.

The hypothesis of a bandlimited signal is hardly verified in biomedical signals due to the signal characteristics or due to the effect of superimposed wideband noise. It is worth noting that filtering

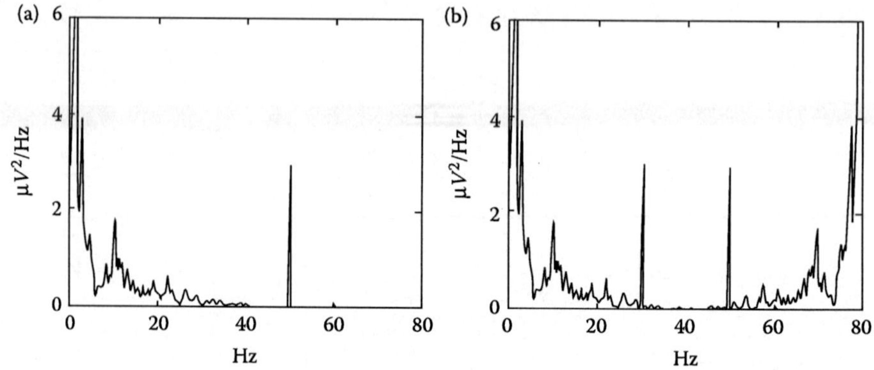

FIGURE 1.3 Power spectrum of an EEG signal (originally bandlimited up to 40 Hz). The presence of 50 Hz mains noise (a) causes aliasing error in the 30 Hz component (i.e., in the b diagnostic band) in the sampled signal (b) if $f_s = 80$ Hz.

before sampling is always needed even if we assume the incoming signal to be bandlimited. Let us consider the following example of an EEG signal whose frequency content of interest ranges between 0.5 and 40 Hz (the usual diagnostic bands are δ, 0.5–4 Hz; ϑ, 4–7 Hz; α, 8–13 Hz; β, 13–40 Hz). We may decide to sample it at 80 Hz, thus, literally respecting the Shannon theorem. If we do it without prefiltering, we could find some unpleasant results. Typically, the 50-Hz mains noise will replicate itself in the signal band (30 Hz, i.e., the β band), thus, corrupting irreversibly the information, which is of great interest from a physiologic and clinical point of view. The effect is shown in Figure 1.3a (before sampling) and Figure 1.3b (after sampling). Generally, it is advisable to sample at a frequency $>2f_b$ (Gardenhire, 1964) in order to take into account the nonideal behavior of the filter or the other preprocessing devices. Therefore, the prefiltering block of Figure 1.1 is always required to bandlimit the signal before sampling and to avoid aliasing errors.

1.1.2 Quantization Effects

The quantization produces a discrete signal (we indicate by n the discrete-time variable) whose samples can assume only certain values according to the way they are coded. Typical step functions for a uniform quantizer are reported in Figure 1.4a and b, where the quantization interval Δ between two quantization levels is evidenced in two cases, rounding and truncation, respectively.

Quantization is a heavily nonlinear procedure, but fortunately its effects can be statistically modeled. Figure 1.4c and d shows it; the nonlinear quantization block is substituted by a statistical model in which the error induced by quantization is treated as an additive noise $e(n)$ (*quantization error*) to the signal $x(n)$.

The following hypotheses are considered in order to deal with a simple mathematical problem:

1. $e(n)$ is supposed to be a white noise with uniform distribution
2. $e(n)$ and $x(n)$ are uncorrelated

First of all, it should be noted that the probability density of $e(n)$ changes according to the adopted coding procedure. If we decide to round the real sample to the nearest quantization level, we have $-\Delta/2 < \Psi e(n) < \Delta/2$, while if we decide to truncate the sample amplitude, we have $-\Delta\Psi e(n) < 0$. The two probability densities are plotted in Figure 1.4e and f.

The two ways of coding yield processes with different statistical properties. In the first case, the mean and variance value of $e(n)$ are

$$m_e = 0 \quad \sigma_e^2 = \Delta^2/12$$

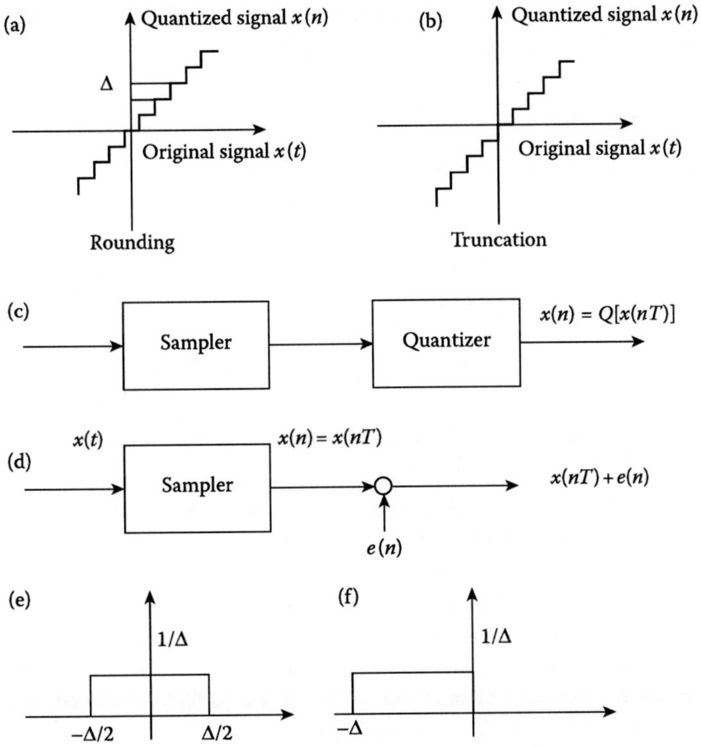

FIGURE 1.4 Nonlinear relationships for rounding (a) and truncation (b) quantization procedures. Description of quantization block (c) by a statistical model (d) and probability densities for the quantization noise $e(n)$ for rounding (e) and truncation (f). Δ is the quantization interval.

while in the second case, $m_e = -\Delta/2$, and the variance is still the same. Variance reduces in the presence of a reduced quantization interval as expected.

Finally, it is possible to evaluate the signal-to-noise ratio (SNR) for the quantization process:

$$\mathrm{SNR} = 10\log_{10}\left(\frac{\sigma_x^2}{\sigma_e^2}\right) = 10\log_{10}\left(\frac{\sigma_x^2}{2^{-2b}/12}\right) = 6.02b + 10.79 + 10\log_{10}(\sigma_x^2) \tag{1.4}$$

having set $\Delta = 2^{-2b}$ and where σ_x^2 is the variance of the signal and b is the number of bits used for coding. It should be noted that the SNR increases by almost 6 dB for each added bit of coding. Several forms of quantization are usually employed: uniform, nonuniform (preceding the uniform sampler with a nonlinear block), or roughly (small number of quantization levels and high quantization step). Details can be found in Carassa (1983), Jaeger (1982), and Widrow (1956).

1.2 Signal Processing

A brief review of different signal-processing techniques will be given in this section. They include traditional filtering, averaging techniques, and spectral estimators.

Only the main concepts of analysis and design of digital filters are presented, and a few examples are illustrated in the processing of the ECG signal. Averaging techniques will then be described briefly and their usefulness evidenced when noise and signal have similar frequency contents but different statistical properties; an example for evoked potentials enhancement from EEG background noise is illustrated.

Finally, different spectral estimators will be considered and some applications shown in the analysis of RR fluctuations (i.e., the heart rate variability (HRV) signal).

1.2.1 Digital Filters

A digital filter is a discrete-time system that operates some transformation on a digital input signal $x(n)$ generating an output sequence $y(n)$, as schematically shown by the block diagram in Figure 1.5. The characteristics of transformation $T[\cdot]$ identify the filter. The filter will be time-variant if $T[\cdot]$ is a function of time or time-invariant otherwise, while it is said to be *linear* if, and only if, having $x_1(n)$ and $x_2(n)$ as inputs producing $y_1(n)$ and $y_2(n)$, respectively, we have

$$T[ax_1 + bx_2] = aT[x_1] + bT[x_2] = ay_1 + by_2 \tag{1.5}$$

In the following, only linear, time-invariant filters will be considered, even if several interesting applications of nonlinear (Glaser and Ruchkin, 1976; Tompkins, 1993) or time-variant (Huta and Webster, 1973, 1987; Widrow et al., 1975; Cohen, 1983; Thakor, 1987; Sayed, 2003) filters have been proposed in the literature for the analysis of biologic signals.

The behavior of a filter is usually described in terms of input–output relationships. They are usually assessed by exciting the filter with different inputs and evaluating which is the response (output) of the system. In particular, if the input is the impulse sequence $\delta(n)$, the resulting output, the impulse response, has a relevant role in describing the characteristic of the filter. Such a response can be used to determine the response to more complicated input sequences. In fact, let us consider a generic input sequence $x(n)$ as a sum of weighted and delayed impulses

$$x(n) = \sum_{k=-\infty,\infty} x(k) \cdot \delta(n-k) \tag{1.6}$$

and let us identify the response to $\delta(n-k)$ as $h(n-k)$. If the filter is time-invariant, each delayed impulse will produce the same response, but time-shifted; due to the linearity property, such responses will be summed at the output:

$$y(n) = \sum_{k=-\infty,\infty} x(k) \cdot h(n-k) \tag{1.7}$$

This convolution product links input and output and defines the property of the filter. Two of them should be recalled: *stability* and *causality*. The former ensures that bounded (finite) inputs will produce bounded outputs (also called BIBO stability). Such a property can be deduced by the impulse response; it can be proved that the filter is stable if and only if

$$\sum_{k=-\infty,\infty} |h(k)| < \infty \tag{1.8}$$

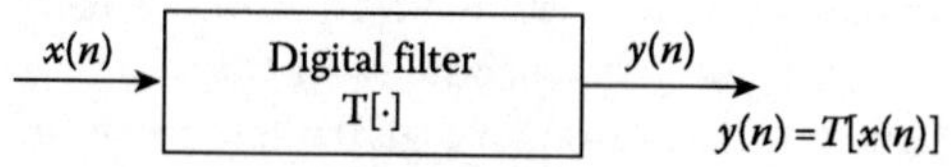

FIGURE 1.5 General block diagram of a digital filter. The output digital signal $y(n)$ is obtained from the input $x(n)$ by means of a transformation $T[\cdot]$ which identifies the filter.

Causality means that the filter will not respond to an input before the input is applied. This is in agreement with our physical concept of a system, but it is not strictly required for a digital filter that can be implemented in a noncausal form. A filter is causal if and only if

$$h(k) = 0 \quad \text{for } k < 0 \tag{1.8a}$$

Even if Equation 1.7 completely describes the properties of the filter, most often it is necessary to express the input–output relationships of linear discrete-time systems under the form of the z-transform operator, which allows one to express Equation 1.7 in a more useful, operative, and simpler form.

1.2.1.1 z-Transform

The z-transform of a sequence $x(n)$ is defined by (Rainer et al., 1972)

$$X(z) = \sum_{k=-\infty,\infty} x(k) \cdot z^{-k} \tag{1.9}$$

where z is a complex variable. This series will converge or diverge for different z values. The set of z values which makes Equation 1.9 converge is the *region of convergence*, and it depends on the series $x(n)$ considered.

Among the properties of the z-transform, we recall

- The delay (shift) property:

$$\text{If } w(n) = x(n-T), \quad \text{then } W(z) = X(z) \cdot z^{-T} \tag{1.9a}$$

- The product of convolution:

$$\text{If } w(n) = \sum_{k=-\infty,\infty} x(k) \cdot y(n-k), \quad \text{then } W(z) = X(z) \cdot Y(z) \tag{1.9b}$$

1.2.1.2 Transfer Function in z Domain

Thanks to the previous properties, we can express Equation 1.7 in the z domain as a simple multiplication:

$$Y(z) = H(z) \cdot X(z) \tag{1.10}$$

where $H(z)$, known as the *transfer function* of the filter, is the z-transform of the impulse response. $H(z)$ plays a relevant role in the analysis and design of digital filters. The response to input sinusoids can be evaluated as follows: assume a complex sinusoid $x(n) = e^{j\omega nT_s}$ as input; the corresponding filter output will be

$$y(n) = \sum_{k=0,\infty} h(k)e^{j\omega T_2(n-k)} = e^{-j\omega nT_s} \sum_{k=0,\infty} h(k)e^{-j\omega kT_s} = x(n) \cdot H(z)\big|_{z=e^{j\omega T_s}} \tag{1.11}$$

Then a sinusoid in input is still the same sinusoid at the output, but multiplied by a complex quantity $H(\omega)$. Such a complex function defines the response of the filter for each sinusoid of ω pulse in input, and it is known as the frequency response of the filter. It is evaluated in the complex z plane by computing $H(z)$ for $z = e^{j\omega nT_s}$, namely, on the point locus that describes the unitary circle on the z plane ($|e^{j\omega nT_s}| = 1$).

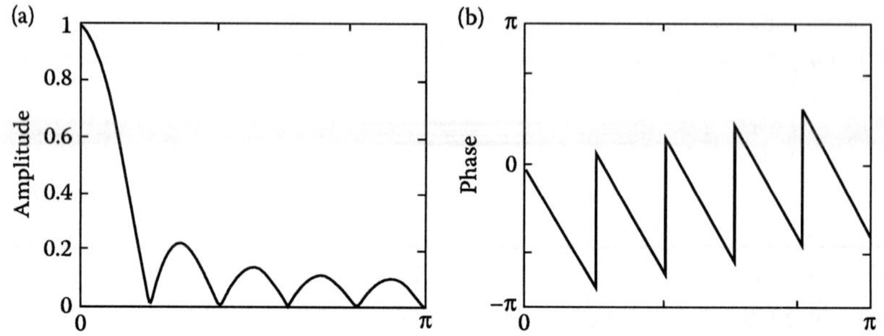

FIGURE 1.6 Modulus (a) and phase (b) diagrams of the frequency response of a moving average filter of order 5. Note that the frequency plots are depicted up to π. In fact, taking into account that we are dealing with a sampled signal whose frequency information is up to $f_s/2$, we have $\omega_{max} = 2\pi f_s/2 = \pi f_s$ or $\hat{\omega}_{max} = \pi$ if normalized with respect to the sampling rate, f_s.

As a complex function, $H(\omega)$ will be defined by its module $|H(\omega)|$ and by its phase $\angle H(\omega)$ functions, as shown in Figure 1.6 for a moving average filter of order 5. The figure indicates that the lower-frequency components will come through the filter almost unaffected, while the higher-frequency components will be drastically reduced. It is usual to express the horizontal axis of frequency response from 0 to π. This is obtained because only pulse frequencies up to $\omega_s/2$ are reconstructable (due to the Shannon theorem), and therefore, in the horizontal axis, the value of ωT_s is reported which goes from 0 to π. Furthermore, Figure 1.6b demonstrates that the phase is piecewise linear, and in correspondence with the zeroes of $|H(\omega)|$, there is a change in phase of π value. According to their frequency response, the filters are usually classified as (1) low-pass, (2) high-pass, (3) bandpass, or (4) bandstop filters. Figure 1.7 shows the ideal frequency response for such filters with the proper low- and high-frequency cutoffs.

For a large class of linear, time-invariant systems, $H(z)$ can be expressed in the following general form:

$$H(z) = \frac{\sum_{m=0,M} b_m z^{-m}}{1+\sum_{k=1,N} a_k z^{-k}} \tag{1.12}$$

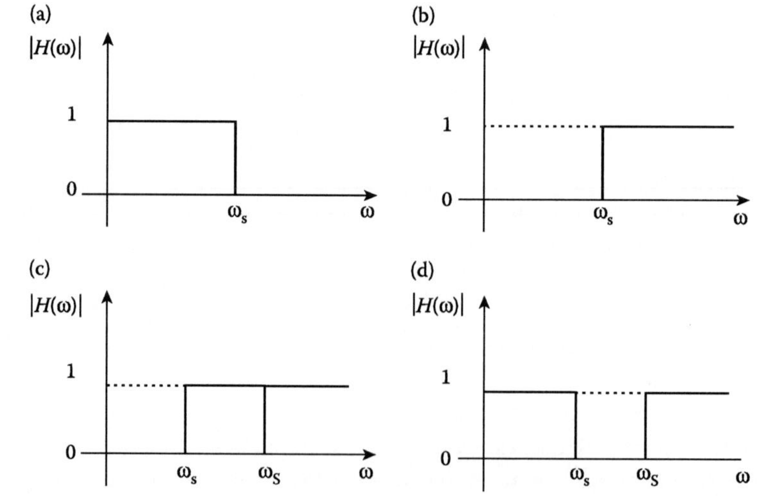

FIGURE 1.7 Ideal frequency–response moduli for low-pass (a), high-pass (b), bandpass (c), and bandstop filters (d).

which describes in the z domain the following *difference equation* in this discrete-time domain:

$$y(n) = -\sum_{k=1,N} a_k y(n-k) + \sum_{m=0,M} b_m x(n-m) \tag{1.13}$$

When at least one of the a_k coefficients is different from zero, some output values contribute to the current output. The filter contains some feedback, and it is said to be implemented in a recursive form. On the other hand, when the a_k values are all zero, the filter output is obtained only from the current or previous inputs, and the filter is said to be implemented in a *nonrecursive* form.

The transfer function can be expressed in a more useful form by finding the roots of both numerator and denominator:

$$H(z) = \frac{b_0 z^{N-M} \prod_{m=1,M} (z - z_m)}{\prod_{k=1,N} (z - p_k)} \tag{1.14}$$

where z_m are the zeroes and p_k are the poles. It is worth noting that $H(z)$ presents $N - M$ zeroes in correspondence with the origin of the z plane and M zeroes elsewhere (N zeroes totally) and N poles. The pole-zero form of $H(z)$ is of great interest because several properties of the filter are immediately available from the geometry of poles and zeroes in the complex z plane. In fact, it is possible to easily assess stability and by visual inspection to roughly estimate the frequency response without making any calculations.

Stability is verified when all poles lie inside the unitary circle, as can be proved by considering the relationships between the z-transform and the Laplace s-transform and by observing that the left side of the s plane is mapped inside the unitary circle (Oppenheim and Schafer, 1975; Jackson, 1986).

The frequency response can be estimated by noting that $(z - z_m)|_{z=e^{j\omega n T_s}}$ is a vector joining the mth zero with the point on the unitary circle identified by the angle ωT_s. Defining

$$\begin{aligned} \vec{B}_m &= (z - z_m)\,|_{z=e^{j\omega T_s}} \\ \vec{A}_k &= (z - p_k)\,|_{z=e^{j\omega T_s}} \end{aligned} \tag{1.15}$$

we obtain

$$\begin{aligned} |H(\omega)| &= \frac{b_0 \prod_{m=1,M} |\vec{B}_m|}{\prod_{k=1,N} |\vec{A}_k|} \\ \angle H(\omega) &= \sum_{m=1,M} \angle \vec{B}_m - \sum_{k=1,N} \angle \vec{A}_k + (N - M)\omega T_s \end{aligned} \tag{1.16}$$

Thus, the modulus of $H(\omega)$ can be evaluated at any frequency ω° by computing the distances between poles and zeroes and the point on the unitary circle corresponding to $\omega = \omega^{\circ}$, as evidenced in Figure 1.8, where a filter with two pairs of complex poles and three zeroes is considered.

To obtain the estimate of $H(\omega)$, we move around the unitary circle and roughly evaluate the effect of poles and zeroes by keeping in mind a few rules (Challis and Kitney, 1982) (1) when we are close to a zero, $|H(\omega)|$ will approach zero, and a positive phase shift will appear in $\angle H(\omega)$ as the vector from the zero reverses its angle; (2) when we are close to a pole, $|H(\omega)|$ will tend to peak, and a negative phase change is found in $\angle H(\omega)$ (the closer the pole to unitary circle, the sharper is the peak until it reaches infinite and the filter becomes unstable); and (3) near a closer pole-zero pair, the response modulus will

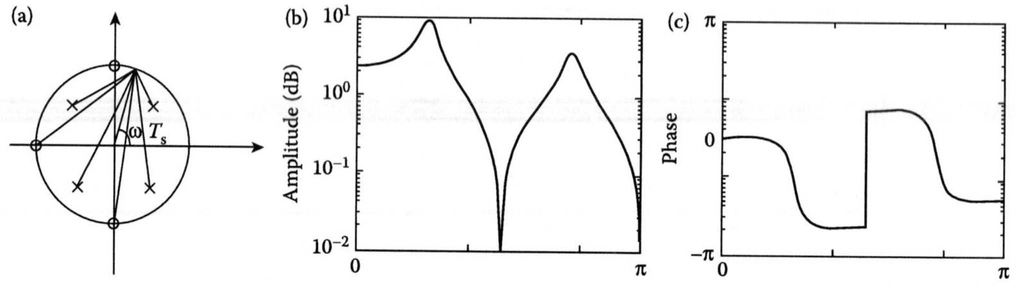

FIGURE 1.8 Poles and zeroes geometry (a); relative frequency response modulus (b); and phase (c) characteristics. Moving around the unitary circle a rough estimation of $|H(\omega)|$ and $\angle H(\omega)$ can be obtained. Note the zeroes' effects at π and $\pi/2$ and modulus rising in proximity of the poles. Phase shifts are clearly evident in part (c) closer to zeroes and poles.

tend to zero or infinity if the zero or the pole is closer, while far from this pair, the modulus can be considered unitary. As an example, it is possible to compare the modulus and phase diagram of Figure 1.8b and c with the relative geometry of the poles and zeroes of Figure 1.8a.

1.2.1.3 FIR and IIR Filters

A common way of classifying digital filters is based on the characteristics of their impulse response. For finite impulse response (FIR) filters, $h(n)$ is composed of a finite number of nonzero values, while for infinite impulse response (IIR) filters, $h(n)$ oscillates up to infinity with nonzero values. It is clearly evident that in order to obtain an infinite response to an impulse in input, the IIR filter must contain some feedback that sustains the output as the input vanishes. The presence of feedback paths requires putting particular attention to the filter stability.

Even if FIR filters are usually implemented in a nonrecursive form and IIR filters in a recursive form, the two ways of classification are not coincident. In fact, as shown by the following example, an FIR filter can be expressed in a recursive form:

$$H(z) = \sum_{k=0,N-1} z^{-k} = \sum_{k=0,N-1} z^{-k}\frac{(1-z^{-1})}{(1-z^{-1})} = \frac{1-z^{-N}}{1-z^{-1}} \tag{1.17}$$

for a more convenient computational implementation.

As shown previously, two important requirements for filters are stability and linear phase response. FIR filters can be easily designed to fulfill such requirements; they are always stable (having no poles outside the origin), and the linear phase response is obtained by constraining the impulse response coefficients to have symmetry around their midpoint. Such constrain implies

$$b_m = \pm b^{*}_{M-m} \tag{1.18}$$

where the b_m are the M coefficients of an FIR filter. The sign + or – stays in accordance with the symmetry (even or odd) and M value (even or odd). This is a necessary and sufficient condition for FIR filters to have linear phase response. Two cases of impulse response that yield a linear phase filter are shown in Figure 1.9.

It should be noted that Equation 1.18 imposes geometric constrains to the zero locus of $H(z)$. Taking into account Equation 1.12, we have

$$z^M H(z) = H\left(\frac{1}{z^*}\right)z \tag{1.19}$$

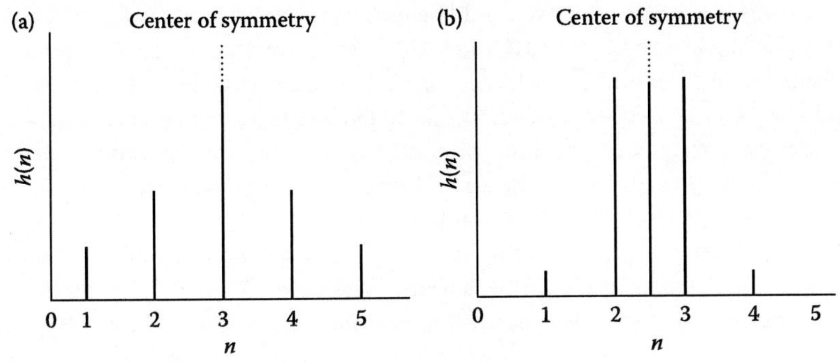

FIGURE 1.9 Examples of impulse response for linear phase FIR filters: odd (a) and even (b) number of coefficients.

Thus, both z_m and $1/z_m^*$ must be zeroes of $H(z)$. Then the zeroes of linear phase FIR filters must lie on the unitary circle, or they must appear in pairs and with inverse moduli.

1.2.1.4 Design Criteria

In many cases, the filter is designed in order to satisfy some requirements, usually on the frequency response, which depend on the characteristic of the particular application the filter is intended for. It is known that ideal filters, like those reported in Figure 1.7, are not physically realizable (they would require an infinite number of coefficients of impulse response); thus, we can design FIR or IIR filters that can only mimic, with an acceptable error, the ideal response. Figure 1.10 shows a frequency response of a nonideal low-pass filter. Here, there are ripples in passband and in stopband, and there is a transition band from passband to stopband, defined by the interval $\omega_s - \omega_p$.

Several design techniques are available, and some of them require heavy computational tasks, which are capable of developing filters with defined specific requirements. They include window technique, frequency-sampling method, or equiripple design for FIR filters. Butterworth, Chebychev, elliptical design, and impulse-invariant or bilinear transformation are instead employed for IIR filters. For detailed analysis of digital filter techniques, see Antoniou (1979), Cerutti (1983), and Oppenheim and Schafer (1975).

1.2.1.5 Examples

A few examples of different kinds of filters will be presented in the following, showing some applications on ECG signal processing. It is shown that the ECG contains relevant information over a wide range of

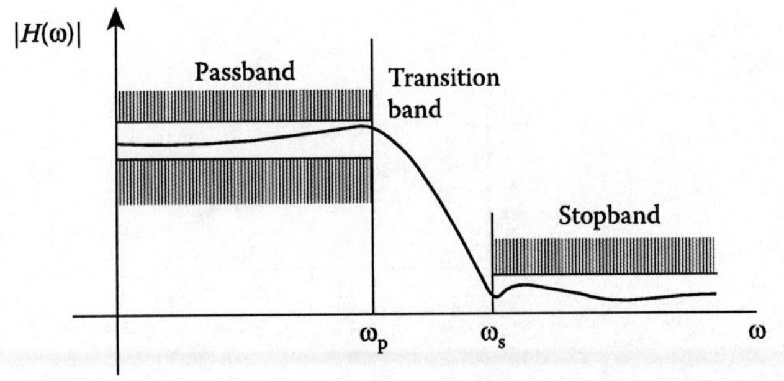

FIGURE 1.10 Amplitude response for a real low-pass filter. Ripples are admitted in both passband and stopband, but they are constrained into restricted areas. Limitations are also imposed to the width of the transition band.

frequencies; the lower-frequency contents should be preserved for correct measurement of the slow ST displacements, while higher-frequency contents are needed to correctly estimate amplitude and duration of the faster contributions, mainly at the level of the QRS complex. Unfortunately, several sources of noise are present in the same frequency band, such as higher-frequency noise due to muscle contraction (EMG noise), the lower-frequency noise due to motion artifacts (baseline wandering), the effect of respiration or the low-frequency noise in the skin–electrode interface, and others.

In the first example, the effect of two different low-pass filters will be considered. An ECG signal corrupted by an EMG noise (Figure 1.11a) is low-pass filtered by two different low-pass filters whose frequency responses are shown in Figure 1.11b and c. The two FIR filters have cutoff frequencies at 40 and 20 Hz, respectively, and were designed through window techniques (Weber–Cappellini window, filter length = 256 points) (Cappellini et al., 1978), and result more aggressive in respect to the recommended diagnostic bandwidth (0.5–200 Hz).

The output signals are shown in Figure 1.11d and e. The two drastic filterings here indicated reduce the superimposed noise but at the same time alter the original ECG waveform. In particular, the *R* wave amplitude is progressively reduced by decreasing the cutoff frequency, and the QRS width is progressively increased as well. On the other hand, *P* waves appear almost unaffected, having frequency components generally lower than 20 Hz. At this point, it is worth noting that an increase in QRS duration is generally associated with various pathologies, such as ventricular hypertrophy or bundle-branch block. It is, therefore, necessary to check that an excessive band limitation does not introduce a false-positive indication in the diagnosis of the ECG signal.

An example of an application for stopband filters (*notch filters*) is presented in Figure 1.12. It is used to reduce the 50-Hz mains noise on the ECG signal, and it was designated by placing a zero in corresponding to the frequency we want to suppress.

Finally, an example of a high-pass filter is shown for the detection of the QRS complex. Detecting the time occurrence of a fiducial point in the QRS complex is indeed the first task usually performed in ECG signal analysis. The QRS complex usually contains the higher-frequency components with respect to the other ECG waves, and thus, such components will be enhanced by a high-pass filter. Figure 1.13 shows

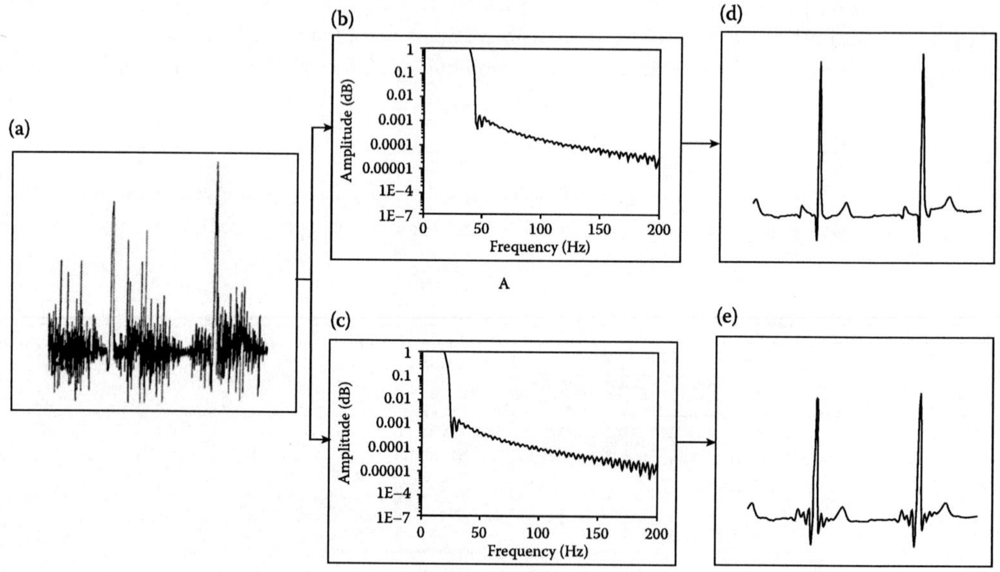

FIGURE 1.11 Effects of two different low-pass filters (b) and (c) on an ECG trace (a) corrupted by EMG noise. The resulting filtered signal is shown in panel (d) and (e). Both amplitude reduction and variation in the QRS induced by too drastic low-pass filtering are evidenced.

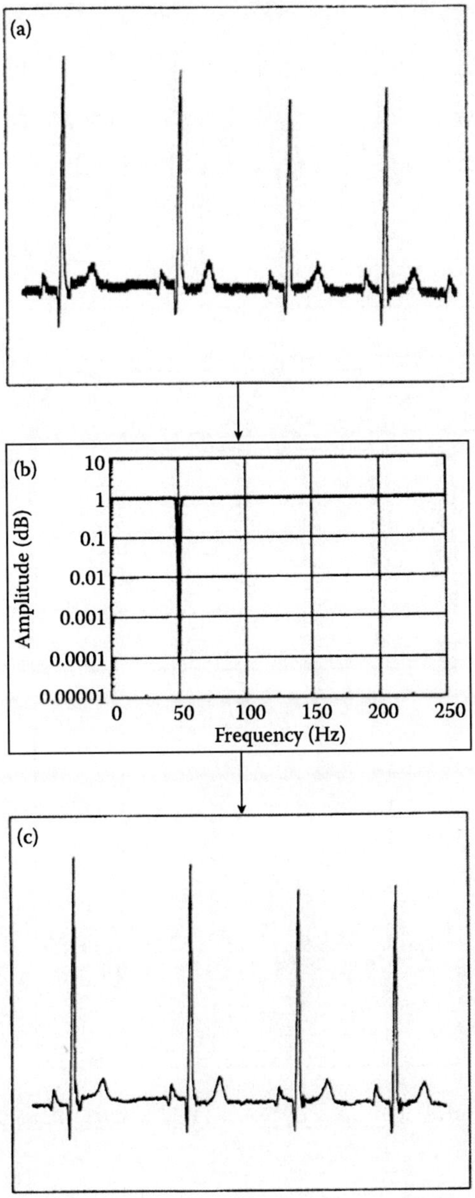

FIGURE 1.12 A 50-Hz noisy ECG signal (a); a 50-Hz rejection filter (b); and a filtered signal (c).

how QRS complexes (Figure 1.13a) can be identified by a derivative high-pass filter with a cutoff frequency to decrease the effect of the noise contributions at high frequencies (Figure 1.13b). The filtered signal (Figure 1.13c) presents sharp and well-defined peaks that are easily recognized as QRS occurrences by a threshold value.

1.2.2 Signal Averaging

Traditional filtering performs very well when the frequency content of signal and noise do not overlap. When the noise bandwidth is completely separated from the signal bandwidth, the noise can be

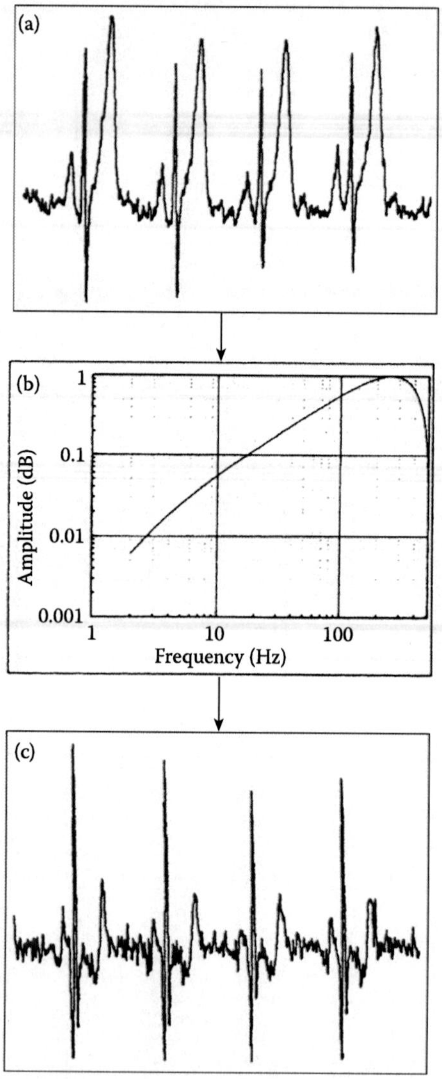

FIGURE 1.13 Effect of a derivative high-pass filter (b) on an ECG lead (a). The output of the filter (c).

decreased easily by means of a linear filter according to the procedures described earlier. On the other hand, when the signal and noise bandwidth overlap and the noise amplitude is enough to seriously corrupt the signal, a traditional filter, designed to cancel the noise, also will introduce signal cancellation or, at least, distortion. As an example, let us consider the brain potentials evoked by a sensory stimulation (visual, acoustic, or somatosensory) generally called evoked potentials (EP). Such a response is very difficult to be determined because its amplitude is generally much lower than the background EEG activity. Both EP and EEG signals contain information in the same frequency range; thus, the problem of separating the desired response cannot be approached via traditional digital filtering (Aunon et al., 1981). Another typical example is in the detection of ventricular late potentials (VLP) in the ECG signal. These potentials are very small in amplitude and are comparable with the noise superimposed on the signal and also for what concerns the frequency content (Simson, 1981). In such cases, an increase in the SNR may be achieved on the basis of different statistical properties of signal and noise.

When the desired signal repeats identically at each iteration (i.e., the EP at each sensory stimulus, the VLP at each cardiac cycle), the averaging technique can satisfactorily solve the problem of separating signal from noise. This technique sums a set of temporal epochs of the signal together with the superimposed noise. If the time epochs are properly aligned, through efficient trigger-point recognition, the signal waveforms directly sum together. If the signal and the noise are characterized by the following statistical properties:

1. All the signal epochs contain a deterministic signal component $x(n)$ that does not vary for all the epochs.
2. The superimposed noise $w(n)$ is a broadband stationary process with zero mean and variance σ^2 so that

$$\begin{aligned} E[w(n)] &= 0 \\ E[w^2(n)] &= \sigma^2 \end{aligned} \qquad (1.20)$$

3. Signal $x(n)$ and noise $w_i(n)$ are uncorrelated so that the recorded signal $y(n)$ at the ith iteration can be expressed as

$$y(n)_i = x(n) + w_i(n) \qquad (1.21)$$

then the averaging process yields y_t:

$$y_t(n) = \frac{1}{N}\sum_{i=1}^{N} y_i = x(n) + \sum_{i=1}^{N} w_i(n) \qquad (1.22)$$

The noise term is an estimate of the mean by taking the average of N realizations. Such an average is a new random variable that has the same mean of the sum terms (zero in this case) and which has a variance of σ^2/N. The effect of the coherent averaging procedure is then to maintain the amplitude of the signal and reduce the variance of the noise by a factor of N. In order to evaluate the improvement in the SNR (in rms value) in respect to the SNR (at the generic ith sweep):

$$\text{SNR} = \text{SNR}_i \cdot \sqrt{N} \qquad (1.23)$$

Thus, signal averaging improves the SNR by a factor of $\sqrt{N}$ in rms value.

A coherent averaging procedure can be viewed as a digital filtering process, and its frequency characteristics can be investigated. From Equation 1.17 through the z-transform, the transfer function of the filtering operation results in

$$H(z) = \frac{1 + z^{-h} + z^{-2h} + L + z^{-(N-1)h}}{N} \qquad (1.24)$$

where N is the number of elements in the average and h is the number of samples in each response. An alternative expression for $H(z)$ is

$$H(z) = \frac{1}{N}\frac{1 - z^{Nh}}{1 - z^{h}} \qquad (1.25)$$

This is a moving average low-pass filter as discussed earlier, where the output is a function of the preceding value with a lag of h samples; in practice, the filter operates not on the time sequence but in the sweep sequence on corresponding samples.

The frequency response of the filter is shown in Figure 1.14 for different values of the parameter N. In this case, the sampling frequency f_s is the repetition frequency of the sweeps, and we may assume it to be 1 without loss of generality. The frequency response is characterized by a main lobe with the first zero

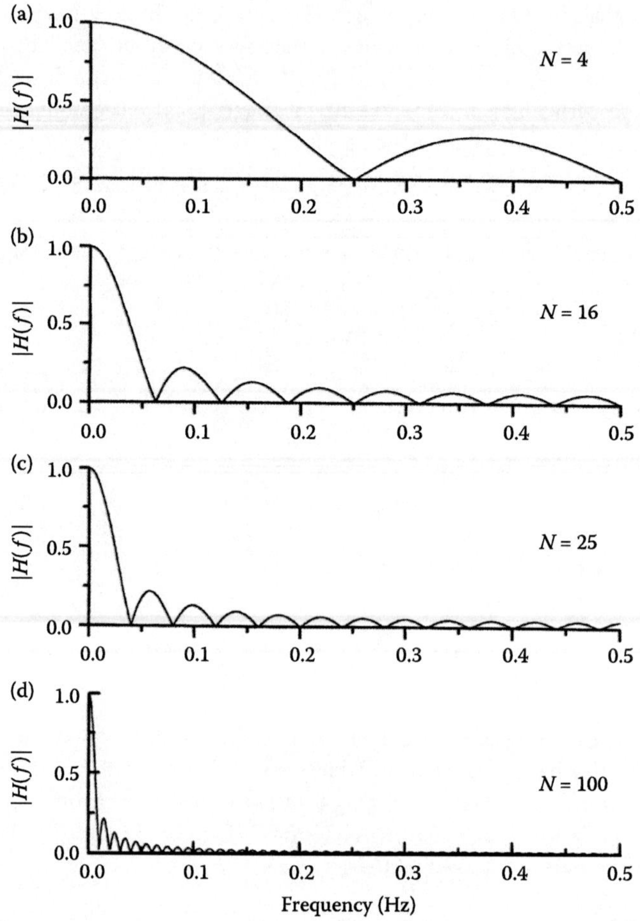

FIGURE 1.14 Equivalent frequency response for the signal-averaging procedure for different values of N. From (a) to (d) N increases.

corresponding to $f = 1/N$ and by successive secondary lobes separated by zeroes at intervals $1/N$. The width of each tooth decreases as well as the amplitude of the secondary lobes when increasing the number N of sweeps.

The desired signal is sweep-invariant, and it will be unaffected by the filter, while the broadband noise will be decreased. Some leakage of noise energy takes place in the center of the sidelobes and, of course, at zero frequency. Under the hypothesis of zero mean noise, the dc component has no effect, and the diminishing sidelobe amplitude implies the leakage to be not relevant for high frequencies. It is important to recall that the average filtering is based on the hypothesis of broadband distribution of the noise and lack of correlation between signal and noise. Unfortunately, these assumptions are not always verified in biologic signals. For example, the assumptions of independence of the background EEG and the evoked potential may be not completely realistic (Gevins and Remond, 1987). In addition, much attention must be paid to the alignment of the sweeps; in fact, slight misalignments (fiducial point jitter) will lead to a low-pass filtering effect of the final result.

1.2.2.1 Example

As mentioned previously, one of the fields in which signal-averaging technique is employed extensively is in the evaluation of cerebral evoked response after a sensory stimulation. Figure 1.15 shows the EEG recorded from the scalp of a normal subject after a somatosensory stimulation released at time $t = 0$. The

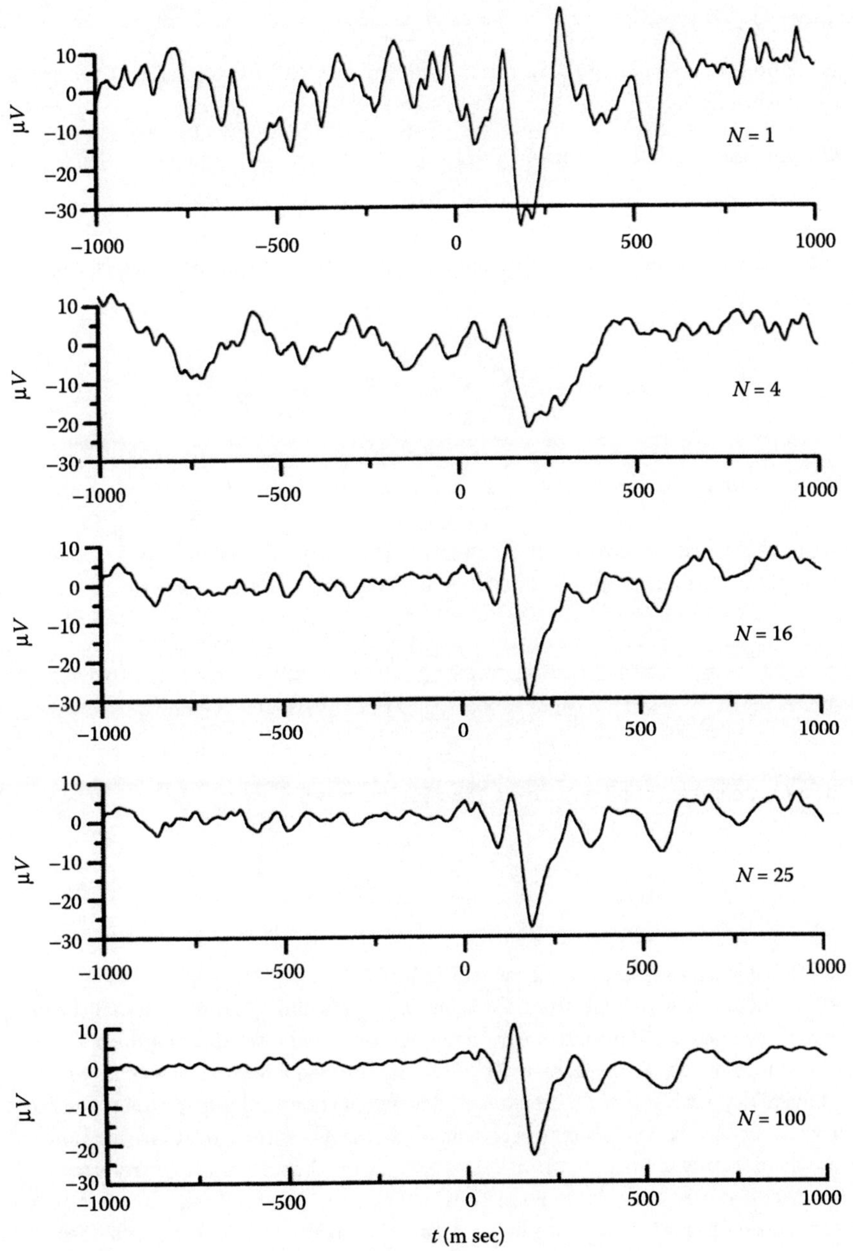

FIGURE 1.15 Enhancement of evoked potential (EP) by means of averaging technique. The EEG noise is progressively reduced, and the EP morphology becomes more recognizable as the number of averaged sweeps (N) is increased.

evoked potential ($N = 1$) is not visible because it is buried in the background EEG (upper panel). In the successive panels, there is the same evoked potential after averaging different numbers of sweeps corresponding to the frequency responses shown in Figure 1.14. As N increases, the SNR is improved by a factor $\sqrt{N}$ (in rms value), and the morphology of the evoked potential becomes more recognizable while the EEG contribution is markedly diminished. In this way, it is easy to evaluate the quantitative indices of clinical interest, such as the amplitude and the latency of the relevant waves.

1.2.3 Spectral Analysis

The various methods to estimate the power spectrum density (PSD) of a signal may be classified as *nonparametric* and *parametric*.

1.2.3.1 Nonparametric Estimators of PSD

This is a traditional method of frequency analysis based on the Fourier transform that can be evaluated easily through the fast Fourier transform (FFT) algorithm (Marple, 1987). The expression of the PSD as a function of the frequency $P(f)$ can be obtained directly from the time series $y(n)$ by using the periodogram expression

$$P(f) = \frac{1}{T_s}\left|T_s\sum_{k=0}^{N-1} y(k)e^{-j2\pi fkT_s}\right|^2 = \frac{1}{NT_s}|Y(f)|^2 \tag{1.26}$$

where T_s is the sampling period, N is the number of samples, and $Y(f)$ is the discrete-time Fourier transform of $y(n)$.

On the basis of the Wiener–Khintchin theorem, PSD is also obtainable in two steps from the FFT of the autocorrelation function $\hat{R}_{yy}(k)$ of the signal, which is estimated by means of the following expression:

$$\hat{R}_{yy}(k) = \frac{1}{N}\sum_{i=0}^{N-k-1} y(i)y^*(i+k) \tag{1.27}$$

where * denotes the complex conjugate. Thus, the PSD is expressed as

$$P(f) = T_s \cdot \sum_{k=-N}^{N} \hat{R}_{yy}(k)e^{-j2\pi fkT_s} \tag{1.28}$$

based on the available lag estimates $\hat{R}_{yy}(k)$, where $-(1/2T_s) \le f \le (1/2T_s)$.

FFT-based methods are widely diffused, for their easy applicability, computational speed, and direct interpretation of the results. Quantitative parameters are obtained by evaluating the power contribution at different frequency bands. This is achieved by dividing the frequency axis in ranges of interest and by integrating the PSD on such intervals. The area under this portion of the spectrum is the fraction of the total signal variance due to the specific frequencies. However, autocorrelation function and Fourier transform are theoretically defined on infinite data sequences. Thus, errors are introduced by the need to operate on finite data records in order to obtain estimators of the true functions. In addition, for the finite data set, it is necessary to make assumptions, sometimes not realistic, about the data outside the recording window; commonly, they are considered to be zero. This implicit rectangular windowing of the data results in a special leakage in the PSD. Different windows that smoothly connect the side samples to zero are most often used in order to solve this problem, even if they may introduce a reduction in the frequency resolution (Harris, 1978). Furthermore, the estimators of the signal PSD are not statistically consistent, and various techniques are needed to improve their statistical performances. Various methods are mentioned in the literature; the methods of Dariell (1946), Bartlett (1948), and Welch (1970) are the most diffused ones. Of course, all these procedures cause a further reduction in frequency resolution.

1.2.3.2 Parametric Estimators

Parametric approaches assume the time series under analysis to be the output of a given mathematical model, and no drastic assumptions are made about the data outside the recording window. The

PSD is calculated as a function of the model parameters according to appropriate expressions. A critical point in this approach is the choice of an adequate model to represent the data sequence. The model is completely independent of the physiologic, anatomic, and physical characteristics of the biologic system but simply provides the input–output relationships of the process in the so-called black-box approach.

Among the numerous possibilities of modeling, linear models, characterized by a rational transfer function, are able to describe a wide number of different processes. In the most general case, they are represented by the following linear equation that relates the input-driving signal $w(k)$ and the output of an autoregressive moving average (ARMA) process:

$$y(k) = -\sum_{i=1}^{p} a_i y(k-i) + \sum_{j=1}^{q} b_j w(k-j) + w(k) \tag{1.29}$$

where $w(k)$ is the input white noise with zero mean value and variance λ^2, p and q are the orders of AR and MA parts, respectively, and a_i and b_j are the proper coefficients.

The ARMA model may be reformulated as an AR or an MA if the coefficients b_j or a_i are, respectively, set to zero. Since the estimation of the AR parameters results in linear equations, AR models are usually employed in place of ARMA or MA models, also on the basis of the Wold decomposition theorem (Marple, 1987) that establishes that any stationary ARMA or MA process of finite variance can be represented as a unique AR model of appropriate order, even infinite; likewise, any ARMA or AR process can be represented by an MA model of sufficiently high order.

The AR PSD is then obtained from the following expression:

$$P(f) = \frac{\lambda T^2}{\left|1 + \sum_1^p a_k z^{-k}\right|^2_{\exp(j2\pi f T_s)}} = \frac{\lambda T^2}{\left|\prod_1^p (z - z_l)\right|^2_{\exp(j2\pi f T_s)}} \tag{1.30}$$

The right side of the relation puts into evidence the poles of the transfer function that can be plotted in the z-transform plane. Figure 1.16b shows the PSD function of the HRV signal depicted in Figure 1.16a, while Figure 1.16c displays the corresponding pole diagram obtained according to the procedure described in the preceding section.

Parametric methods are methodologically and computationally more complex than the nonparametric ones since they require an *a priori* choice of the structure and of the order of the model of the signal-generation mechanism. Some tests are required *a posteriori* to verify the whiteness of the prediction error, such as the Anderson test (autocorrelation test) (Box and Jenkins, 1976) in order to test the reliability of the estimation.

Postprocessing of the spectra can be performed as well for nonparametric approaches by integrating the $P(f)$ function in predefined frequency ranges; however, the AR modeling has the advantage of allowing a spectral decomposition for a direct and automatic calculation of the power and frequency of each spectral component. In the z-transform domain, the autocorrelation function (ACF) $R(k)$ and the $P(z)$ of the signal are related by the following expression:

$$R(k) = \frac{1}{2\pi j} \int_{|z|=1} P(z) z^{k-1}\, dz \tag{1.31}$$

If the integral is calculated by means of the residual method, the ACF is decomposed into a sum of dumped sinusoids, each one related to a pair of complex conjugate poles, and of dumped exponential functions, related to the real poles (Zetterberg, 1969). The Fourier transform of each one of these terms

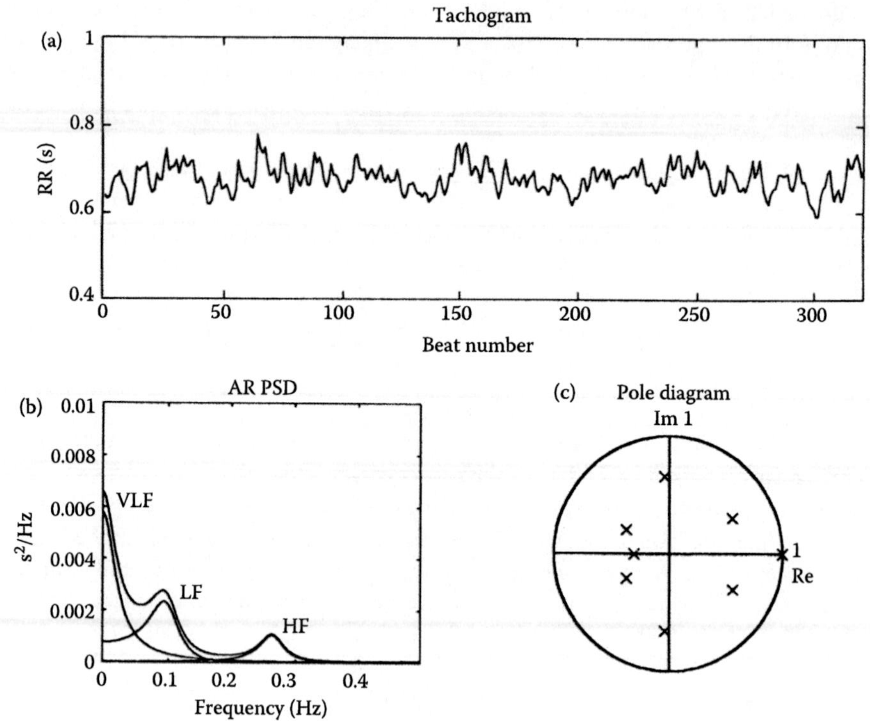

FIGURE 1.16 (a) Interval tachogram obtained from an ECG recording as the sequence of the RR time intervals expressed in seconds as a function of the beat number. (b) PSD of the signal (a) evaluated by means of an AR model (see text). (c) Pole diagram of the PSD shown in (b).

gives the expression of each spectral component that fits the component related to the relevant pole or pole pair. The argument of the pole gives the central frequency of the component, while the ith spectral component power is the residual γ_i in the case of real poles and $2\text{Re}(\gamma_i)$ in case of conjugate pole pairs. γ_i is computed from the following expression:

$$\gamma_i = z^{-1}(z - z_i)P(z)\,|_{z=z_i}$$

It is advisable to point out the basic characteristics of the two approaches that have been described above: the nonparametric and the parametric. The latter (parametric) has evident advantages with respect to the former, which can be summarized in the following:

- It has a more statistical consistency even on short segments of data, that is, under certain assumptions, a spectrum estimated through autoregressive modeling is a maximum entropy spectrum (MES).
- The spectrum is more easily interpretable with an "implicit" filtering of what is considered random noise.
- An easy and more reliable calculation of the spectral parameters (postprocessing of the spectrum), through the spectral decomposition procedure, is possible. Such parameters are directly interpretable from a physiologic point of view.
- There is no need to window the data in order to decrease the spectral leakage.
- The frequency resolution does not depend on the number of data.

On the other hand, the parametric approach

- Is more complex from a methodologic and computational point of view
- Requires an *a priori* definition of the kind of model (AR, MA, ARMA, or other) to be fitted and mainly its complexity defined (i.e., the number of parameters)

Some figures of merit introduced in the literature may be of help in determining their value (Akaike, 1974). Still, this procedure may be difficult in some cases.

1.2.3.3 Example

As an example, let us consider the frequency analysis of the HRV signal. In Figure 1.16a, the time sequence of the RR intervals obtained from an ECG recording is shown. The RR intervals are expressed in seconds as a function of the beat number in the so-called interval tachogram. It is worth noting that the RR series is not constant but is characterized by oscillations of up to 10% of its mean value. These oscillations are not causal but are the effect of the action of the autonomic nervous system in controlling heart rate. In particular, the frequency analysis of such a signal (Figure 1.16b shows the PSD obtained by means of an AR model) has evidenced three principal contributions in the overall variability of the HRV signal. A very low frequency (VLF) component is due to the long-term regulation mechanisms that cannot be resolved by analyzing a few minutes of signal (3–5 min are generally studied in the traditional spectral analysis of the HRV signal). Other techniques are needed for a complete understanding of such mechanisms. The low-frequency (LF) component is centered around 0.1 Hz, in a range between 0.03 and 0.15 Hz. An increase in its power has always been observed in relation to sympathetic activations. Finally, the high-frequency (HF) component, in synchrony with the respiration rate, is due to the respiration activity mediated by the vagus nerve; thus, it can be a marker of vagal activity. In particular, LF and HF power, both in absolute and in normalized units (i.e., as percentage value on the total power without the VLF contribution), and their ratio LF/HF are quantitative indices widely employed for the quantification of the sympathovagal balance in controlling heart rate (Malliani et al., 1991; Task Force, 1996).

1.3 Conclusion

The basic aspects of signal acquisition and processing have been illustrated, intended as fundamental tools for the treatment of biologic signals. A few examples also were reported relative to the ECG signal, as well as EEG signals and EPs. Particular processing algorithms have been described that use digital filtering techniques, coherent averaging, and power spectrum analysis as reference examples on how traditional or innovative techniques of digital signal processing may impact the phase of informative parameter extraction from biologic signals. They may improve the knowledge of many physiologic systems as well as help clinicians in dealing with new quantitative parameters that could better discriminate between normal and pathologic cases.

Defining Terms

Aliasing: Phenomenon that takes place when, in A/D conversion, the sampling frequency f_s is lower than twice the frequency content f_b of the signal; frequency components above $f_s/2$ are folded back and are summed to the lower-frequency components, distorting the signal.

Averaging: Filtering technique based on the summation of N stationary waveforms buried in casual broadband noise with a synchronization trigger. The SNR is improved by a factor of $\sqrt{N}$.

Frequency response: A complex quantity that, multiplied by a sinusoid input of a linear filter, gives the output sinusoid. It completely characterizes the filter and is the Fourier transform of the impulse response.

Impulse reaction: Output of a digital filter when the input is the impulse sequence $d(n)$. It completely characterizes linear filters and is used for evaluating the output corresponding to different kinds of inputs.

Notch filter: A stopband filter whose stopped band is very sharp and narrow.

Parametric methods: Spectral estimation methods based on the identification of a signal-generating model. The power spectral density is a function of the model parameters.

Quantization error: Error added to the signal, during the A/D procedure, due to the fact that the analog signal is represented by a digital signal that can assume only a limited and predefined set of values.

Region of convergence: In the z-transform plane, the ensemble containing the z complex points that makes a series converge to a finite value.

References

Akaike H. 1974. A new look at the statistical model identification. *IEEE Trans. Autom. Contr.* (AC-19): 716.

Antoniou A. 1979. *Digital Filters: Analysis and Design.* New York, McGraw-Hill.

Aunon J.L., McGillim C.D., and Childers D.G. 1981. Signal processing in evoked potential research: Averaging and modeling. *CRC Crit. Rev. Bioeng.* 5: 323.

Bartlett M.S. 1948. Smoothing periodograms from time series with continuous spectra. *Nature* 61: 686.

Box G.E.P. and Jenkins G.M. 1976. *Time Series Analysis: Forecasting and Control.* San Francisco, Holden-Day.

Cappellini V., Constantinides A.G., and Emiliani P. 1978. *Digital Filters and Their Applications.* London, Academic Press.

Carassa F. 1983. *Comunicazioni Elettriche.* Torino, Boringhieri.

Cerutti S. 1983. *Filtri numerici per l'eleborazione di segnali biologici.* Milano, CLUP.

Challis R.E. and Kitney R.I. 1982. The design of digital filters for biomedical signal processing: 1. Basic concepts. *J. Biomed. Eng.* 5: 267.

Cobbold R.S.C. 1988. *Transducers for Biomedical Measurements.* New York, John Wiley & Sons.

Cohen A. 1983. *Biomedical Signal Processing: Time and Frequency Domains Analysis.* Boca Raton, FL, CRC Press.

Dariell P.J. 1946. On the theoretical specification and sampling properties of autocorrelated time-series (discussion). *J. R. Stat. Soc.* 8: 88.

Gardenhire L.W. 1964. Selecting sample rate. *ISA J.* 4:59.

Gevins A.S. and Remond A. (eds). 1987. *Handbook of Electrophysiology and Clinical Neurophysiology.* Amsterdam, Elsevier.

Glaser E.M. and Ruchkin D.S. 1976. *Principles of Neurophysiological Signal Processing.* New York, Academic Press.

Harris F.J. 1978. On the use of windows for harmonic analysis with the discrete Fourier transform. *Proc. IEEE* 64: 51.

Huta K. and Webster J.G. 1973. 60-Hz interference in electrocardiography. *IEEE Trans. Biomed. Eng.* 20: 91.

Jackson L.B. 1986. *Digital Signal Processing.* Hingham, MA, Kluwer Academic.

Jaeger R.C. 1982. Tutorial: Analog data acquisition technology: II. Analog to digital conversion. *IEEE Micro.* 8: 46.

Malliani A., Pagani M., Lombardi F., and Cerutti S. 1991. Cardiovascular neural regulation explored in the frequency domain. *Circulation* 84: 482.

Marple S.L. 1987. *Digital Spectral Analysis with Applications.* Englewood Cliffs, NJ, Prentice-Hall.

Oppenheim A.V. and Schafer R.W. 1975. *Digital Signal Processing.* Englewood Cliffs, NJ, Prentice-Hall.

Rabiner L., Cooley J., Helms H., Jackson L., Kaiser J., Rader C., Schafer R., Steiglitz K., and Weinstein C. 1972. Terminology in digital signal processing. *IEEE Trans. Audio Electroac.* AU-20: 322.

Sayed A.H. 2003. *Fundamentals of Adaptive Filtering*, Hoboken, NJ, Wiley & Sons.
Shannon C.E. 1949. Communication in presence of noise. *Proc. IRE* 37: 10.
Simson M.B. 1981. Use of signals in the terminal QRS complex to identify patients with ventricular tachycardia after myocardial infarction. *Circulation* 64: 235.
Task Force of the European Society of Cardiology the North American Society of Pacing Electrophysiology. 1996. *Heart Rate Variability: Standards of Measurement, Physiological Interpretation, and Clinical Use*. 93: 1043.
Thakor N.V. 1987. Adaptive filtering of evoked potential. *IEEE Trans. Biomed. Eng.* 34: 1706.
Tompkins W.J. (ed). 1993. *Biomedical Digital Signal Processing*. Englewood Cliffs, NJ, Prentice-Hall.
Tompkins W.J. and Webster J.G. (eds). 1981. *Design of Microcomputer-Based Medical Instrumentation*. Englewood Cliffs, NJ, Prentice-Hall.
Webster J.G. (ed). 2009. *Medical Instrumentation Application and Design*, 4th ed. Somerset, NJ, John Wiley & Sons.
Welch D.P. 1970. The use of fast Fourier transform for the estimation of power spectra: A method based on time averaging over short modified periodograms. *IEEE Trans. Acoust.* AU-15: 70.
Widrow B. 1956. A study of rough amplitude quantization by means of Nyquist sampling theory. *IRE Trans. Cric. Theory* 3: 266.
Widrow B., Glover J.R., Jr., McCool J.M., Kaunitz J., Williams C.S., Hearn R.H., Zeidler J.R., Eugene Dong, Jr., and Goodlin R.C. 1975. Adaptive noise cancelling: Principles and applications. *Proc. IEEE* 63: 1692.
Zetterberg L.H. 1969. Estimation of parameters for a linear difference equation with application to EEG analysis. *Math. Biosci.* 5: 227.

Further Information

A book that provides a general overview of basic concepts in biomedical signal processing is *Digital Biosignal Processing*, by Rolf Weitkunat (ed) (Elsevier Science Publishers, Amsterdam, 1991). Contributions by different authors provide descriptions of several processing techniques and many applicative examples on biologic signal analysis.

A fair introduction to biomedical signal processing topics is provided by the book *Introduction to Applied Statistical Signal Analysis: Guide to Biomedical and Electrical Engineering Applications*, by R. Shiavi (CRC Press, 3rd edition, 2007).

Readers who are interested in advanced applications of biomedical signal processing methodologies can refer to the book *Bioelectrical Signal Processing in Cardiac and Neurological Applications* by L. Sornmo and P. Laguna (Academic Press, 2005) and to the book *Advanced Methods of Biomedical Signal Processing* (Wiley IEEE Press Series on Biomedical Engineering, 2009) by S. Cerutti and C. Marchesi.

Advances in signal processing are published monthly in the journal *IEEE Transactions on Signal Processing*, while the *IEEE Transaction on Biomedical Engineering* provides examples of applications in biomedical engineering fields.

2

Time–Frequency Signal Representations for Biomedical Signals

G. Faye Boudreaux-Bartels
University of Rhode Island

Robin Murray
University of Rhode Island
Naval Undersea Warfare Center

The Fourier transform of a signal $x(t)$

$$X(f) = \int x(t)e^{-j2\pi ft}\,dt \tag{2.1}$$

is a useful tool for analyzing the spectral content of a stationary signal and for transforming difficult operations such as convolution, differentiation, and integration into very simple algebraic operations in the Fourier dual domain. The inverse Fourier transform equation

$$x(t) = \int X(f)e^{j2\pi ft}\,df \tag{2.2}$$

is a linear combination of complex sinusoids of infinite duration which implicitly assumes that each sinusoidal component is present at all times and, hence, the spectral content of the signal does not change with time. However, many signals in bioengineering are produced by biological systems whose spectral characteristics can change rapidly with time. To analyze these rapid spectral changes, one needs a two-dimensional, mixed time–frequency signal representation (TFR) that is analogous to a musical score with time represented along one axis and frequency along the other, indicating which frequency components (notes) are present at each time instant.

The first purpose of this chapter is to review several TFRs defined in Table 2.1 and to describe many of the desirable properties listed in Table 2.2 that an ideal TFR should satisfy. TFRs will be grouped into classes satisfying similar properties to provide a more intuitive understanding of their similarities, advantages, and disadvantages. Further, each TFR within a given class is completely characterized by a unique set of kernels that provide valuable insight into whether or not a given TFR (1) satisfies other ideal TFR properties, (2) is easy to compute, and (3) reduces nonlinear cross-terms. The

TABLE 2.1 List of Time–Frequency Representations of a Signal $x(t)$ Whose Fourier Transform Is $X(f)$

Ackroyd distribution	$\mathrm{ACK}_x(t,f)=\mathrm{Re}\left\{x^*(t)X(f)e^{j2\pi ft}\right\}$
Affine Wigner distribution	$\mathrm{AWD}_X(t,f;G,F)=\int G\left(\frac{\nu}{f}\right)X\left(fF\left(\frac{\nu}{f}\right)+\frac{\nu}{2}\right)X^*\left(fF\left(\frac{\nu}{f}\right)-\frac{\nu}{2}\right)e^{j2\pi t\nu}d\nu$
Altes–Marinovic distribution	$\mathrm{AM}_X(t,f)=\lvert f\rvert\int X(fe^{u/2})X^*(fe^{-u/2})e^{j2\pi tfu}du=\lvert f\rvert\iint \mathrm{WAF}_X(\tau,e^{\beta})e^{j2\pi(tf\beta-f\tau)}d\tau d\beta$
(Narrowband) ambiguity function	$\mathrm{AF}_x(\tau,\nu)=\int x\left(t+\frac{\tau}{2}\right)x^*\left(t-\frac{\tau}{2}\right)e^{-j2\pi\nu t}dt=\int X\left(f+\frac{\nu}{2}\right)X^*\left(f-\frac{\nu}{2}\right)e^{j2\pi\tau f}df$
Andrieux et al. distribution	$\mathrm{AND}_x(t,f)=\iint\frac{1}{\sigma_{(t-t')}\sigma_{(f-f')}}\exp\left[-\left(\frac{(t-t')^2}{2\sigma^2_{(t-t')}}+\frac{(f-b_{(t-t')}(t-t'))^2}{2\sigma^2_{(f-f')}}\right)\right]\times\mathrm{WD}_x(t',f')dt'df'$ where for $x(t)=e^{j2\pi\varphi(t)}$, then $b_t=\frac{d^2}{dt^2}\varphi(t),\ \sigma_t=\left\lvert\frac{d^3}{dt^3}\varphi(t)\right\rvert^{-1/3}$, and $2\pi\sigma_t\sigma_f=\frac{1}{2}$
Autocorrelation function	
Temporal	$\mathrm{act}_x(\tau)=\int x^*(t)x(t+\tau)dt=\int\lvert X(f)\rvert^2e^{j2\pi f\tau}df$
Spectral	$\mathrm{ACF}_X(\nu)=\int X^*(f)X(f+\nu)df=\int\lvert x(t)\rvert^2e^{-j2\pi t\nu}dt$
Bertrand P_k distribution	$BkD_x(t,f;\mu_k)=\lvert f\rvert\int X(f\lambda_k(u))X^*(f\lambda_k(-u))\mu_k(u)e^{j2\pi tf(\lambda_k(u)-\lambda_k(-u))}du$
	with $\lambda_0(u)=\frac{u/2e^{u/2}}{\sinh(u/2)},\ \lambda_1(u)=\exp\left[1+\left(\frac{ue^{-u}}{e^{-u}-1}\right)\right],\lambda_k(u)=\left[k\frac{e^{u}-1}{e^{-ku}-1}\right]^{1/(k-1)}$ $k\neq 0,1,\mu_k(u)=\mu_k(-u)>0$
Born–Jordon distribution	$\mathrm{BJD}_x(t,f)=\int\frac{1}{\tau}\left[\int_{t-\lvert\tau\rvert/2}^{t+\lvert\tau\rvert/2}x\left(t'+\frac{\tau}{2}\right)x^*\left(t'-\frac{\tau}{2}\right)dt'\right]e^{-j2\pi f\tau}d\tau$
Butterworth distribution	$\mathrm{BUD}_x(t,f)=\iint\left(1+\left(\frac{\tau}{\tau_0}\right)^{2M}\left(\frac{\nu}{\nu_0}\right)^{2N}\right)^{-1}\mathrm{AF}_x(\tau,\nu)e^{j2\pi(t\nu-f\tau)}d\tau d\nu$
Choi–Williams exponential distribution	$\mathrm{CWD}_x(t,f)=\iint\sqrt{\frac{\sigma}{4\pi}}\frac{1}{\lvert\tau\rvert}\exp\left[-\frac{\sigma}{4}\left(\frac{t-t'}{\tau}\right)^2\right]x\left(t'+\frac{\tau}{2}\right)x^*\left(t'-\frac{\tau}{2}\right)e^{-j2\pi f\tau}dt'd\tau$

TABLE 2.1 (continued) List of Time–Frequency Representations of a Signal $x(t)$ Whose Fourier Transform Is $X(f)$

Cohen's nonnegative distribution	$\mathrm{CND}_x(t,f)=\frac{\lvert x(t)\rvert^2\lvert X(f)\rvert^2}{E_x}\left[1+c\rho(\xi_x(t),\eta_x(f))\right]$ with $\xi_x(t)=\frac{1}{E_x}\int_{-\infty}^{t}\lvert x(\tau)\rvert^2\,\mathrm{d}\tau,\ \eta_x(f)=\frac{1}{E_x}\int_{-\infty}^{f}\lvert X(f')\rvert^2\,\mathrm{d}f',\ E_x=\int\lvert x(t)\rvert^2\,\mathrm{d}t$
Cone–Kernel distribution	$\mathrm{CKD}_x(t,f)=\int g(\tau)\left[\int_{t-\lvert\tau\rvert/2}^{t+\lvert\tau\rvert/2}x\left(t'+\frac{\tau}{2}\right)x^*\left(t'-\frac{\tau}{2}\right)\mathrm{d}t'\right]\mathrm{e}^{-j2\pi f\tau}\mathrm{d}\tau$
Cumulative attack spectrum	$\mathrm{CAS}_x(t,f)=\left\lvert\int_{-\infty}^{t}x(\tau)\mathrm{e}^{-j2\pi f\tau}\mathrm{d}\tau\right\rvert^2$
Cumulative decay spectrum	$\mathrm{CDS}_x(t,f)=\left\lvert\int_{t}^{\infty}x(\tau)\mathrm{e}^{-j2\pi f\tau}\mathrm{d}\tau\right\rvert^2$
Flandrin *D*-distribution	$\mathrm{FD}_X(t,f)=\lvert f\rvert\int X\left(f\left[1+\frac{u}{4}\right]^2\right)X^*\left(f\left[1-\frac{u}{4}\right]^2\right)\left[1-\left(\frac{u}{4}\right)^2\right]\mathrm{e}^{j2\pi tfu}\mathrm{d}u$
Gabor expansion, $\mathrm{GE}_x(n,k;g)$	$x(t)=\Sigma_n\Sigma_k\mathrm{GE}_x(n,k;g)g(t-n\Delta T)\mathrm{e}^{j2\pi(k\Delta F)t}$
Generalized Altes distribution	$\mathrm{GAM}_X(t,f;\alpha)=\lvert f\rvert\int\mathrm{e}^{-\alpha u}X\left(f\mathrm{e}^{((1/2)-\alpha)u}\right)X^*\left(f\mathrm{e}^{-((1/2)+\alpha)u}\right)\mathrm{e}^{j2\pi tfu}\mathrm{d}u$
Generalized exponential distribution	$\mathrm{GED}_x(t,f)=\iint\exp\left[-\left(\frac{\tau}{\tau_0}\right)^{2M}\left(\frac{\nu}{\nu_0}\right)^{2N}\right]\mathrm{AF}_x(\tau,\nu)\mathrm{e}^{j2\pi(t\nu-f\tau)}\mathrm{d}\tau\mathrm{d}\nu$
Generalized rectangular distribution	$\mathrm{GRD}_x(t,f)=\iint rect_1\left(\frac{\lvert\tau\rvert^{\frac{M}{N}}\lvert\nu\rvert}{\sigma}\right)\mathrm{AF}_x(\tau,\nu)\mathrm{e}^{j2\pi(t\nu-f\tau)}\mathrm{d}\tau\mathrm{d}\nu$, where $rect_b(t)=\begin{cases}1, & \lvert t\rvert<\lvert b\rvert\\ 0, & \lvert t\rvert>\lvert b\rvert\end{cases}$
Generalized Wigner distribution	$\mathrm{GWD}_x(t,f;\tilde{\alpha})=\int x\left(t+\left(\frac{1}{2}+\tilde{\alpha}\right)\tau\right)x^*\left(t-\left(\frac{1}{2}-\tilde{\alpha}\right)\tau\right)\mathrm{e}^{-j2\pi f\tau}\mathrm{d}\tau$
Hyperbolic ambiguity function	$\mathrm{HAF}_X(\zeta,\beta)=\int_0^{\infty}X(f\mathrm{e}^{\beta/2})X^*(f\mathrm{e}^{-\beta/2})\mathrm{e}^{j2\pi\zeta\ln(f/f_r)}\mathrm{d}f$
Hyperbolic wavelet transform	$\mathrm{HWT}_X(t,f;\Gamma)=\sqrt{\frac{f_r}{f}}\int_0^{\infty}X(\xi)\Gamma^*\left(\frac{f_r}{f}\xi\right)\mathrm{e}^{j2\pi tf\ln(\xi/f_r)}\mathrm{d}\xi$
Hyperbologram	$\mathrm{HYP}_X(t,f;\Gamma)=\left\lvert\sqrt{\frac{f_r}{f}}\int_0^{\infty}X(\xi)\Gamma^*\left(\frac{f_r}{f}\xi\right)\mathrm{e}^{j2\pi tf\ln(\xi/f_r)}\mathrm{d}\xi\right\rvert^2=\lvert\mathrm{HWT}_X(t,f;\Gamma)\rvert^2$
Levin distribution	$\mathrm{LD}_x(t,f)=-\frac{\mathrm{d}}{\mathrm{d}t}\left\lvert\int_t^{\infty}x(\tau)\mathrm{e}^{-j2\pi f\tau}\mathrm{d}\tau\right\rvert^2$
Margineau–Hill distribution	$\mathrm{MH}_x(t,f)=\mathrm{Re}\left\{x(t)X^*(f)\mathrm{e}^{-j2\pi ft}\right\}$
Multiform, tiltable distributions	Let $\tilde{\mu}(\tilde{\tau},\tilde{\nu};\alpha,r,\beta,\gamma)=\left((\tilde{\tau})^2\left((\tilde{\nu})^2\right)^{\alpha}+\left((\tilde{\tau})^2\right)^{\alpha}(\tilde{\nu})^2+2r\left((\tilde{\tau}\tilde{\nu})^{\beta}\right)^{\gamma}\right)$

continued

TABLE 2.1 (continued) List of Time–Frequency Representations of a Signal $x(t)$ Whose Fourier Transform Is $X(f)$

Butterworth	$\mathrm{MTBD}_x(t,f)=\iint\left[1+\tilde{\mu}^{2\lambda}\left(\frac{\tau}{\tau_0},\frac{\nu}{\nu_0};\alpha,r,\beta,\gamma\right)\right]^{-1}\mathrm{AF}_x(\tau,\nu)e^{j2\pi(t\nu-f\tau)}d\tau d\nu$
Exponential	$\mathrm{MTED}_x(t,f)=\iint\exp\left\{-\pi\tilde{\mu}^{2\lambda}\left(\frac{\tau}{\tau_0},\frac{\nu}{\nu_0};\alpha,r,\beta,\gamma\right)\right\}\mathrm{AF}_x(\tau,\nu)e^{j2\pi(t\nu-f\tau)}d\tau d\nu$
(Inverse) Chebyshev	$\mathrm{MT}(I)C_x(t,f)=\iint\left[1+\varepsilon^2C_\lambda^{\pm 2}\left(\tilde{\mu}\left(\frac{\tau}{\tau_0},\frac{\nu}{\nu_0};\alpha,r,\beta,\gamma\right)^{\pm 1}\right)\right]^{-1}\mathrm{AF}_x(\tau,\nu)e^{j2\pi(t\nu-f\tau)}d\tau d\nu$ where $C_\lambda(a)$ is a Chebyshev polynomial of order λ
Nutall–Griffin distribution	$\mathrm{ND}_x(t,f)=\iint\exp\left\{-\pi\left[\left(\frac{\tau}{\tau_0}\right)^2+\left(\frac{\nu}{\nu_0}\right)^2+2r\left(\frac{\tau\nu}{\tau_0\nu_0}\right)\right]\right\}\mathrm{AF}_x(\tau,\nu)e^{j2\pi(t\nu-f\tau)}d\tau d\nu$
Page distribution	$2\,\mathrm{Re}\left\{x^*(t)\,e^{j2\pi tf}\int_{-\infty}^{t}x(\tau)e^{-j2\pi f\tau}d\tau\right\}$
*k*th Power	
Ambiguity function	$B_X^{(\kappa)}(\zeta,\beta)=\mathrm{AF}_{\mathcal{W}_\kappa X}\left(\frac{\zeta}{f_r},f_r\beta\right),\quad(\mathcal{W}_\kappa X)(f)=\frac{1}{\sqrt{f_r\,\lvert\tau_\kappa(f_r\xi_\kappa^{-1}(f/f_r))\rvert}}X\left(f_r\xi_\kappa^{-1}\left(\frac{f}{f_r}\right)\right)$
Central member	$\mathrm{AM}_X^{(\kappa)}(t,f)=\mathrm{WD}_{\mathcal{W}_\kappa X}\left(\frac{t}{f_r\tau_\kappa(f)},f_r\xi_\kappa\left(\frac{f}{f_r}\right)\right),\quad\tau_\kappa(f)=\frac{d}{df}\xi_\kappa\left(\frac{f}{f_r}\right)$ where $\xi_\kappa(b)=\begin{cases}\mathrm{sgn}(b)\lvert b\rvert^\kappa, & b\in\mathcal{R}\text{ for }\kappa\neq 0\\ \ln(b), & b>0\text{ for }\kappa=0\end{cases}$ and $\xi_\kappa^{-1}(b)=\begin{cases}\mathrm{sgn}(b)\lvert b\rvert^{1/\kappa}, & b\in\mathcal{R},\kappa\neq 0\\ e^b, & b>0,\kappa=0\end{cases}$
Power spectral density	$\mathrm{PSD}_x(f)=\lvert X(f)\rvert^2=\int\mathrm{act}_x(\tau)e^{-j2\pi f\tau}d\tau$
Pseudo-Altes distribution	$\mathrm{PAD}_X(t,f;\Gamma)=f_r\int_0^\infty\mathrm{AM}_\Gamma\left(0,\frac{f_rf}{f'}\right)\mathrm{AM}_X\left(\frac{tf}{f'},f'\right)\frac{df'}{f'}$
Pseudo-Wigner distribution	$\mathrm{PWD}_x(t,f;\eta)=\int x\left(t+\frac{\tau}{2}\right)x^*\left(t-\frac{\tau}{2}\right)\eta\left(\frac{\tau}{2}\right)\eta^*\left(-\frac{\tau}{2}\right)e^{-j2\pi f\tau}d\tau$
Radially adaptive Gaussian distribution	$\mathrm{RAGD}_x(t,f)=\iint\exp\left[\frac{-(\tau/\tau_0)^2+(\nu/\nu_0)^2}{2\sigma_x^2(\theta)}\right]\mathrm{AF}_x(\tau,\nu)e^{j2\pi(t\nu-f\tau)}d\tau d\nu$ where $\theta=\arctan\left[\frac{\nu/\nu_0}{\tau/\tau_0}\right]$
Real generalized Wigner distribution	$\mathrm{RGWD}_x(t,f;\tilde{\alpha})=\mathrm{Re}\left\{\int x\left(t+\left(\frac{1}{2}+\tilde{\alpha}\right)\tau\right)x^*\left(t-\left(\frac{1}{2}-\tilde{\alpha}\right)\tau\right)e^{-j2\pi f\tau}d\tau\right\}$

TABLE 2.1 (continued) List of Time–Frequency Representations of a Signal $x(t)$ Whose Fourier Transform Is $X(f)$

Reduced interference distribution	$\mathrm{RID}_x(t,f;S_{\mathrm{RID}}) = \iint \frac{1}{\lvert\tau\rvert} S_{\mathrm{RID}}\left(\frac{t-t'}{\tau}\right) x\left(t'+\frac{\tau}{2}\right) x^*\left(t'-\frac{\tau}{2}\right) \mathrm{e}^{-j2\pi f\tau}\mathrm{d}t'\mathrm{d}\tau$ with $S_{\mathrm{RID}}(\beta)\in\mathcal{R},\ S_{\mathrm{RID}}(0)=1, \left\{\frac{\mathrm{d}}{\mathrm{d}\beta}S_{\mathrm{RID}}(\beta)\Big\vert_{\beta=0}=0\right\}, \left\{S_{\mathrm{RID}}(\alpha)=0 \text{ for } \lvert\alpha\rvert>\frac{1}{2}\right\}$
Rihaczek distribution	$\mathrm{RD}_x(t,f) = x(t)X^*(f)\mathrm{e}^{-j2\pi tf}$
Running spectrum, past	$\mathrm{RSP}_x(t,f) = \int_{-\infty}^{t} x(u)\mathrm{e}^{-j2\pi fu}\mathrm{d}u,$
Running spectrum, future	$\mathrm{RSF}_x(t,f) = \int_{t}^{\infty} x(u)\mathrm{e}^{-j2\pi fu}\mathrm{d}u$
Scalogram	$\mathrm{SCAL}_x(t,f;\gamma) = \left\lvert \int x(\tau)\sqrt{\left\lvert\frac{f}{f_r}\right\rvert}\gamma^*\left(\frac{f}{f_r}(\tau-t)\right)\mathrm{d}\tau \right\rvert^2 = \lvert \mathrm{WT}_x(t,f;\gamma)\rvert^2$
Short-time Fourier transform	$\mathrm{STFT}_x(t,f;\gamma) = \int x(\tau)\gamma^*(\tau-t)\mathrm{e}^{-j2\pi f\tau}\mathrm{d}\tau = \mathrm{e}^{-j2\pi tf}\int X(f')\Gamma^*(f'-f)\mathrm{e}^{j2\pi tf'}\mathrm{d}f'$
Smoothed Pseudo-Altes distribution	$\mathrm{SPAD}_X(t,f;\Gamma,g) = \int g(tf-c)\mathrm{PAD}_X\left(\frac{c}{f},f;\Gamma\right)\mathrm{d}c$
Smoothed Pseudo-Wigner distribution	$\mathrm{SPWD}_x(t,f;\gamma,\eta) = \iint \gamma(t-t')\eta\left(\frac{\tau}{2}\right)\eta^*\left(-\frac{\tau}{2}\right)x\left(t'+\frac{\tau}{2}\right)x^*\left(t'-\frac{\tau}{2}\right)\mathrm{e}^{-j2\pi f\tau}\mathrm{d}t'\mathrm{d}\tau$
Spectrogram	$\mathrm{SPEC}_x(t,f;\gamma) = \left\lvert \int x(\tau)\gamma^*(\tau-t)\mathrm{e}^{-j2\pi f\tau}\mathrm{d}\tau \right\rvert^2 = \lvert \mathrm{STFT}_x(t,f;\gamma)\rvert^2$
Unterberger active distribution	$\mathrm{UAD}_X(t,f) = f\int_0^{\infty} X(fu)X^*(f/u)[1+u^{-2}]\mathrm{e}^{j2\pi tf(u-1/u)}\mathrm{d}u$
Unterberger passive distribution	$\mathrm{UPD}_X(t,f) = 2f\int_0^{\infty} X(fu)X^*(f/u)[u^{-1}]\mathrm{e}^{j2\pi tf(u-1/u)}\mathrm{d}u$
Wavelet transform	$\mathrm{WT}_x(t,f;\gamma) = \int x(\tau)\sqrt{\left\lvert\frac{f}{f_r}\right\rvert}\gamma^*\left(\frac{f}{f_r}(\tau-t)\right)\mathrm{d}\tau = \int X(f')\sqrt{\left\lvert\frac{f_r}{f}\right\rvert}\Gamma^*\left(\frac{f_r}{f}f'\right)\mathrm{e}^{j2\pi tf'}\mathrm{d}f'$
Wideband ambiguity function	$\mathrm{WAF}_X(\tau,\alpha) = \int_0^{\infty} X(f\sqrt{\alpha})X^*(f/\sqrt{\alpha})\mathrm{e}^{j2\pi\tau f}\mathrm{d}f$
Wigner distribution	$\mathrm{WD}_x(t,f) = \int x\left(t+\frac{\tau}{2}\right)x^*\left(t-\frac{\tau}{2}\right)\mathrm{e}^{-j2\pi f\tau}\mathrm{d}\tau = \int X\left(f+\frac{\nu}{2}\right)X^*\left(f-\frac{\nu}{2}\right)\mathrm{e}^{j2\pi t\nu}\mathrm{d}\nu$

second goal of this chapter is to discuss applications of TFRs to signal analysis and detection problems in bioengineering. Unfortunately, none of the current TFRs is ideal; some give erroneous information when the signal's spectrum is rapidly time-varying. Researchers often analyze several TFRs side by side, keeping in mind the relative strengths and weaknesses of each TFR before drawing any conclusions.

TABLE 2.2 List of Desirable Properties for Time–Frequency Representations and Their Corresponding Kernel Constraints for Cohen's Class and the Hyperbolic Class

Property Name	TFR Property	Kernel Constraints for Cohen's Class	Kernel Constraints for Hyperbolic Class
P_1: Frequency-shift covariant	$T_y(t,f)=T_x(t,f-f_0)$ for $y(t)=x(t)e^{j2\pi f_0 t}$	Always satisfied	
P_2: Time-shift covariant	$T_y(t,f)=T_x(t-t_0,f)$ for $y(t)=x(t-t_0)$	Always satisfied	$\Psi_H(\zeta,\beta)=B_H(\beta)e^{-j2\pi\zeta\ln G(\beta)}$ with $G(\beta)=\dfrac{\beta/2}{\sinh(\beta/2)}$
P_3: Scale covariant	$T_y(t,f)=T_x(at,f/a)$ for $y(t)=\sqrt{\lvert a\rvert}x(at)$	$\Psi_C(\tau,\nu)=S_C(\tau\nu)$	Always satisfied
P_4: Hyperbolic time shift	$T_y(t,f)=T_x(t-c/f,f)$ if $Y(f)=\exp\left(-j2\pi c\ln\frac{f}{f_r}\right)X(f)$		Always satisfied
P_5: Convolution covariant	$T_y(t,f)=\int T_h(t-\tau,f)T_x(\tau,f)d\tau$ for $y(t)=\int h(t-\tau)x(\tau)d\tau$	$\Psi_C(\tau_1+\tau_2,\nu)=\Psi_C(\tau_1,\nu)\cdot\Psi_C(\tau_2,\nu)$	$\Phi_H(b_1,\beta)\Phi_H(b_2,\beta)=$ $e^{b_1}\Phi_H(b_1,\beta)\delta(b_1-b_2)$
P_6: Modulation covariant	$T_y(t,f)=\int T_h(t,f-f')T_x(t,f')df'$ for $y(t)=h(t)x(t)$	$\Psi_C(\tau,\nu_1+\nu_2)=\Psi_C(\tau,\nu_1)\cdot\Psi_C(\tau,\nu_2)$	
P_7: Real-valued	$T_x^*(t,f)=T_x(t,f)$	$\Psi_C^*(-\tau,-\nu)=\Psi_C(\tau,\nu)$	$\Psi_H^*(-\zeta,-\beta)=\Psi_H(\zeta,\beta)$
P_8: Positivity	$T_x(t,f)\geq 0$	$\Psi_C(\tau,\nu)=AF_\gamma(-\tau,-\nu)$	$\Psi_H(\zeta,\beta)=HAF_\Gamma(-\zeta,-\beta)$
P_9: Time marginal	$\int T_x(t,f)df = \lvert x(t)\rvert^2$	$\Psi_C(0,\nu)=1$	
P_{10}: Frequency marginal	$\int T_x(t,f)dt = \lvert X(f)\rvert^2$	$\Psi_C(\tau,0)=1$	$\Psi_H(\zeta,0)=1$
P_{11}: Energy distribution	$\iint T_x(t,f)dt\,df=\int \lvert X(f)\rvert^2 df$	$\Psi_C(0,0)=1$	$\Psi_H(0,0)=1$
P_{12}: Time moments	$\iint t^n T_x(t,f)dt\,df=\int t^n \lvert x(t)\rvert^2 dt$	$\Psi_C(0,\nu)=1$	
P_{13}: Frequency moments	$\iint f^n T_x(t,f)dt\,df=\int f^n \lvert X(f)\rvert^2 df$	$\Psi_C(\tau,0)=1$	

P_{14}: Finite time support	$T_x(t,f)=0$ for $t \notin (t_1,t_2)$ if $x(t)=0$ for $t \notin (t_1,t_2)$	$\varphi_C(t,\tau)=0, \left\|\frac{t}{\tau}\right\| > \frac{1}{2}$	
P_{15}: Finite frequency support	$T_x(t,f)=0$ for $f \notin (f_1,f_2)$ if $X(f)=0$ for $f \notin (f_1,f_2)$	$\Phi_C(f,\nu)=0, \left\|\frac{f}{\nu}\right\| > \frac{1}{2}$	$\Phi_H(c,\zeta)=0, \left\|\frac{c}{\zeta}\right\| > \frac{1}{2}$
P_{16}: Instantaneous frequency	$\frac{\int f\,T_x(t,f)\mathrm{d}f}{\int T_x(t,f)\mathrm{d}f}=\frac{1}{2\pi}\frac{\mathrm{d}}{\mathrm{d}t}\arg\{x(t)\}$	$\Psi_C(0,\nu)=1$ and $\frac{\partial}{\partial\tau}\Psi_C(\tau,\nu)\|_{\tau=0}=0$	
P_{17}: Group delay	$\frac{\int tT_x(t,f)\mathrm{d}t}{\int T_x(t,f)\mathrm{d}t}=-\frac{1}{2\pi}\frac{\mathrm{d}}{\mathrm{d}f}\arg\{X(f)\}$	$\Psi_C(\tau,0)=1$ and $\frac{\partial}{\partial\nu}\Psi_C(\tau,\nu)\|_{\nu=0}=0$	$\Psi_H(\zeta,0)=1$ and $\frac{\partial}{\partial\beta}\Psi_H(\zeta,\beta)\|_{\beta=0}=0$
P_{18}: Fourier transform	$T_y(t,f)=T_x(-f,t)$ for $y(t)=X(t)$	$\Psi_C(-\nu,\tau)=\Psi_C(\tau,\nu)$	
P_{19}: Frequency localization	$T_x(t,f)=\delta(f-f_0)$ for $X(f)=\delta(f-f_0)$	$\Psi_C(\tau,0)=1$	$\Psi_H(\zeta,0)=1$
P_{20}: Time localization	$T_x(t,f)=\delta(t-t_0)$ for $x(t)=\delta(t-t_0)$	$\Psi_C(0,\nu)=1$	
P_{21}: Linear chirp localization	$T_x(t,f)=\delta(t-cf)$ for $X(f)=\mathrm{e}^{-j\pi cf^2}$	$\Psi_C(\tau,\nu)=1$	
P_{22}: Hyperbolic localization	$T_{X_c}(t,f)=\frac{1}{f}\delta\left(t-\frac{c}{f}\right), f>0$ if $X_c(f)=\frac{1}{\sqrt{f}}\mathrm{e}^{-j2\pi c\ln(f/f_r)}, f>0$		$\Psi_H(0,\beta)=1$
P_{23}: Chirp convolution	$T_y(t,f)=T_x(t-f/c,f)$ for $y(t)=\int x(t-\tau)\sqrt{\|c\|}\mathrm{e}^{j\pi c\tau^2}\mathrm{d}\tau$	$\Psi_C\left(\tau-\frac{\nu}{c},\nu\right)=\Psi_C(\tau,\nu)$	
P_{24}: Chirp multiplication	$T_y(t,f)=T_x(t,f-ct)$ for $y(t)=x(t)\mathrm{e}^{j\pi ct^2}$	$\Psi_C(\tau,\nu-c\tau)=\Psi_C(\tau,\nu)$	
P_{25}: Moyal's formula	$\iint T_x(t,f)T_y^*(t,f)\mathrm{d}t\,\mathrm{d}f=\left\|\int x(t)y^*(t)\mathrm{d}t\right\|^2$	$\|\Psi_C(\tau,\nu)\|=1$	$\|\Psi_H(\zeta,\beta)\|=1$

2.1 One-Dimensional Signal Representations

The instantaneous frequency and the group delay of a signal are one-dimensional representations that attempt to represent temporal and spectral signal characteristics simultaneously. The instantaneous frequency of the signal

$$f_x(t) = \frac{1}{2\pi}\frac{\mathrm{d}}{\mathrm{d}t}\arg\{x(t)\} \tag{2.3}$$

has been used in communication theory to characterize the time-varying frequency content of narrowband and frequency-modulated signals. It is a generalization of the fact that the frequency f_0 of a complex sinusoidal signal $x(t) = \exp(j2\pi f_0 t)$ is proportional to the derivative of the signal's phase. A dual concept used in filter analysis is the group delay

$$\tau_H(f) = -\frac{1}{2\pi}\frac{\mathrm{d}}{\mathrm{d}f}\arg\{H(f)\} \tag{2.4}$$

which can be interpreted as the time delay or distortion introduced by the filter's frequency response $H(f)$ at each frequency. Group delay is a generalization of the fact that time translations are coded in the derivative of the phase of the Fourier transform. Unfortunately, if the signal contains several signal components that overlap in time or frequency, then $f_x(t)$ or $\tau_H(f)$ only provides average spectral characteristics, which are not very useful.

2.2 Desirable Properties of Time–Frequency Representations

Mixed TFRs map a one-dimensional signal into a two-dimensional function of time and frequency in order to analyze the time-varying spectral content of the signal. Before discussing any particular TFR in Table 2.1, it is helpful to first investigate what types of properties an "ideal" time–frequency representation should satisfy. The list of desirable TFR properties in Table 2.2 can be broken up conceptually into the following categories: covariance, statistics, signal analysis, localization, and inner products (Claasen and Mecklenbräuker, 1980; Cohen, 1989; Boashash, 1991; Hlawatsch and Boudreaux-Bartels, 1992; Flandrin, 1993). The covariance properties P_1 to P_6 basically state that certain operations on the signal, such as translations, dilations, or convolution, should be preserved, that is, produce exactly the same operation on the signal's TFR. The second category of properties originates from the desire to generalize the concepts of the one-dimensional instantaneous signal energy $|x(t)|^2$ and power spectral density $|X(f)|^2$ into a two-dimensional statistical energy distribution $T_x(t_0, f_0)$ that provides a measure of the local signal energy or the probability that a signal contains a sinusoidal component of frequency f_0 at time t_0. Properties P_7 to P_{13} state that such an energy-distribution TFR should be real and nonnegative, have its marginal distributions equal to the signal's temporal and spectral energy densities $|x(t)|^2$ and $|X(f)|^2$, respectively, and preserve the signal energy, mean, variance, and other higher-order moments of the instantaneous signal energy and power spectral density. The next category of properties, P_{14} to P_{18}, arises from signal-processing considerations. A TFR should have the same duration and bandwidth as the signal under analysis. At any given time t, the average frequency should equal the instantaneous frequency of the signal, while the average or center of gravity in the time direction should equal the group delay of the signal. These two properties have been used to analyze the distortion of audio systems and the complex FM sonar signals used by bats and whales for echolocation. Property P_{18} is the TFR equivalent of the duality property of Fourier transforms. The group of properties P_{19} to P_{24} constitutes ideal TFR localization properties that are desirable for high-resolution capabilities. Here, $d(a)$ is the Dirac function. These properties state that if a signal is perfectly concentrated in time or frequency, that is, an impulse or a sinusoid, then its TFR also should be perfectly concentrated at the same time or

TABLE 2.3 List of Desirable Properties Satisfied by Time–Frequency Representations

TFR	ACK	AM	B0D	BJD	BUD	CWD	CKD	CAS	CDS	FD	GAM	GED	GRD	GWD	HYP	LD	MH	MTED	ND	PD	AMκ	PAD	PWD	RID	RD	SCAL	SPAD	SPWD	SPEC	UAD	UPD	WD
Class(es)	c a	h	a h	c a	c	c a	c	c	c	a	h	c	c	c a	h	c	c a	c	c	c	p	h	c	c a	c a	a	h	c	c	a	a	c a
Property																																
1. Frequency shift	✓			✓	✓	✓	✓	✓	✓			✓	✓	✓		✓	✓	✓	✓	✓			✓	✓	✓			✓	✓			✓
2. Time shift	✓		✓	✓	✓	✓	✓	✓	✓	✓		✓	✓	✓		✓	✓	✓	✓	✓			✓	✓	✓	✓		✓	✓	✓	✓	✓
3. Scale covariance	✓	✓	✓	✓	✓1	✓				✓	✓	✓1	✓1	✓	✓		✓	✓9			✓	✓		✓	✓	✓	✓			✓	✓	✓
4. Hyperbolic time shift		✓	✓								✓				✓						✓	✓		✓	✓	✓	✓			✓	✓	✓
5. Convolution												✓6		✓				✓10							✓					✓		
6. Modulation												✓7		✓		✓		✓10		✓					✓							✓
7. Real-valued	✓	✓	✓	✓	✓	✓	✓4	✓	✓	✓		✓	✓		✓	✓	✓	✓	✓	✓	✓	✓	✓	✓		✓	✓17	✓18	✓	✓	✓	✓
8. Positivity															✓											✓			✓			
9. Time marginal	✓			✓	✓	✓				✓		✓	✓	✓		✓	✓	✓11		✓			✓13	✓	✓						✓	✓
10. Frequency marginal	✓	✓	✓	✓	✓	✓				✓	✓	✓	✓	✓		✓	✓	✓11		✓	✓			✓	✓					✓	✓	✓
11. Energy distribution	✓	✓	✓	✓	✓	✓				✓	✓	✓	✓	✓	✓8	✓	✓	✓	✓	✓	✓	✓12		✓	✓	✓16	✓12	✓19	✓20	✓	✓	✓
12 Time moments	✓			✓	✓	✓						✓	✓	✓		✓	✓	✓11		✓			✓13	✓	✓							✓
13. Frequency moments	✓			✓	✓	✓						✓	✓	✓		✓	✓	✓11		✓				✓	✓							✓
14. Finite time support				✓			✓							✓5		✓				✓			✓	✓	✓							✓
15. Finite frequency support		✓	✓	✓							✓5			✓5							✓			✓	✓					✓	✓	✓
16. Instantaneous frequency	✓			✓	✓2	✓						✓2	✓			✓	✓	✓11		✓			✓14	✓								✓
17. Group delay	✓	✓	✓	✓	✓3	✓				✓		✓3	✓				✓	✓11			✓			✓						✓	✓	✓
18. Fourier transform	✓			✓	✓1	✓						✓1	✓1				✓	✓9						✓15								✓

continued

TABLE 2.3 (continued) List of Desirable Properties Satisfied by Time–Frequency Representations

TFR	ACK	AM	B0D	BJD	BUD	CWD	CKD	CAS	CDS	FD	GAM	GED	GRD	GWD	HYP	LD	MHD	MTED	ND	PD	AMκ	PAD	PWD	RID	RD	SCAL	SPAD	SPWD	SPEC	UAD	UPD	WD
Class(es)	c a	h	a h	c a	c	c a	c	c	c	a	h	c	c	c a	h	c	c a	c	c	c	p	h	c	c a	c a	a	h	c	c	a	a	c a
Property																																
19. Frequency localization	✓	✓	✓	✓	✓	✓				✓	✓	✓	✓	✓		✓	✓	✓11		✓	✓			✓	✓					✓	✓	✓
20. Time localization	✓			✓	✓	✓				✓		✓	✓	✓		✓	✓	✓11		✓			✓13	✓	✓					✓	✓	✓
21. Linear chirp localization																																✓
22. Hyperbolic localization		✓	✓								✓																					
23. Chirp convolution																																✓
24. Chirp multiplication																																✓
25. Moyal's formula		✓	✓								✓			✓		✓				✓	✓				✓							✓

Note: A ✓ indicates that the TFR can be shown to satisfy the given property. A number following the ✓ indicates that the TFR defined in Table 2.1 requires additional constraints to satisfy the property. The constraints are as follows: (1): $M = N$; (2): $M > 1/2$; (3): $N > 1/2$; (4): $g(\tau)$ even; (5): $|\alpha| < 1/2$; (6): $M = 1/2$; (7): $N = 1/2$; (8): $\int_0^\infty |\Gamma(f)|^2\, df = 1$; (9): $\alpha = 1$; (10): $r = 0$, $\alpha = 1$, $\gamma = 1/4$; (11): $\alpha \neq 1$; (12): $|\rho_\Gamma(0)|^2 = (1/f_r)$; (13): $|\eta(0)| = 1$; (14): $\eta(0) = 1$; (15): $s_{RID}(\beta)$ even; (16): $\int |\Gamma(b)|^2 db/|b| = 1$; (17): $g(c) \in \Re$; (18): $\gamma(t) \in \Re$; (19): $\Gamma(0)|\eta(0)|^2 = 1$; (20): $\int |\gamma(t)|^2 dt = 1$. In the second row, the letters *c*, *a*, *h*, and *p* indicate that the corresponding TFR is a member of the Cohen, Affine, Hyperbolic, and κth Power class, respectively. The meanings of the TFR acronyms listed in the column head are given in Table 2.1.

frequency. Properties P_{21} and P_{22} state that the TFRs of linear or hyperbolic spectral FM chirp signals should be perfectly concentrated along the chirp signal's group delay. Property P_{24} states that a signal modulated by a linear FM chirp should have a TFR whose instantaneous frequency has been sheared by an amount equal to the linear instantaneous frequency of the chirp. The last property, known as *Moyal's formula* or the *unitarity property*, states that TFRs should preserve the signal projections, inner products, and orthonormal signal basis functions that are used frequently in signal detection, synthesis, and approximation theory. Table 2.3 indicates which properties are satisfied by the TFRs listed in Table 2.1.

A TFR should be relatively easy to compute and interpret. Interpretation is greatly simplified if the TFR is linear, that is

$$T_y(t,f) = \sum_{n=1}^{N} T_{x_n}(t,f) \quad \text{for } y(t) = \sum_{n=1}^{N} x_n(t). \tag{2.5}$$

However, energy is a quadratic function of the signal, and hence, so too are many of the TFRs in Table 2.1. The nonlinear nature of TFRs gives rise to troublesome cross-terms. If $y(t)$ contains N signal components or auto-terms $x_n(t)$ in Equation 2.5, then a quadratic TFR of $y(t)$ can have as many nonzero cross-terms as there are unique pairs of auto-terms, that is, $N(N-1)/2$. For many TFRs, these cross-terms are oscillatory and overlap with auto-terms, obscuring visual analysis of TFRs.

Two common methods used to reduce the number of cross-terms are to reduce any redundancy in the signal representation and to use local smoothing or averaging to reduce oscillating cross-terms. TFR analysis of real, bandpass signals should be carried out using the analytic signal representation, that is, the signal added to $\sqrt{-1}$ times its Hilbert transform, in order to remove cross-terms between the positive- and negative-frequency axis components of the signal's Fourier transform. As we will see in upcoming sections, cross-term reduction by smoothing is often achieved at the expense of significant auto-term distortion and loss of desirable TFR properties.

2.3 TFR Classes

This section will briefly review Cohen's class of shift covariant TFRs, the Affine class of affine covariant TFRs, the Hyperbolic class (developed for signals with hyperbolic group delay), and the Power class (which is useful for signals with polynomial group delay). Each class is formed by grouping TFRs that satisfy two properties. They provide very helpful insight as to which types of TFRs will work best in different situations. Within a class, each TFR is completely characterized by a unique set of TFR-dependent kernels which can be compared against a class-dependent list of kernel constraints in Tables 2.2 and 2.6 to quickly determine which properties the TFR satisfies.

2.3.1 Cohen's Class of TFRs

Cohen's class consists of all quadratic TFRs that satisfy the frequency-shift and time-shift covariance properties, that is, those TFRs with a check in the first two property rows in Table 2.3 (Claasen and Mecklenbräuker, 1980; Cohen, 1989; Hlawatsch and Boudreaux-Bartels, 1992; Flandrin, 1993). Time- and frequency-shift covariances are very useful properties in the analysis of speech, narrowband Doppler systems, and multipath environments. Any TFR in Cohen's class can be written in one of the four equivalent "normal forms":

$$C_x(t,f;\Psi_C) = \iint \varphi_C(t-t',\tau)\, x\!\left(t'+\frac{\tau}{2}\right) x^*\!\left(t'-\frac{\tau}{2}\right) e^{-j2\pi f\tau}\, dt'\, d\tau \tag{2.6}$$

$$= \iint \Phi_C(f-f',\nu)\, X\!\left(f'+\frac{\nu}{2}\right) X^*\!\left(f'-\frac{\nu}{2}\right) e^{j2\pi t\nu}\, df'\, d\nu \tag{2.7}$$

$$= \iint \psi_C(t-t', f-f')\mathrm{WD}_x(t', f')dt'df' \tag{2.8}$$

$$= \iint \Psi_C(\tau, \nu)\mathrm{AF}_x(\tau, \nu)e^{j2\pi(t\nu - f\tau)}d\tau d\nu. \tag{2.9}$$

Each normal form is characterized by one of the four kernels $\varphi_C(t, \tau)$, $\varphi_C(f, \nu)$, $\psi_C(t, f)$, and $\Psi_C(\tau, \nu)$ which are interrelated by the following Fourier transforms:

$$\varphi_C(t,\tau) = \iint \Phi_C(f,\nu)e^{j2\pi(f\tau+\nu t)}df\,d\nu = \int \Psi_C(\tau,\nu)e^{j2\pi\nu t}d\nu \tag{2.10}$$

$$\psi_C(t,f) = \iint \Psi_C(\tau,\nu)e^{j2\pi(\nu t - f\tau)}d\tau d\nu = \int \Phi_C(f,\nu)e^{j2\pi\nu t}d\nu \tag{2.11}$$

The kernels for the TFRs in Cohen's class are given in Table 2.4.

The four normal forms offer various computational and analysis advantages. For example, the first two normal forms can be computed directly from the signal $x(t)$ or its Fourier transform $X(f)$ via a one-dimensional convolution with $\varphi_C(t, \tau)$ or $\Phi_C(f, \nu)$. If $\varphi_C(t, \tau)$ is of fairly short duration, then it may be possible to implement Equation 2.6 on a digital computer in real time using only a small number of signal samples. The third normal form indicates that any TFR in Cohen's shift covariant class can be computed by convolving the TFR-dependent kernel $\psi_C(t, f)$ with the Wigner distribution (WD) of the signal, defined in Table 2.1. Hence the WD is one of the key members of Cohen's class, and many TFRs correspond to smoothed WDs, as seen in the top of Table 2.5. Equation 2.11 and the fourth normal form in Equation 2.9 indicates that the two-dimensional convolution in Equation 2.8 transforms to multiplication of the Fourier transform of the kernel $\psi_C(t, f)$ with the ambiguity function (AF) in Table 2.1; the AF is the Fourier transform of the WD. This last normal form provides an intuitive interpretation that the "AF domain" kernel $\Psi_C(\tau, \nu)$ can be thought of as the frequency response of a two-dimensional filter.

The kernels in Equations 2.6 through 2.11 are signal-independent and provide valuable insight into the performance of each Cohen class TFR, regardless of the input signal. For good cross-term reduction and little auto-term distortion, each TFR kernel $\Psi_C(\tau, \nu)$ given in Table 2.4 should be as close as possible to an ideal low-pass filter. If these kernels satisfy the constraints in the third column of Table 2.2, then the TFR properties in the first column are guaranteed to always hold (Claasen and Mecklenbräuker, 1980; Hlawatsch and Boudreaux-Bartels, 1992). For example, the last row of Table 2.2 indicates that Moyal's formula is satisfied by any TFR whose AF domain kernel, listed in the third column of Table 2.4, has unit modulus, for example, the Rihaczek distribution. Since the AF domain kernel of the WD is equal to one, that is, $\Psi_{WD}(\tau, \nu) = 1$, then the WD automatically satisfies the kernel constraints in Table 2.2 for properties P_9 to P_{13} and P_{16} to P_{21} as well as 12pt Moyal's formula. However, it also acts as an all-pass filter, passing all cross-terms. The Choi–Williams Gaussian kernel in Table 2.4 was formulated to satisfy the marginal property constraints of having an AF domain kernel equal to one along the axes and to be a low-pass filter that reduces cross-terms.

2.3.2 Affine Class of TFRs

TFRs that are covariant to scale changes and time translations, that is, properties P_2 and P_3 in Tables 2.2 and 2.3, are members of the *Affine class* (Bertrand chapter in Boashash, 1991; Flandrin, 1993). The scale covariance property P_3 is useful when analyzing wideband Doppler systems, signals with fractal structure, octave-band systems such as the cochlea of the inner ear, and detecting short-duration "transients." Any Affine class TFR can be written in four "normal form" equations similar to those of Cohen's class:

$$A_x(t, f; \Psi_A) = |f| \iint \varphi_A(f(t'-t), f\tau)x(t'+\tau/2)x^*(t'-\tau/2)dt'd\tau \tag{2.12}$$

TABLE 2.4 Kernels of Cohen's Shift-Invariant Class of Time–Frequency Representations

TFR	$\psi_C(t,f)$	$\Psi_C(\tau,\nu)$	$\varphi_C(t,\tau)$	$\Phi_C(f,\nu)$
ACK	$2\cos(4\pi tf)$	$\cos(\pi\tau\nu)$	$\frac{\delta(t+\tau/2)+\delta(t-\tau/2)}{2}$	$\frac{\delta(f-\nu/2)+\delta(f+\nu/2)}{2}$
BJD		$\frac{\sin(\pi\tau\nu)}{\pi\tau\nu}$	$\begin{cases}\frac{1}{\lvert\tau\rvert}, & \lvert t/\tau\rvert<1/2\\ 0, & \lvert t/\tau\rvert>1/2\end{cases}$	$\begin{cases}\frac{1}{\lvert\nu\rvert}, & \lvert f/\nu\rvert<1/2\\ 0, & \lvert f/\nu\rvert>1/2\end{cases}$
BUD		$\left(1+\left(\frac{\tau}{\tau_0}\right)^{2M}\left(\frac{\nu}{\nu_0}\right)^{2N}\right)^{-1}$		
CWD		$e^{-(2\pi\tau\nu)^2/\sigma}$	$\sqrt{\frac{\sigma}{4\pi}}\frac{1}{\lvert\tau\rvert}\exp\left[-\frac{\sigma}{4}\left(\frac{t}{\tau}\right)^2\right]$	$\sqrt{\frac{\sigma}{4\pi}}\frac{1}{\lvert\nu\rvert}\exp\left[-\frac{\sigma}{4}\left(\frac{f}{\nu}\right)^2\right]$
CKD		$g(\tau)\lvert\tau\rvert\frac{\sin(\pi\tau\nu)}{\pi\tau\nu}$	$\begin{cases}g(\tau), & \lvert t/\tau\rvert<1/2\\ 0, & \lvert t/\tau\rvert>1/2\end{cases}$	
CAS		$\left[\frac{1}{2}\delta(\nu)+\frac{1}{j\nu}\right]e^{-j\pi\lvert\tau\rvert\nu}$		
CDS		$\left[\frac{1}{2}\delta(-\nu)-\frac{1}{j\nu}\right]e^{j\pi\lvert\tau\rvert\nu}$		
GED		$\exp\left[-\left(\frac{\tau}{\tau_0}\right)^{2M}\left(\frac{\nu}{\nu_0}\right)^{2N}\right]$	$\frac{\nu_0}{2\sqrt{\pi}}\left\lvert\frac{\tau_0}{\tau}\right\rvert^M\exp\left[\frac{-\nu_0^2\tau_0^{2M}t^2}{4\tau^{2M}}\right]$ $N=1$ only	$\frac{\tau_0}{2\sqrt{\pi}}\left\lvert\frac{\nu_0}{\nu}\right\rvert^N\exp\left[\frac{-\tau_0^2\nu_0^{2N}f^2}{4\nu^{2N}}\right]$ $M=1$ only
GRD		$\begin{cases}1, & \left\lvert\lvert\tau\rvert^{M/N}\lvert\nu\rvert/r\right\rvert<1\\ 0, & \left\lvert\lvert\tau\rvert^{M/N}\lvert\nu\rvert/r\right\rvert>1\end{cases}$	$\frac{\sin(2\pi\lvert\sigma\rvert t/\lvert\tau\rvert^{M/N})}{\pi t}$	
GWD	$\frac{1}{\lvert\tilde{\alpha}\rvert}e^{j2\pi tf/\tilde{\alpha}}$	$e^{j2\pi\tilde{\alpha}\tau\nu}$	$\delta(t+\tilde{\alpha}\tau)$	$\delta(f-\tilde{\alpha}\nu)$
LD		$e^{j\pi\lvert\tau\rvert\nu}$	$\delta(t+\lvert\tau\rvert/2)$	
MH		$\cos(\pi\tau\nu)$	$\frac{\delta(t+\tau/2)+\delta(t-\tau/2)}{2}$	$\frac{\delta(f-\nu/2)+\delta(f+\nu/2)}{2}$

continued

TABLE 2.4 (continued) Kernels of Cohen's Shift-Invariant Class of Time–Frequency Representations

TFR	$\psi_C(t,f)$	$\Psi_C(\tau,\nu)$	$\varphi_C(t,\tau)$	$\Phi_C(f,\nu)$
MTBD		$\left[1+\tilde{\mu}^{2\lambda}\left(\frac{\tau}{\tau_0},\frac{\nu}{\nu_0};\alpha,r,\beta,\gamma\right)\right]^{-1}$		
MTC		$\left[1+\varepsilon_p^2 C_\lambda^2\left(\tilde{\mu}\left(\frac{\tau}{\tau_0},\frac{\nu}{\nu_0};\alpha,r,\beta,\gamma\right)\right)\right]^{-1}$		
MTED		$\exp\left[-\pi\tilde{\mu}^{2\lambda}\left(\frac{\tau}{\tau_0},\frac{\nu}{\nu_0};\alpha,r,\beta,\gamma\right)\right]$		
MTIC		$\left[1+\varepsilon_s^2 C_\lambda^{-2}\left(\tilde{\mu}^{-1}\left(\frac{\tau}{\tau_0},\frac{\nu}{\nu_0};\alpha,r,\beta,\gamma\right)\right)\right]^{-1}$		
ND		$\exp\left[-\pi\tilde{\mu}\left(\frac{\tau}{\tau_0},\frac{\nu}{\nu_0};0,r,1,1\right)\right]$		
PD		$e^{-j\pi\|\tau\|\nu}$	$\delta(t-\|\tau\|/2)$	
PWD	$\delta(t)WD_\eta(0,f)$	$\eta(\tau/2)\eta^*(-\tau/2)$	$\delta(t)\eta(\tau/2)\eta^*(-\tau/2)$	$WD_\eta(0,f)$
RGWD	$\frac{1}{\|\tilde{\alpha}\|}\cos(2\pi tf/\tilde{\alpha})$	$\cos(2\pi\tilde{\alpha}\tau\nu)$	$\frac{\delta(t+\tilde{\alpha}\tau)+\delta(t-\tilde{\alpha}\tau)}{2}$	$\frac{\delta(f-\tilde{\alpha}\nu)+\delta(f+\tilde{\alpha}\nu)}{2}$
RID	$\int\frac{1}{\tau}s_{RID}\left(\frac{t}{\tau}\right)e^{-j2\pi f\tau}d\tau$	$S_{RID}(\tau\nu)$,	$\frac{1}{\|\tau\|}s_{RID}\left(\frac{t}{\tau}\right)$,	$\frac{1}{\|\nu\|}s_{RID}\left(-\frac{f}{\nu}\right)$,
		$S_{RID}(\beta)\varepsilon\text{Real}, S_{RID}(0)=1$	$s_{RID}(\alpha)=0, \|\alpha\|>\frac{1}{2}$	$s_{RID}(\alpha)=0, \|\alpha\|>\frac{1}{2}$
RD	$2e^{-j4\pi tf}$	$e^{-j\pi\tau\nu}$	$\delta(t-\tau/2)$	$\delta(f+\nu/2)$
SPWD	$\gamma(t)WD_\eta(0,f)$	$\eta\left(\frac{\tau}{2}\right)\eta^*\left(-\frac{\tau}{2}\right)\Gamma(\nu)$	$\gamma(t)\eta\left(\frac{\tau}{2}\right)\eta^*\left(-\frac{\tau}{2}\right)$	$\Gamma(\nu)WD_\eta(0,f)$
SPEC	$WD_\gamma(-t,-f)$	$AF_\gamma(-\tau,-\nu)$	$\gamma\left(-t-\frac{\tau}{2}\right)\gamma^*\left(-t+\frac{\tau}{2}\right)$	$\Gamma\left(f-\frac{\nu}{2}\right)\Gamma^*\left(-f+\frac{\nu}{2}\right)$
WD	$\delta(t)\delta(f)$	1	$\delta(t)$	$\delta(f)$

Note: Here, $\tilde{\mu}(\tilde{\tau},\tilde{\nu};\alpha,r,\beta,\gamma)=((\tilde{\tau})^2((\tilde{\nu})^2)^\alpha+((\tilde{\tau})^2)^\alpha(\tilde{\nu})^2+2r((\tilde{\tau}\tilde{\nu})^\beta)^\gamma)$ and $C_\lambda(a)$ is a Chebyshev polynomial of order λ. Functions with lowercase and uppercase letters, for example, $\gamma(t)$ and $\Gamma(f)$, indicate Fourier transform pairs.

TABLE 2.5 Many TFRs Are Equivalent to Smoothed or Warped Wigner Distributions

TFR Name	TFR Formulation
	Examples of TFRs Equivalent to Smoothed Wigner Distributions
Cohen's class TFR	$C_x(t,f;\psi_C)=\iint \psi_C(t-t',f-f')\mathrm{WD}_x(t',f')\mathrm{d}t'\mathrm{d}f'$
Pseudo-Wigner distribution	$\mathrm{PWD}_x(t,f;\eta)=\int \mathrm{WD}_\eta(0,f-f')\mathrm{WD}_x(t,f')\mathrm{d}f'$
Scalogram	$\mathrm{SCAL}_x(t,f;\gamma)=\iint \mathrm{WD}_\gamma\left(\frac{f}{f_r}(t'-t),f_r\frac{f'}{f}\right)\mathrm{WD}_x(t',f')\mathrm{d}t'\mathrm{d}f'$
Smoothed Pseudo-Wigner distribution	$\mathrm{SPWD}_x(t,f;\gamma,\eta)=\iint \gamma(t-t')\mathrm{WD}_\eta(0,f-f')\mathrm{WD}_x(t',f')\mathrm{d}t'\mathrm{d}f'$
Spectrogram	$\mathrm{SPEC}_x(t,f;\gamma)=\iint \mathrm{WD}_\gamma(t'-t,f'-f)\mathrm{WD}_x(t',f')\mathrm{d}t'\mathrm{d}f'$
	Examples of TFRs Equivalent to Warped Wigner Distributions
Altes distribution	$\mathrm{AM}_X(t,f)=\mathrm{WD}_{\mathcal{W}X}\left(\frac{tf}{f},f_r\ln\frac{f}{f_r}\right)$
κth Power Altes distribution	$\mathrm{AM}_X^{(\kappa)}(t,f)=\mathrm{WD}_{\mathcal{W}_\kappa X}\left(\frac{t}{\kappa\,\lvert f/f_r\rvert^{\kappa-1}},f_r\mathrm{sgn}(f)\lvert f/f_r\rvert^{\kappa}\right),\kappa\neq 0$
Hyperbologram	$\mathrm{HYP}_X(t,f;\Gamma)=\int_{-\infty}^{\infty}\int_0^{\infty}\mathrm{WD}_{\mathcal{W}\Gamma}\left(t'-\frac{tf}{f_r},f'-f_r\ln\frac{f}{f_r}\right)\mathrm{WD}_{\mathcal{W}X}(t',f')\mathrm{d}t'\mathrm{d}f'$
Pseudo-Altes distribution	$\mathrm{PAD}_X(t,f;\Gamma)=f_r\int_0^{\infty}\mathrm{WD}_{\mathcal{W}\Gamma}\left(0,f_r\ln\frac{f}{f'}\right)\mathrm{WD}_{\mathcal{W}X}\left(\frac{tf}{f_r},f_r\ln\frac{f'}{f_r}\right)\frac{\mathrm{d}f'}{f'}$
Smoothed Pseudo-Altes distribution	$\mathrm{SPAD}_X(t,f;\Gamma,g)=f_r\int_{-\infty}^{\infty}\int_0^{\infty}g(tf-c)\mathrm{WD}_{\mathcal{W}\Gamma}\left(0,f_r\ln\frac{f}{f'}\right)\mathrm{WD}_{\mathcal{W}X}\left(\frac{c}{f_r},f_r\ln\frac{f'}{f_r}\right)\frac{\mathrm{d}f'}{f'}\mathrm{d}c$

Note: Where $f_r>0$ is a positive reference frequency, $(\mathcal{W}H)(f)=\sqrt{e^{f/f_r}}\,H(f_r e^{f/f_r}),(\mathcal{W}_\kappa H)(f)\lvert\kappa\rvert(f_r/f)^{\lvert(\kappa-1)/\kappa\rvert^{-1/2}}$ $H(f_r\mathrm{sgn}(f)\lvert f/f_r\rvert^{1/\kappa})$, $\kappa\neq 0$, and $\mathrm{sgn}(f)=\begin{cases}1, & f>0\\ -1, & f<0\end{cases}$.

$$=\frac{1}{\lvert f\rvert}\iint \Phi_A\left(\frac{f'}{f},\frac{\nu}{f}\right)X(f'+\nu/2)X^*(f'-\nu/2)e^{j2\pi t\nu}\mathrm{d}f'\mathrm{d}\nu \tag{2.13}$$

$$=\iint \psi_A\left(f(t-t'),\frac{f'}{f}\right)\mathrm{WD}_x(t',f')\mathrm{d}t'\mathrm{d}f' \tag{2.14}$$

$$=\iint \Psi_A\left(f\tau,\frac{\nu}{f}\right)\mathrm{AF}_x(\tau,\nu)e^{j2\pi t\nu}\mathrm{d}\tau\mathrm{d}\nu \tag{2.15}$$

The Affine class kernels are interrelated by the same Fourier transforms given in Equations 2.10 and 2.11. Note that the third normal form of the Affine class involves an Affine smoothing of the WD. Well-known members of the Affine class are the Bertrands' P_0 distribution, the scalogram, and the Unterberger distributions. All are defined in Table 2.1, and their kernel forms and TFR property constraints are listed in Table 2.6. Because of the scale covariance property, many TFRs in the Affine class exhibit constant-Q behavior, permitting multiresolution analysis.

TABLE 2.6 Affine Class Kernels and Constraints

TFR	$\Psi_A(\zeta,\beta)$	$\Phi_A(b,\beta)$
BOD	$\frac{\beta/2}{\sinh\beta/2} e^{-j2\pi\zeta\left[\frac{\beta}{2}\coth\frac{\beta}{2}\right]}$	$\frac{\beta/2}{\sinh\beta/2}\delta\left(b-\left[\frac{\beta}{2}\coth\frac{\beta}{2}\right]\right)$
FD	$\left[1-\left(\frac{\beta}{4}\right)^2\right] e^{j2\pi\zeta\left[1+(\beta/4)^2\right]}$	$\left[1-\left(\frac{\beta}{4}\right)^2\right]\delta\left(b-\left[1+(\beta/4)^2\right]\right)$
GWD	$e^{-j2\pi\zeta[1-\tilde{\alpha}\beta]}$	$\delta(b-[1-\tilde{\alpha}\beta])$
SCAL	$AF_\gamma(-\zeta/f_r,-f_r\beta)$	$f_r\Gamma(f_r(b-\beta/2))\Gamma^*(f_r(b+\beta/2))$
UAD	$e^{-j2\pi\zeta\sqrt{1+\beta^2/4}}$	$\delta\left(b-\sqrt{1+\beta^2/4}\right)$
UPD	$\left[1+\beta^2/4\right]^{-1/2} e^{-j2\pi\zeta\sqrt{1+\beta^2/4}}$	$\left[1+\beta^2/4\right]^{-1/2}\delta\left(b-\sqrt{1+\beta^2/4}\right)$
WD	$e^{-j2\pi\zeta}$	$\delta(b-1)$

Property	Constraint on Kernel
P_1: Frequency shift	$\Psi_A(\zeta,\beta)=S_{A\cap C}(\zeta\cdot\beta)\,e^{-j2\pi\zeta}$
P_2: Time shift	Always satisfied
P_3: Scale covariance	Always satisfied
P_4: Hyperbolic time shift	$\Phi_A(b,\beta)=G_A(\beta)\delta\left(b-\frac{\beta}{2}\coth\frac{\beta}{2}\right)$
P_5: Convolution	$\Psi_A(\zeta_1+\zeta_2,\beta)=\Psi_A(\zeta_1,\beta)\cdot\Psi_A(\zeta_2,\beta)$
P_7: Real-valued	$\Psi_A(\zeta,\beta)=\Psi_A^*(-\zeta,-\beta)$
P_9: Time marginal	$\int\Phi_A(b,-2b)\frac{db}{\lvert b\rvert}=1$
P_{10}: Frequency marginal	$\Phi_A(b,0)=\delta(b-1)$
P_{11}: Energy distribution	$\int\Phi_A(b,0)\frac{db}{\lvert b\rvert}=1$
P_{14}: Finite time support	$\varphi_A(a,\zeta)=0,\quad\left\lvert\frac{a}{\zeta}\right\rvert>\frac{1}{2}$
P_{15}: Finite frequency support	$\Phi_A(b,\beta)=0,\quad\left\lvert\frac{b-1}{\beta}\right\rvert>\frac{1}{2}$
P_{17}: Group delay	$\Phi_A(b,0)=\delta(b-1)$ and $\frac{\partial}{\partial\beta}\Phi_A(b,\beta)\Big\rvert_{\beta=0}=0$
P_{19}: Frequency localization	$\Phi_A(b,0)=\delta(b-1)$
P_{25}: Moyal's formula	$\int\Phi_A^*(b\beta,\tilde{\eta}\beta)\Phi_A(\beta,\tilde{\eta}\beta)d\beta=\delta(b-1),\ \forall\tilde{\eta}$

Note: Here, $S_{A\cap C}(\cdot)$ is a one-dimensional product kernel characterizing the frequency shift members of the affine class.

2.3.3 Hyperbolic Class of TFRs

The Hyperbolic class of TFRs consists of all TFRs that are covariant to scale changes and hyperbolic time shifts, that is, properties P_3 and P_4 in Table 2.2 (Papandreou et al., 1993). They can be analyzed using the following four normal forms:

$$H_X(t,f;\Psi_H) = \iint \varphi_H(tf - c,\zeta)\upsilon_X(c,\zeta)e^{-j2\pi[\ln(f/f_r)]\zeta}\,dc\,d\zeta \quad (2.16)$$

$$= \iint \Phi_H\left(\ln\frac{f}{f_r} - b,\beta\right) f_r e^b X(f_r e^{b+\beta/2})X^*(f_r e^{b-\beta/2})e^{j2\pi tf\beta}\,db\,d\beta \quad (2.17)$$

$$= \int_{-\infty}^{\infty}\int_{0}^{\infty} \psi_H\left(tf - t'f',\ln\frac{f}{f'}\right)AM_X(t',f')\,dt'df' \quad (2.18)$$

$$= \iint \Psi_H(\zeta,\beta)HAF_X(\zeta,\beta)e^{j2\pi(tf\beta-[\ln(f/f_r)]\zeta)}\,d\zeta\,d\beta \quad (2.19)$$

where $AM_X(t,f)$ is the Altes distribution and $HAF_X(\zeta, \beta)$ is the hyperbolic AF defined in Table 2.1, $\upsilon_X(c, \zeta)$ is defined in Table 2.7, $(\mathcal{W}X)(f) = \sqrt{e^{f/f_r}}\,X(f_r e^{f/f_r})$ is a unitary warping on the frequency axis of the signal, and the kernels are interrelated via the Fourier transforms in Equations 2.10 and 2.11.

Table 2.3 reveals that the Altes–Marinovic, the Bertrands' P_0, and the hyperbologram distributions are members of the Hyperbolic class. Their kernels are given in Table 2.7, and kernel property constraints are given in Table 2.2. The hyperbolic TFRs give highly concentrated TFR representations for signals with hyperbolic group delay. Each Hyperbolic class TFR, kernel, and property corresponds to a warped version of a Cohen's class TFR, kernel, and property, respectively. For example, Table 2.5 shows that the Altes distribution is equal to the WD after both the signal and the time–frequency axes are

TABLE 2.7 Kernels of the Hyperbolic Class of Time–Frequency Representations

TFR	$\psi_H(c,b)$	$\Psi_H(\zeta,\beta)$	$\varphi_H(c,\zeta)$	$\Phi_H(b,\beta)$
AM	$\delta(c)\delta(b)$	1	$\delta(c)$	$\delta(b)$
B0D	$\int \delta(b+\ln\lambda(\beta))e^{j2\pi c\beta}d\beta$	$e^{-j2\pi\zeta\ln\lambda(\beta)}$	$\int e^{j2\pi(c\beta-\zeta\ln\lambda(\beta))}d\beta$	$\delta(b+\ln\lambda(\beta))$
GAM	$\frac{1}{\lvert\tilde{\alpha}\rvert}e^{-j2\pi cb/\tilde{\alpha}}$	$e^{j2\pi\tilde{\alpha}\zeta\beta}$	$\delta(c+\tilde{\alpha}\zeta)$	$\delta(b-\tilde{\alpha}\beta)$
HYP	$AM_\Gamma\left(\frac{-c}{f_r e^{-b}}, f_r e^{-b}\right)$	$HAF_\Gamma(-\zeta,-\beta)$	$\upsilon_\Gamma(-c,-\zeta)$	$V_\Gamma(-b,-\beta)$
PAD	$f_r\delta(c)AM_\Gamma(0, f_r e^b)$	$f_r\upsilon_\Gamma(0,\zeta)$	$f_r\delta(c)\upsilon_\Gamma(0,\zeta)$	$f_r AM_\Gamma(0, f_r e^b)$
SPAD	$f_r g(c)AM_\Gamma(0, f_r e^b)$	$f_r G(\beta)\upsilon_\Gamma(0,\zeta)$	$f_r g(c)\upsilon_\Gamma(0,\zeta)$	$f_r G(\beta)AM_\Gamma(0, f_r e^b)$

Note: Here, $\lambda(\beta) = (\beta/2)/(\sinh\beta/2)$, $V_\Gamma(b,\beta) = f_r e^b\Gamma(f_r e^{b+\beta/2})\Gamma^*(f_r e^{b-\beta/2})$, $\upsilon_\Gamma(c,\zeta) = \rho_\Gamma(c+\zeta/2)\rho_\Gamma^*(c-\zeta/2)$, and $\rho_\Gamma(c) = \int_0^\infty \Gamma(f)(f/f_r)^{j2\pi c}\frac{df}{\sqrt{f}}$.

warped appropriately. The WD's perfect localization of linear FM chirps (P_{21}) corresponds to the Altes distribution's perfect localization for hyperbolic FM chirps (P_{22}). This one-to-one correspondence between the Cohen and Hyperbolic classes greatly facilitates their analysis and gives alternative methods for calculating various TFRs.

2.3.4 κth Power Class

The Power class of TFRs consists of all TFRs that are scale covariant and power time-shift covariant, that is

$$PC_Y^{(\kappa)}(t,f) = PC_X^{(\kappa)}\left(t - c\frac{d}{df}\xi(f/f_r), f\right) \quad \text{for } Y(f) = e^{-j2\pi c \xi_\kappa(f/f_r)}X(f) \tag{2.20}$$

where $\xi_\kappa(f) = \text{sgn}(f)\,|f|^\kappa$, for $\kappa \neq 0$ (Hlawatsch et al., 1999). Consequently, the κth Power class represents well group delay changes in the signal that are powers of frequency. When $\kappa = 1$, the Power class is equivalent to the Affine class. The central member, $AM^{(\kappa)}$ in Table 2.1, is the Power class equivalent to the Altes–Marinovic distribution.

2.4 Common TFRs and Their Use in Biomedical Applications

This section will briefly review some of the TFRs commonly used in biomedical analysis and summarize their relative advantages and disadvantages.

2.4.1 Wigner Distribution

One of the oldest TFRs in Table 2.1 is the WD, which Wigner proposed in quantum mechanics as a two-dimensional statistical distribution relating the Fourier transform pairs of position and momentum of a particle. Table 2.3 reveals that the WD satisfies a large number of desirable TFR properties, P_1 to P_3, P_5 to P_7, P_9 to P_{21}, and P_{23} and P_{25}. It is a member of both the Cohen and the Affine classes. The WD is a high-resolution TFR for linear FM chirps, sinusoids, and impulses. Since the WD satisfies Moyal's formula, it has been used to design optimal signal-detection and synthesis algorithms. The drawbacks of the WD are that it can be negative, it requires the signal to be known for all time, and it is a quadratic TFR with no implicit smoothing to remove cross-terms.

2.4.2 Smoothed Wigner Distributions

Many TFRs are related to the WD by either smoothing or warping, for example, see Equations 2.8 and 2.18 and Table 2.5. An intuitive understanding of the effects of cross-terms on quadratic TFRs can be obtained by analyzing the WD of a multicomponent signal $y(t)$ in Equation 2.5 under the assumption that each signal component is a shifted version of a basic envelope, that is, $x_n(t) = x(t - t_n)\, e^{j2\pi f_n t}$:

$$\begin{aligned} WD_y(t,f) = {} & \sum_{n=1}^{N} WD_x(t - t_n, f - f_n) + 2\sum_{k=1}^{N-1}\sum_{q=k+1}^{N} WD_x(t - \bar{t}_{k,q}, f - \bar{f}_{k,q}) \\ & \cos(2\pi[\Delta f_{k,q}(t - \Delta t_{k,q}) - \Delta t_{k,q}(f - \Delta f_{k,q}) + \Delta f_{k,q}\Delta t_{k,q}]) \end{aligned} \tag{2.21}$$

where $\Delta f_{k,q} = f_k - f_q$ is the difference or "beat" frequency and $\bar{f}_{k,q} = (f_k + f_q)/2$ is the average frequency between the kth and qth signal components. Similarly, $\Delta t_{k,q}$ is the difference time and $\bar{t}_{k,q}$ is the average time. The auto-WD terms in the first summation properly reflect the fact that the WD is a member of Cohen's shift covariant class. Unfortunately, the cross-WD terms in the second summation occur midway in the time–frequency plane between each pair of signal components and oscillate with a spatial frequency proportional to the distance between them. The Pseudo-WD (PWD) and the smoothed PWD (SPWD) defined in Table 2.1 use low-pass smoothing windows $\eta(\tau)$ and $\gamma(t)$ to reduce oscillatory cross-components. However, Table 2.5 reveals that the PWD performs smoothing only in the frequency direction. Short smoothing windows greatly reduce the limits of integration in the PWD and SPWD formulations and hence reduce computation time. However, Table 2.3 reveals that smoothing the WD reduces the number of desirable properties it satisfies from 18 to 7 for the PWD and to only 3 for the SPWD.

2.4.3 Spectrogram

One of the most commonly used TFRs for slowly time-varying or quasi-stationary signals is the spectrogram, defined in Tables 2.1 and 2.5 (Rabiner and Schafer, 1978). It is equal to the squared magnitude of the short-time Fourier transform, performing a local or "short-time" Fourier analysis by using a sliding analysis window $\gamma(t)$ to segment the signal into short sections centered near the output time t before computing a Fourier transformation. The spectrogram is easy to compute, using either FFTs or a parallel bank of filters, and it is often easy to interpret. The quadratic spectrogram smooths away all cross-terms except those which occur when two signal components overlap. This smoothing also distorts auto-terms. The spectrogram does a poor job representing rapidly changing spectral characteristics or resolving two closely spaced components because there is an inherent trade-off between good time resolution, which requires a short analysis window, and good frequency resolution, which requires a long analysis window. The spectrogram satisfies only three TFR properties listed in Tables 2.2 and 2.3, that is, it is a nonnegative member of Cohen's shift invariant class.

2.4.4 Choi–Williams Exponential and Reduced Interference Distributions

The Choi–Williams exponential distribution (CWD) and the reduced interference distribution (RID) in Table 2.1 are often used as a compromise between the high-resolution but cluttered WD versus the smeared but easy to interpret spectrogram (Williams and Jeong, 1992). Since they are members of both the Cohen class and the Affine class, their AF domain kernels in Table 2.4 have a very special form, that is, $\Psi_C(\tau, \nu) = S_c(\tau\nu)$, called a product kernel, which is a one-dimensional kernel evaluated at the product of its time–frequency variables (Hlawatsch and Boudreaux-Bartels, 1992). The CWD uses a Gaussian product kernel in the AF plane to reduce cross-terms, while the RID typically uses a classic window function that is time-limited and normalized to automatically satisfy many desirable TFR properties (see Table 2.3). The CWD has one scaling factor σ that allows the user to select either good cross-term reduction or good auto-term preservation but, unfortunately, not always both. The generalized exponential distribution in Table 2.1 is an extension of the CWD that permits both (Hlawatsch and Boudreaux-Bartels, 1992). Because the CWD and RID product kernels have hyperbolic isocontours in the AF plane, they always pass cross-terms between signal components that occur at either the same time or frequency, and they can distort auto-terms of linear FM chirp signals whose instantaneous frequency has a slope close to 1. The multiform tiltable exponential distribution (MTED) (Costa and Boudreaux-Bartels, 1995), another extension of the CWD, works well for any linear FM chirp.

2.4.5 Scalogram or Wavelet Transform Squared Magnitude

The scalogram (Flandrin, 1993), defined in Tables 2.1 and 2.5, is the squared magnitude of the wavelet transform (WT) (Rioul and Vetterli, 1991; Daubechies, 1992; Meyer, 1993) and is a member of the Affine class. It uses a special sliding analysis window $\gamma(t)$, called the mother wavelet, to analyze local spectral information of the signal $x(t)$. The mother wavelet is either compressed or dilated to give a multiresolution signal representation. The scalogram can be thought of as the multiresolution output of a parallel bank of octave band-filters. High-frequency regions of the WT domain have very good time resolution, whereas low-frequency regions of the WT domain have very good spectral resolution. The WT has been used to model the middle- to high-frequency range operation of the cochlea, to track transients such as speech pitch and the onset of the QRS complex in electrocardiogram (ECG) signals, and to analyze fractal and chaotic signals. One drawback of the scalogram is its poor temporal resolution at low-frequency regions of the time–frequency plane and poor spectral resolution at high frequencies. Moreover, many "classical" windows do not satisfy the conditions needed for a mother wavelet. The scalogram cannot remove cross-terms when signal components overlap. Further, many discrete WT implementations do not preserve the important time-shift covariance property.

2.4.6 Biomedical Applications

The ECG signal is a recording of the time-varying electrical rhythm of the heart. The short-duration QRS complex is the most predominant feature of the normal ECG signal. Abnormal heart rhythms can be identified on the ECG by detecting the QRS complex from one cycle to the next. The transient detection capability of the WT has been exploited for detection of the QRS complex (Li and Zheng, 1995; Kadambe et al., 1999). The WT exhibits local maxima that align across successive (dyadic) scales at the location of transient components, such as QRS complexes. The advantage of using the WT is that it is robust both to noise and to nonstationarities in the QRS complex.

Other pathological features in the heart's electrical rhythm that appear only in high-resolution signal-averaged ECG signals are ventricular late potentials (VLPs). VLPs are small-amplitude, short-duration micropotentials that occur after the QRS complex and are precursors to dangerous, life-threatening cardiac arrhythmias. Tuteur (1989) used the peak of the WT at a fixed scale to identify simulated VLPs. Jones et al. (1992) and Khadra et al. (2003) compared different time–frequency techniques, such as the spectrogram, the smoothed WD, and the WT, in their ability to discriminate between normal patients and patients susceptible to dangerous arrhythmias. Morlet et al. (1993) used the transient detection capability of the WT to identify VLPs.

The WT has also been applied to the ECG signal in the context of ECG analysis and compression by Crowe et al. (1992). Furthermore, Crowe et al. (1992) exploited the capability of the WT to analyze fractal-like signals to study heart rate variability (HRV) data, which have been described as having fractal-like properties.

The recording of heart sounds, or phonocardiogram (PCG) signal, has been analyzed using many time–frequency techniques. Bulgrin et al. (1993) compared the short-time Fourier transform and the WT for the analysis of abnormal PCGs. Picard et al. (1991) analyzed the sounds produced by different prosthetic valves using the spectrogram. The binomial RID, which is a fast approximation to the CWD, was used to analyze the short-time, narrow-bandwidth features of first heart sound in mongrel dogs by Wood et al. (1992).

TFRs have also been applied to nonstationary brain wave signals, including the electroencephalogram (EEG), the electrocorticogram (ECoG), and evoked potentials (EPs). Zaveri et al. (1992) characterized the nonstationary behavior of the ECoG of epileptic patients using the spectrogram, the WD, and the CWD, with the CWD exhibiting superior results. The WT was used to identify the onset of epileptic seizures in the EEG by Schiff and Milton (1993), to extract a single EP by Bartnik et al. (1992), and to characterize changes in somatosensory EPs due to brain injury caused by oxygen deprivation by Thakor et al. (1993). A principal component analysis data reduction method to extract representative features from TFRs of ERPs was examined by Bernat et al. (2005).

Crackles are lung sounds indicative of pathological conditions. Verreault (1989) used AR models of slices of the WD to discriminate crackles from normal lung sounds.

The electrogastrogram (EGG) is a noninvasive measure of the time-varying electrical activity of the stomach. Promising results regarding abnormal EGG rhythms and the frequency of the EGG slow wave were obtained using the CWD by Lin and Chen (1994).

Widmalm et al. (1991) analyzed temporo mandibular joint (TMJ) clicking using the spectrogram, the WD, and the RID. The RID allowed for better time–frequency resolution of the TMJ sounds than the spectrogram while reducing the cross-terms associated with the WD. TMJ signals were also modeled using nonorthogonal Gabor logons by Brown et al. (1994). The primary advantage of this technique, which optimizes the location and support of each Gabor logon, is that only a few such logons were needed to represent the TMJ clicks.

Auditory applications of TFRs are intuitively appealing because the cochlea exhibits constant-bandwidth behavior at low frequencies and constant-Q behavior at middle to high frequencies. Applications include a wavelet-based model of the early stages of acoustic signal processing in the auditory system (Yang et al., 1992), a comparison of the WD and Rihaczek distribution on the response of auditory neurons to wideband noise stimulation (Eggermont and Smith, 1990), and spectrotemporal analysis of dorsal cochlear neurons in the guinea pig (Backoff and Clopton, 1991).

The importance of mammography, x-ray examination of the breast, lies in the early identification of tumors. Kaewlium and Longbotham (1993) used the spectrogram with a Gabor window as a texture discriminator to identify breast masses. Laine et al. (1994) applied multiresolution techniques, including the dyadic and hexagonal WT, for adaptive feature enhancement of mammograms blended with synthetic clinical features of interest. This technique shows promise for enhancing the visualization of mammographic features of interest without additional cost or radiation.

Magnetic resonance imaging (MRI) allows for the imaging of the soft tissues in the body. Weaver et al. (1992) reduced the long processing time of traditional phase encoding of MRI images by WT encoding. Moreover, unlike phase-encoded images, Gibb's ringing phenomena and motion artifacts are localized in WT-encoded images.

The Doppler ultrasound signal is the reflection of an ultrasonic beam due to moving red blood cells and provides information regarding blood vessels and heart chambers. Doppler ultrasound signals in patients with narrowing of the aortic valve were analyzed using the spectrogram by Cloutier et al. (1991). Guo and colleagues (1994) examined and compared the application of five different time–frequency representations (the spectrogram, short-time AR model, CWD, RID, and Bessel distributions) with simulated Doppler ultrasound signals of the femoral artery. Promising results were obtained from the Bessel distribution, the CWD, and the short-time AR model.

Another focus of bioengineering applications of TFRs has concerned the analysis of biological signals of interest, including the sounds generated by marine mammals, such as dolphins and whales, and the sonar echolocation systems used by bats to locate and identify their prey. The RID was applied to sperm whale acoustic signals by Williams and Jeong (1992) and revealed an intricate time–frequency structure that was not apparent in the original time-series data. Buck et al. (2000) developed a synthetic dolphin whistle algorithm to investigate acoustic features dolphins may use to discriminate signature whistle vocalizations. The complicated time–frequency characteristics of dolphin whistles were analyzed by Tyack et al. (1992) using the spectrogram, the WD, and the RID, with the RID giving the best results. Flandrin (1988) analyzed the time–frequency structure of the different signals emitted by bats during hunting, navigation, and identifying prey using the smoothed PWD. In addition, the instantaneous frequency of the various signals was estimated using time–frequency representations. To model the bat's ability to track amidst clutter, Saillant et al. (1993) proposed the spectrogram correlation and transformation (SCAT) receiver model of the bat's echolocation system which decomposes the bat's return echoes into a monaural temporal representation. Limitations of the SCAT model in the laboratory environment were examined in Peremans and Halam (1998). The most common application of the spectrogram is the analysis and modification of quasi-stationary speech signals (Rabiner and Schafer, 1978).

Acknowledgments

The authors would like to acknowledge the use of the personal notes of Franz Hlawatsch and Antonia Papandreou-Suppappola on TFR kernel constraints as well as the help given by Antonia Papandreou-Suppappola in critiquing the chapter and its tables.

References

Backoff P.M. and Clopton B.M. 1991. A spectrotemporal analysis of DCN single unit responses to wide-band noise in guinea pig. *Hear. Res.* 53: 28.

Bartnik E.A., Blinowska K.J., and Durka P.J. 1992. Single evoked potential reconstruction by means of a wavelet transform. *Biol. Cybern.* 67: 175.

Bernat E.M., Williams W.J., and Gehring W.J. 2005. Decomposing ERP time-frequency using PCA. *Clinical Neurophysiology* 116: 1314.

Boashash B. (ed). 1991. *Time–Frequency Signal Analysis—Methods and Applications.* Melbourne, Australia, Longman-Chesire.

Brown M.L., Williams W.J., and Hero A.O. 1994. Non-orthogonal Gabor representation for biological signals. In *Proceedings of the IEEE 1994 International Conference on Acoustics, Speech and Signal Processing,* Australia, pp. 305–308.

Buck J.R., Morgenbesser, H.B., and Tyack, P.L. 2000. Synthesis and modification of the whistles of the bottlenose dolphin, *Tursiops truncates. JASA* 108: 407.

Bulgrin J.R., Rubal B.J., Thompson C.R., and Moody J.M. 1993. Comparison of short-time Fourier transform, wavelet and time-domain analyses of intracardiac sounds. *Biol. Sci. Instrum.* 29: 465.

Claasen T.A.C.M. and Mecklenbräuker W.F.G. 1980. The Wigner distribution: A tool for time-frequency signal analysis, parts I–III. Philips *J. Res.* 35: 217, 276, 372.

Cloutier G., Lemire F., Durand L., Latour Y., Jarry M., Solignac A., and Langlois Y.E. 1991. Change in amplitude distributions of Doppler spectrograms recorded below the aortic valve in patients with a valvular aortic stenosis. *IEEE Trans. Biomed. Eng.* 39: 502.

Cohen L. 1989. Time–frequency distributions—A review. *Proc. IEEE* 77: 941.

Costa A. and Boudreaux-Bartels G.F. 1995. Design of time-frequency representations using multiform, tiltable kernels. *IEEE Trans. SP* 43: 2283.

Crowe J.A., Gibson N.M., Woolfson M.S., and Somekh M.G. 1992. Wavelet transform as a potential tool for ECG analysis and compression. *J. Biomed. Eng.* 14: 268.

Daubechies I. 1992. *Ten Lectures on Wavelets.* Montpelier, VT, Capital City Press.

Eggermont J.J. and Smith G.M. 1990. Characterizing auditory neurons using the Wigner and Rihaczek distributions: A comparison. *JASA* 87: 246.

Flandrin P. 1993. *Temps-Fréquence.* Hermes, Paris, France.

Flandrin P. 1988. Time-frequency processing of bat sonar signals. In Nachtigall P.E. and Moore P.W.B., (eds.), *Animal Sonar: Processes and Performance,* pp. 797–802. New York, Plenum Press.

Guo Z., Durand L.G., and Lee H.C. 1994. Comparison of time-frequency distribution techniques for analysis of simulated Doppler ultrasound signals of the femoral artery. *IEEE Trans. Biomed. Eng.* 41: 332.

Hlawatsch F. and Boudreaux-Bartels G.F. 1992. Linear and quadratic time–frequency signal representations. *IEEE Sig. Proc. Mag.* March: 21.

Hlawatsch F., Papandreou-Suppappola A., and Boudreaux-Bartels G.F. 1999. The power classes—quadratic time-frequency representations with scale covariance and dispersive time-shift covariance. *IEEE Trans. SP* 47: 3067.

Jones D.L., Tovannas J.S., Lander P., and Albert D.E. 1992. Advanced time–frequency methods for signal averaged ECG analysis. *J. Electrocardiol.* 25: 188.

Kadambe S., Murray R., and Boudreaux-Bartels G.F. 1999. Wavelet transform based QRS complex detector. *IEEE Trans. Biomed. Eng.* 46: 838.

Kaewlium A. and Longbotham H. 1993. Application of Gabor transform as texture discriminator of masses in digital mammograms. *Biol. Sci. Instrum.* 29: 183.

Khadra, L., Dickhaus, H., and Lipp, A. 2003. Representations of ECG—late potentials in the time frequency plane. *Med. Eng. Technol.* 17: 228.

Laine A., Schuler S., and Fan J. 1994. Mammographic feature enhancement by multiscale analysis. *IEEE Trans. Med. Imag.* 13: 725

Li C. and Zheng C. 1995. Detection of ECG characteristic points using wavelet transforms. *IEEE Trans. Biomed. Eng.* 42: 21.

Lin Z.Y. and Chen J.D.Z. 1994. Time–frequency representation of the electrogastrogram: Application of the exponential distribution. *IEEE Trans. Biomed. Eng.* 41: 267.

Meyer Y. 1993. *Wavelets–Algorithms and Applications*. SIAM, Philadelphia.

Morlet D., Peyrin F., Desseigne P., Touboul P., and Rubel P. 1993. Wavelet analysis of high resolution signal averaged ECGs in postinfarction patients. *J. Electrocardiol.* 26: 311.

Murray R. 1995. Summary of biomedical applications of time-frequency representations. Technical report no. 0195-0001, University of Rhode Island, Department of Electrical Engineering, Kingston, RI, 02881.

Papandreou A., Hlawatsch F., and Boudreaux-Bartels G.F. 1993. The Hyperbolic class of quadratic time–frequency representations: I. Constant-Q warping, the hyperbolic paradigm, properties, and members. *IEEE Trans. SP* 41: 3425.

Papandreou-Suppappola A. (ed.) 2003. *Applications in Time-Frequency Signal Processing*. Boca Raton, FL, Taylor & Francis.

Peremans H. and Halam, J 1998. The spectrogram and transformation receiver, revisited. *JASA* 104: 1101.

Picard D., Charara J., Guidoin F., Haggag Y., Poussart D., Walker D., and How T. 1991. Phonocardiogram spectral analysis simulator of mitral valve prostheses. *J. Med. Eng. Technol.* 15: 222.

Rabiner L.R. and Schafer R.W. 1978. *Digital Processing of Speech Signals*. Englewood Cliffs, NJ, Prentice-Hall.

Rioul O. and Vetterli M. 1991. Wavelets and signal processing. *IEEE Sig. Proc. Mag.* October: 14.

Saillant P.A., Simmons J.A., Dear S.P., and McMullen T.A. 1993. A computational model of echo processing and acoustic imaging in frequency-modulated echo-locating bats: The spectrogram correlation and transformation receiver. *JASA* 94: 2691.

Schiff S.J. and Milton J.G. 1993. Wavelet transforms for electroencephalographic spike and seizure detection. In *Proc. SPIE—Intl. Soc. Opt. Eng.* San Diego '93, SPIE Proceedings, Vol. 2036, pp. 50–56.

Thakor N.V., Xin Rong G., Yi Chun S., and Hanley D.F. 1993. Multiresolution wavelet analysis of evoked potentials. *IEEE Trans. BME* 40: 1085.

Tuteur F.B. 1989. Wavelet transformations in signal detection. In *Proc. Intl. Conf. ASSP*, ICASSP-88, New York, NY, pp. 1435–1438.

Tyack P.L., Williams W.J., and Cunningham G. 1992. Time-frequency fine structure of dolphin whistles. In *Proc. IEEE—SP Intl. Symp. T-F and T-S Anal.* Victoria, BC, Canada, pp. 17–20.

Verreault E. 1989. Détection et Caractérisation des Rales Crépitants (French). PhD thesis, l'Université Laval, Faculte des Sciences et de Genie.

Weaver J.B., Xu Y., Healy D.M., and Driscoll J.R. 1992. Wavelet encoded MR imaging. *Magnet Reson. Med.* 24: 275.

Widmalm W.E., Williams W.J., and Zheng C. 1991. Time frequency distributions of TMJ sounds. *J. Oral. Rehabil.* 18: 403.

Williams W.J. and Jeong J. 1992. Reduced interference time–frequency distributions. In Boashash B. (ed.), *Time–Frequency Signal Analysis—Methods and Applications*, pp. 74–97. Melbourne/NY, Longman—Chesire/Wiley.

Wood J.C., Buda A.J., and Barry D.T. 1992. Tme-frequency transforms: A new approach to first heart sound dynamics. *IEEE Trans. Biomed. Eng.* 39: 730.

Yang Z., Wang K., and Shamma S. 1992. Auditory representations of acoustic signals. *IEEE Trans. Info. Theory* 38: 824.

Zaveri H.P., Williams W.J., Iasemidis L.D., and Sackellares J.C. 1992. Time–frequency representations of electrocorticograms in temporal lobe epilepsy. *IEEE Trans. Biomed. Eng.* 39: 502.

Further Information

Several TFR tutorials exist on the Cohen class (Cohen, 1989; Hlawatsch and Boudreaux-Bartels, 1992; Boashash, 1991; Flandrin, 1993), Affine class (Bertrand chapter in Boashash, 1991; Flandrin, 1993), Hyperbolic class (Papandreou et al., 1993), and Power class (Hlawatsch et al., 1999). Several special conferences or issues of IEEE journals devoted to TFRs and the WT include *Proceedings of the IEEE-SP Time Frequency and Time-Scale Workshop*, 1992, *IEEE Sig. Proc. Soc.*; Special issue on wavelet transforms and multiresolution signal analysis, *IEEE Trans. Info. Theory*, 1992; and Special issue on wavelets and signal processing, *IEEE Trans. SP*, 1993. A wide variety of TFR applications, including tutorials and pseudo-code, can be found in (Papandreou-Suppappola, 2010). An extended list of references on the application of TFRs to problems in biomedical or bioengineering can be found in Murray (1995).

3

Multivariate Spectral Analysis of Electroencephalogram: Power, Coherence, and Second-Order Blind Identification

Ramesh Srinivasan
University of California, Irvine

Siyi Deng
University of California, Irvine

3.1 Introduction

Clinical or research electroencephalogram (EEG) records typically consist of time series of potentials recorded with 64–256 electrodes placed on the scalp locations. This large volume of data contains information that is both redundant and difficult to interpret. A natural question is—how can we compress this information into a more concise format and extract features that can be meaningfully related to cognitive processes or clinical disease states? Because the spatial and temporal properties of EEG can vary widely, no universal answer to this question is expected. However, cognitive neuroscience research and clinical neuroscience applications of EEG including brain–computer interfaces (BCIs) almost always benefit from some form of spectral analysis in which temporal waveforms are decomposed into their discrete frequency components. Indeed, this simple approach has revealed many robust connections between different EEG frequency bands and cognitive functions or clinical diseases (Petsche and Etlinger, 1998; Pfurtsheller and Lopes da Silva, 1999; Murias et al., 2007). Spectral analysis is the obvious entry point for studying EEG dynamics, and most EEG scientists use the *power spectrum* as an essential first step in processing EEG signals.

Neuronal dynamics can be considered a stochastic (random) process having statistical properties in time and space. This general framework has important advantages over viewpoints that may prejudge the nature of EEG dynamics, for instance that one location in the brain generates the EEG observed in one frequency band. A more general (and realistic) conceptual model considers that the spatiotemporal statistics of EEG signals contain information that reflect something about the spatiotemporal statistics of current source activity in the brain. While spectral analysis is widely used to analyze the times series at each EEG channel, analyses of spatial properties of EEG are equally important to characterize statistical properties of the underlying source distribution. Across a broad range of cognitive and clinical studies, measures of phase synchronization between electrodes located over different brain regions appear especially promising approaches to identify brain networks. Brain networks are cell assemblies that coordinate neuronal action across brain regions supporting complex cognition, behavior, and consciousness. This coordination is at least partly reflected in the synchronization of EEG signals in one frequency band. *Coherence* measures the consistency of the phase difference between two channels in one frequency band. Many brain diseases, including schizophrenias, attention deficit disorders, and autism are associated with inadequate or inappropriate cell assembly formation, reflected in the strength and spatial pattern of the coherence of EEG signals.

How can we relate power and coherence measured with EEG electrodes on the scalp to statistical properties of the source activity in the brain? Mathematical models of volume conduction in the head are used to *investigate theoretical limitations on EEG dynamic properties as estimates of brain dynamics.* The resulting mathematical models provide a conceptual framework for understanding the EEG data. In this chapter, we provide a theoretical framework with which we can interpret EEG power and coherence. The effect of current flow through tissues of the head is to spatially low pass filter the signal generated in the brain. As a consequence, power at one EEG electrode depends on both the strength and spatial properties of the source activity in the brain. Coherence between electrodes also reflects this spatial filtering; as a consequence only coherence between widely spaced electrodes can be easily interpreted.

The spatial filtering due to volume conduction can be understood as a linear mixing process. Each electrode sums the activity over many sources in the brain and each electrode represented a different mixture of sources. This has led to a great deal of interest in using blind source separation (BSS) techniques to process EEG data, separating source processes according to various statistical criteria. Perhaps the most well known of these techniques, Independent Component Analysis (ICA) has been implemented using a variety of statistical criteria to separate sources from the mixtures at each electrode without any other prior information (Makeig et al., 2004). Spectral analysis can then be performed on these components. However, the source separation achieved by ICA is not optimal for spectral analysis. While ICA usually makes use of features of the joint probability density of the EEG records, the analysis is insensitive to the temporal order in which the multichannel EEG was observed. That is, if the order in which the potentials (at all electrodes) is recorded was randomized there would no effect on ICA. Second-order blind identification (SOBI) is a BSS method developed for time-series analysis (Belouchrani et al., 1997) in array processing which explicitly incorporates the temporal structure of the second-order statistics (covariance) of the signals in developing a BSS from the EEG electrode. When applied to EEG signals, they can be used to obtain a multivariate spectral analysis that can identify brain networks operating in different (or even the same) frequency bands.

3.2 Synaptic Action Generates EEG

Scalp potentials are believed to be generated by *millisecond-scale modulations* of synaptic current sources at the surfaces of neurons (Lopes da Silva and Storm van Leeuwen, 1978; Nunez, 1981, 1995, 2000a,b; Lopes da Silva, 1999).

While cortical and scalp potentials are generated by these microsources associated with synaptic action, potentials are more conveniently modeled in terms of *dipole moment per unit volume* $\mathbf{P}(\mathbf{r}, t)$ where $\mathbf{r}$ spans the volume of the brain. For convenience of this discussion, the brain volume may be parceled into N tissue masses or voxels of volume ΔV, each producing its vector dipole moment. The potential anywhere in the brain or scalp surface is then expressed as a weighted sum (or integral) of contributions from all these sources

$$\Phi_S(\mathbf{r},t) = \int_{B'} G_H(\mathbf{r},\mathbf{r}')\mathbf{P}(\mathbf{r}',t)dV(\mathbf{r}') \tag{3.1}$$

If the volume element $dV(\mathbf{r}')$ is defined in terms of cortical columns, the volume integral may be reduced to an integral over the folded cortical surface. The weighting coefficients G_H is the *Green's function* which depends on the properties of the volume conductor and the locations of source r' and measurement location $\mathbf{r}$. The Green's function is essentially the *impulse response function* between sources and surface measurement locations. For some locations, for example, deep tissues like the thalamus or other subcortical structures, G_H is expected to be very small, while for superficial sources in the gyral crowns of the cortex, G_H is large. G_H contains all geometric and conductive information about the head volume conductor. The most common head models consist of three or four concentric spherical shells, representing brain, cerebrospinal fluid (four sphere), skull and scalp tissue with different electrical conductivities as shown in Figure 3.1 for which analytic solutions have been obtained (Nunez and Srinivasan, 2006). Numerical methods such as the boundary element method (BEM) may also be used to estimate G_H, by employing MRI to determine tissue boundaries, resulting in a more accurate geometrical model. However, the accuracy of these models may be severely limited by incomplete knowledge of tissue conductivities—they may be less accurate conductivity models (Nunez and Srinivasan, 2006; Srinivasan et al., 2007). For the purposes of the article, we make use of the analytic spherical model to estimate GH. The results have been confirmed using ellipsoidal models fit to MRI images (Srinivasan et al., 2007).

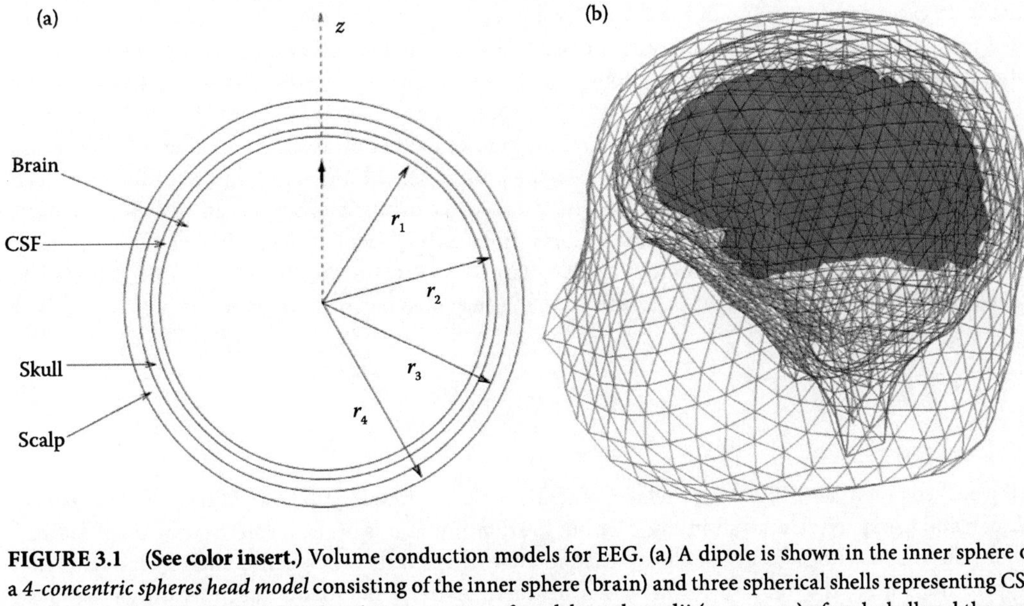

FIGURE 3.1 **(See color insert.)** Volume conduction models for EEG. (a) A dipole is shown in the inner sphere of a *4-concentric spheres head model* consisting of the inner sphere (brain) and three spherical shells representing CSF (cerebrospinal fluid), skull and scalp. The parameters of model are the radii (r_1, r_2, r_3, r_4) of each shell and the conductivity ratios (σ_1/σ_2, σ_1/σ_3, σ_1/σ_4). Typical values are: radii (8, 8.1, 8.6, 9.2 cm) and conductivity ratios (0.2, 40, 1). (b) A realistic shaped BEM of the head. The brain and scalp boundaries were found by segmenting the images with a threshold, and opening and closing operation, respectively, while the outer skull boundary was obtained by dilation of the brain boundary (ASA, Netherlands). Although geometrically more accurate that the spherical model, the (geometrically) realistic BEM is potentially a less accurate model than concentric spheres because tissue resistivity is poorly known.

3.3 Time Domain Spectral Analysis

In EEG applications, spectral analysis provides a means to assess *statistical properties* of oscillations in different frequency bands. It is customary to view any experimental data record as one *realization of a random process* (or *stochastic process*) (Bendat and Piersol, 2001). In this context, the word "random" does not imply that lack of statistical structure or deterministic origins of the signals, only that its statistical properties are yet to be discovered. The spectrum obtained by applying the fast Fourier transform (FFT) to a single EEG epoch provides information about the frequency content of that particular epoch. A number of important issues in practical FFT analysis are detailed in several texts (e.g., Bendat and Piersol, 2001). For our purposes, the estimation of the Fourier coefficients for each epoch is the starting point for the development of various statistical tools based on *spectral analysis.* A number of new approaches to Fourier analysis including wavelet analysis (Lachaux et al., 2002), multitaper analysis (Percival and Walden, 1993), autoregressive models (Ding et al., 2006) and Hilbert transforms (Bendat and Piersol, 2001; Le Van Quyen et al., 2001; Deng and Srinivasan, 2010) have potential applications in EEG, particularly in the analysis of short data epochs or characterizing the variation of the spectrum during a time period following a sensory stimulus or preceding movement. All such methods yield estimates of "Fourier coefficients" that reflect the amplitude and phase of the oscillations within one frequency band (and perhaps localized to one window in time). Any of these Fourier coefficients can be used to carry out spectral analysis of time series. However, interpretations using different techniques depend on the assumptions and parameter choices built in to the specific methods chosen to estimate Fourier coefficients. These limitations are probably not as widely appreciated as those associated with conventional FFT methods, suggesting advantages of comparing multiple methods applied to the same data.

Any observed time series is just one physical realization (sample) of the underlying stochastic process, but is not sufficient to *represent* the stochastic process. Thus, the amplitude spectrum of one epoch of EEG is an exact representation of the frequency content of that particular signal epoch, but only provides one observation about the random process. An ensemble of K observations $\{V_k(t)\}$ can be used to estimate statistical properties of the random process. An important question is whether the stochastic process is stationary, that is, the statistical properties of the random process are invariant to shifts in the time where the sample records are obtained. Many studies have contrasted the EEG in different brain states such as eyes closed resting, eyes open resting, during mental calculations, and different sleep stages under the assumption that within these states the EEG can be reasonably assumed to be stationary. By contrast, EEG data collected following a sensory stimulus clearly violate the stationarity assumption—the time at which each sample record $V_k(t)$ is obtained relative to the stimulus can be expected to influence the observed EEG statistics. In this case, the ensemble mean of observations

$$\mu(t) = \frac{1}{K}\sum_{k=1}^{K} V_k(t) \tag{3.2}$$

is the evoked potential (EP) or event-related potential which varies as a function of time over the epoch. We can still use spectral analysis in this case but the interpretations of the results may be more difficult if conventional methods like the FFT are used to analyze the interval. Spectral analysis methods that capture the temporal evolution of the signal in different frequency bands, such as wavelet analysis (Lachaux et al., 2002) are then preferred.

A random process is weakly stationary if the mean (Equation 3.2) and the *power spectrum* are invariant to shifts in the time at which the sample records are obtained. The *power spectrum* (*autospectral density function*) of an EEG signal provides a decomposition of the *variance* of the signal as a function of frequency. As in the case of any other statistical measure, we can never know the *actual* power spectrum of a stochastic process. Rather, we find *estimates* of the power spectrum. The *power spectrum* may be estimated from an ensemble of observations by applying a Fourier transform and summing over K epochs, that is

$$P(f_n) = \frac{2}{K}\sum_{k=1}^{K} F_k(f_n)F_k(f_n)^* = \frac{2}{K}\sum_{k=1}^{K}\left|F_k(f_n)\right|^2 \quad n = 0,1,2,\ldots(N-1)/2 \tag{3.3}$$

For each sample epoch $V_k(t_n)$, Fourier coefficients $F_k(f_n)$ can be obtained using the FFT. In Equation 3.3, the frequencies f_n are discrete, and depend on the length of each observation (T) as $f_n = n/T$. The factor of two occurs because we use only positive frequencies. The form of the power spectrum estimate in Equation 3.3 does not depend on the specific algorithm used to estimate the Fourier coefficients (although the discretization of frequencies does depend on the method). If the mean value of the signal is zero, the power spectrum summed over all frequencies is equal to the variance in the signal, a relationship known as *Parseval's theorem* (Bendat and Piersol, 2001). If the EEG time series is recorded in units of μV, Equation 3.3 provides a definition of the EEG power spectrum in units that depend on the bandwidth Δf. The power spectrum is sometimes normalized with respect to the bandwidth to express power in units of $\mu V^2/Hz$. The *amplitude spectrum*, the square root of the power spectrum, places more emphasis on nondominant spectral peaks and is often our measure of choice for visualization.

Prior to the widespread availability of the FFT and fast computers, the autospectral density function or in the more common parlance, "power spectrum" of a time series was obtained by first estimating the autocorrelation function:

$$R_{VV}(\tau) = E\left[V(t)^* V(t-\tau)\right] \tag{3.4}$$

Here the expectation operator indicates averaging over observations, and the lag variable τ can take positive or negative values. The autocorrelation function is the covariance of the signal with a delayed copy of the same signal. If τ spans $[-T/2, T/2]$, R_{VV} contains exactly the same information as the power spectrum defined by Equation 3.3. The Fourier transform of the autocorrelation function is the power spectrum of the signal. Modern spectral analysis methods rarely involve direct computation of the autocorrelation function. However, note that later in this chapter we will make use of this formulation of the signal statistics as the basis of a multivariate decomposition of the spectra in multichannel EEG recordings.

Implementation of Equation 3.3 forces tradeoffs involving frequency resolution, statistical power, and putative stationarity. For example, consider the choices involved in analyzing a 60 s EEG record. Figure 3.2 demonstrates power spectra of two EEG channels, one occipital and one frontal, recorded with the subject's eyes closed and at rest. The power spectral estimates were obtained using an epoch length $T = 60$ s ($\Delta f = 0.017$ Hz) and no epoch averaging ($K = 1$ epochs). With this choice, the FFT of the entire record is obtained (exact spectra of the two EEG signals), but no information about the statistical properties of the underlying random process is gained. Note that the power spectrum of the occipital channel (Figure 3.2a) contains two peaks, one below 10 Hz and a larger peak above 10 Hz. The frontal channel (Figure 3.2b) shows a larger peak below 10 Hz. By examining the other channels it was found that the two peaks have distinct spatial distributions over the scalp, suggesting they have different source distributions. Each peak is surrounded by power in sidebands (adjacent frequency bins) of the two peak frequencies. *The signals are stochastic processes occupying relatively narrow bands in the frequency spectrum.*

To analyze the 60 s signal properly, we must decide how to divide the record into epochs to implement Equation 3.3. The choice is a compromise between the advantage of good frequency resolution yielded by long epochs (large T and small K) and the statistical power of our estimate gained by using a larger number of epochs (small T small and large K). If a frequency resolution of $\Delta f = 0.5$ Hz is chosen, the

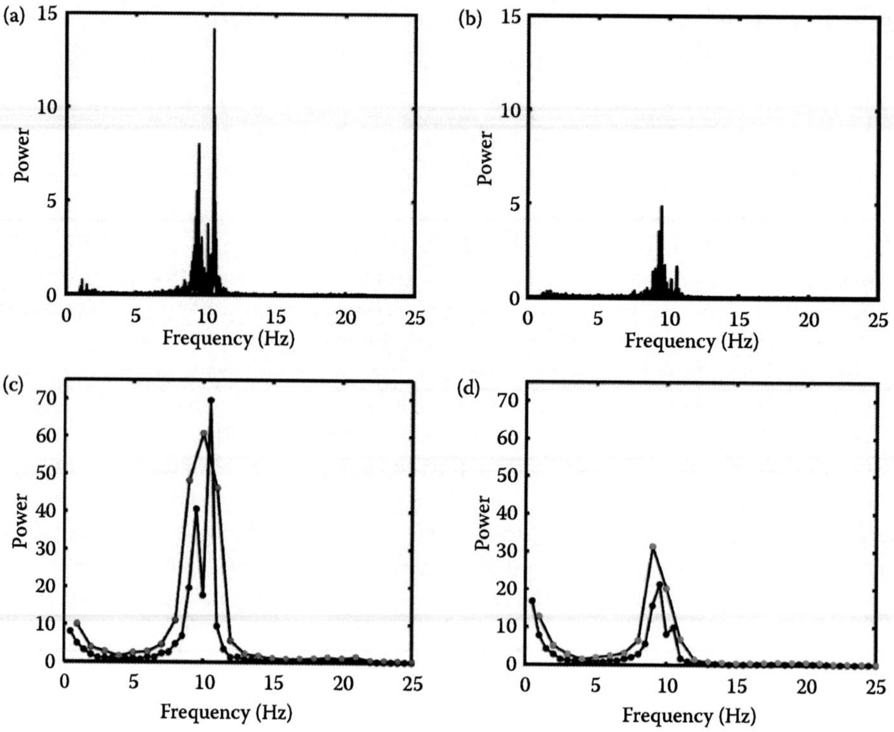

FIGURE 3.2 Example power spectra from a single subject (female, 22 years). The subject is at rest with eyes closed. (a) Power spectrum of a midline occipital channel with epoch length $T = 60$ s and $K = 1$ epochs. The power spectrum appears to have two distinct peaks one below 10 Hz and one above 10 Hz. (b) Power spectrum at a midline frontal channel with epoch length $T = 60$ s and $K = 1$ epochs. Here only the peak below 10 Hz is visible. (c) Power spectra of a midline occipital channel calculated with two different choices of epoch length T and number of epochs K. The gray circles indicate the power spectrum with $T = 1$ s and $K = 60$ epochs. The black circles indicate the power spectrum with $T = 2$ s and $K = 30$ epochs. (d) Power spectra of a midline frontal channel calculated as in Part (c).

record is segmented into $K = 30$ epochs of length $T = 2$ s. If frequency resolution is reduced to $\Delta f = 1$ Hz, we divide the record into $K = 60$ epochs of length $T = 1$ s. Figure 3.2c and d shows the power spectra of the frontal and occipital channels with $\Delta f = 1$ Hz (gray circles) and $\Delta f = 0.5$ Hz (black circles). The power spectra at the occipital and frontal channels are both dominated by alpha rhythm oscillations. At the occipital electrode (Figure 3.2c) two separate peak frequencies are at 9.5 and 10.5 Hz are evident with $\Delta f = 0.5$ Hz, but this is not revealed with $\Delta f = 1$ Hz, where only a single peak frequency at 10 Hz is evident. Lowering frequency resolution has a similar effect at the frontal channel (Figure 3.2d), but since there is very little power at 10.5 Hz, the only clear peak appears at 9 Hz. Thus, by choosing lower frequency resolution we see a signal representation having different (single) peak frequencies at the two sites, while choosing higher frequency resolution results in pairs of frequency peaks at both sites but with different relative magnitudes.

By examining the power spectra for the occipital (Figure 3.3a) and frontal sites (Figure 3.3b) for individual epochs with $\Delta f = 0.5$ Hz, support for two different oscillations within the alpha band is obtained. At the occipital channel individual epochs display two distinct peaks at 9.5 and 10.5 Hz. The first 15 epochs show a strong response at 10.5 Hz but the later epochs show a stronger response at 9.5 Hz. The dominant frequency in each epoch is summarized in the peak power histograms in Figure 3.3c showing that individual epochs displayed peak frequencies at both 9.5 and 10.5 Hz. By contrast, very few epochs have a peak frequency of 10.5 Hz at the frontal site (Figure 3.3d); most epochs have peak

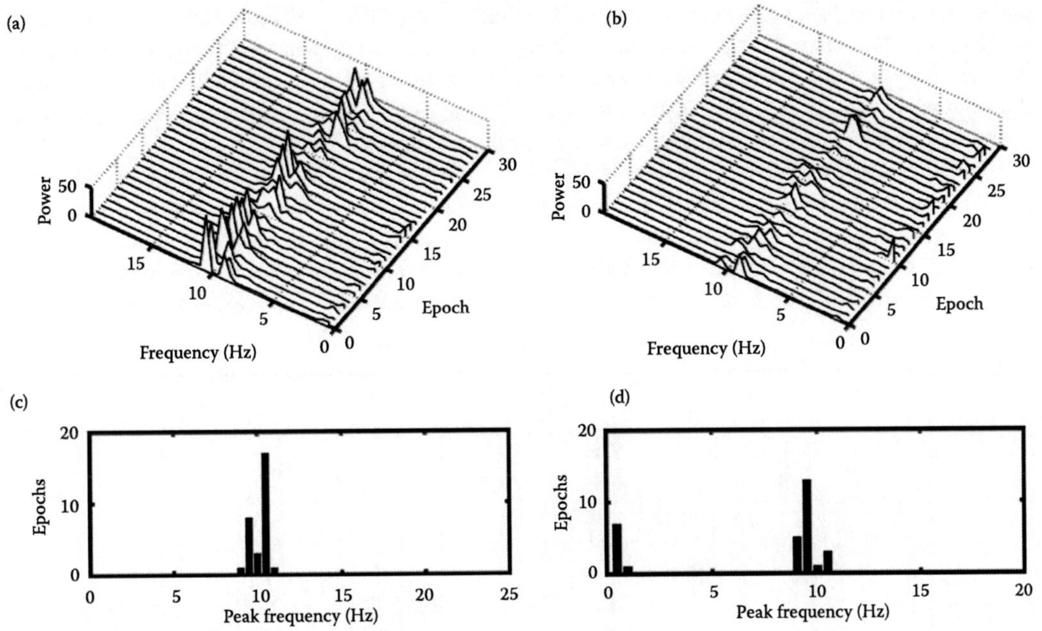

FIGURE 3.3 (a) Plots of 30 (individual epoch) power spectra for the occipital channel shown in Figure 3.2a and c. (b) Plots of the same 30 individual epoch spectra for the frontal channel. (c) Peak power histograms show the distribution of peak frequencies for the 30 epochs shown in Part (a). (d) Peak power histograms for the 30 epochs shown in Part (b).

frequencies either at 9.5 Hz or in the delta band (<2 Hz). Note that during most epochs with strong delta activity in Figure 3.3d the alpha peaks are attenuated.

In summary, estimating the *power spectrum* from an ensemble of epochs provides a decomposition of the variance of the signal as a function of frequency. This is a particularly useful approach because EEG contains oscillatory activity in distinct frequency bands that are associated with different brain states. In the simple example, we presented here of the alpha rhythm in Figures 3.2 and 3.3, electrodes at different locations show different magnitudes of two distinct oscillations with center frequencies at 9.5 and 10.5 Hz. In the next section, factors that determine the magnitude of peaks in the EEG power spectrum are considered. In later sections, methods to quantify spatial properties of EEG rhythms, which are evidently different for the two peak frequencies in this example, are investigated.

3.4 Impact of Spatial Filtering on EEG Power Spectra

Scalp potential amplitude at any frequency can change for several reasons related to "synchronization" of neurons. The large changes in scalp amplitude that occur when brain state changes are believed to be due mostly to such changes in the correlation of the synaptic activity. EEG scientists and clinicians have adopted the label *desynchronization* to indicate large amplitude reductions, particularly in the alpha band (Pfurtscheller and Lopes da Silva, 1999). However, synchronization among neurons may occur in different directions and at different spatial scales, and may occur with zero phase lag or with finite phase differences. In this section, we consider how synchronization of the underlying sources determines EEG power.

There are several (possibly overlapping) means by which synchronization can influence the EEG power spectrum. For convenience of this, we can divide the brain into several thousand volume elements (e.g., macrocolumns, 3 mm in each dimension) located along the folded gray-matter surface of the brain each having a (vector) dipole moment per unit volume **P**(**r**, *t*). Volume elements in the white matter, ventricles, and other tissues of the head have very little current source activity. The strength of the dipoles (magnitude of the moment) depends strongly on the synchronization of the synapses within the volume element (Nunez and Srinivasan, 2006). As the source strength increases, we expect scalp potential to increase proportionately if there are no other changes.

A small region of the cortex, for example a gyral crown of surface area 2 cm^2, is composed of around 25 volume elements. Thus, it is more realistic to consider the EEG signals to be generated by dipole layer, consisting of many adjacent dipole sources. Figure 3.4 shows examples of dipole layers of diameter ranging from 3 to 5 cm composed only of radially oriented dipole sources in a concentric spheres model of the head. Each dipole layer is composed of dipole sources with time series that are constructed by adding

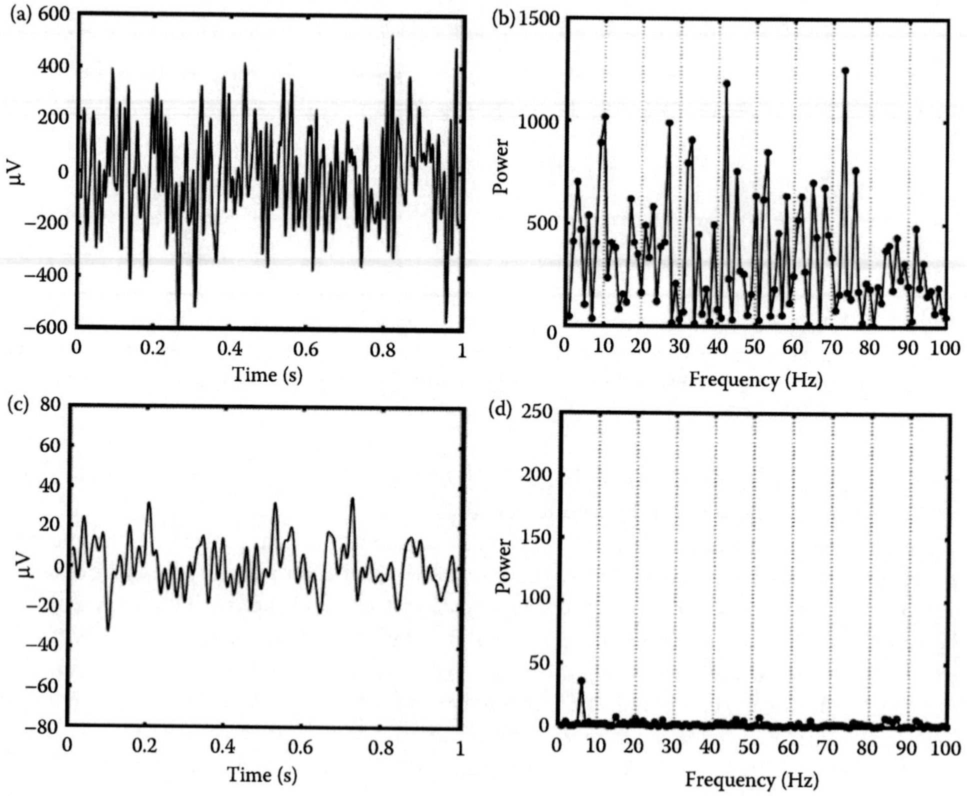

FIGURE 3.4 (a) Time series of a dipole meso-source **P**(**r**, *t*) composed of a 15 µV sine wave added to Gaussian random noise with standard deviation σ = 150 µV. The Gaussian random noise was low pass filtered at 100 Hz. The sine wave has variance (power) equal 1% of the noise. (b) Power spectrum of the time series shown in Part (a). The power spectrum has substantial power at frequencies other than 6 Hz. (c) Time series recorded by an electrode on the outer sphere (scalp) of a four concentric spheres model above the center of a dipole layer of diameter 3 cm. The dipole layer is composed of 32 dipole sources **P**(**r**, *t*) with time series constructed similar to Part (a) with independent Gaussian noise (uncorrelated) at each dipole source. Scalp potential was calculated for a dipole layer at a radius $r_z = 7.8$ cm in a four concentric spheres model. The model parameters were radii $(r_1, r_2, r_3, r_4) = (8, 8.1, 8.6, 9.2)$ and conductivity ratios $(\sigma_1/\sigma_2, \sigma_1/\sigma_3, \sigma_1/\sigma_4) = (0.2, 40, 1)$. Notice the time series is smoother than in the case of the individual dipole source. (d) Power spectrum of the time series shown in Part (c). Note the peak at 6 Hz. (e) Time series similar to Part (c), but due to a dipole layer of diameter of 4 cm composed of 68 dipole sources. (f) Power spectrum of the time series shown in Part (e). (g) Similar time series to Part (c), but with a dipole layer of diameter 5 cm composed of 112 dipole sources. The presence of the 6 Hz sinusoid is obvious from the time series. (h) Power spectrum of the time series shown in Part (g). Large spectral peak at 6 Hz is evident.

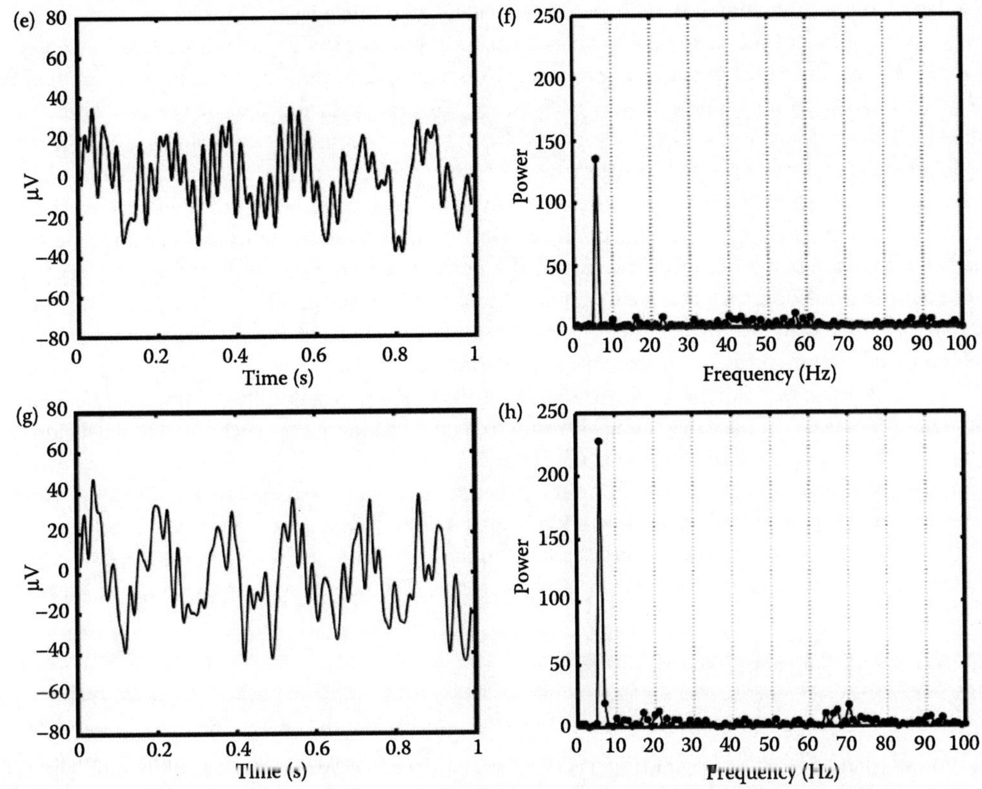

FIGURE 3.4 Continued.

a 6 Hz sinusoid of fixed amplitude $A = 15$ μV to a Gaussian random processes with mean $\mu = 0$ and standard deviation $\sigma = 150$ μV. *The 6 Hz components are phase locked across the dipoles, whereas all other components have random phases.* Each source signal is an independent random time series representing transcortical potential across the dipole layer. The source time series of a single dipole source (dipole layer of very small size) is plotted in Figure 3.4a and the corresponding power spectrum is plotted in Figure 3.4b. The power spectrum shows that the source signal is broadband, with some power at 6 Hz but even higher power at other frequencies. The power of the 6 Hz sinusoid is only 1% of the total power of each dipole source, and does not stand out in either the time series or the power spectrum. Figure 3.4c and d shows the estimated potential on the scalp directly above the center of a superficial dipole layer of diameter 3 cm, based on four concentric spheres model of the head. The time series shows considerably less power at higher frequencies because of cancellation of potential from asynchronous sources and exhibits a smooth appearance compared to the source time series. The corresponding power spectrum (Figure 3.4d) shows a clear peak at 6 Hz and no other peak frequencies. As the diameter of the dipole layer is increased from 3 to 4 to 5 cm, the calculated surface potential becomes more obviously sinusoidal (Figure 3.4e–h). The power substantially increases at 6 Hz, but the power distributed across the rest of the spectrum is essentially unchanged. Another factor that potentially influences the power spectrum is the relative phases of the 6 Hz sources within the dipole layer. In this example, the 6 Hz oscillation is at the same phase in every source. Variability in the phases of the sources would reduce the power.

Clearly, source synchrony is as important as source strength and source size in the generation of scalp potentials. Most (99%) of the source activity in this examples is uncorrelated; as a result, sources contribute minimally to scalp potential even as the size of the source region increases. By contrast, relatively small magnitude (1%) source activity that is synchronous across all sources in the dipole layer generates a large scalp potential that increases dramatically as dipole layer diameter increases. We have quantified this effect of the size of a dipole layer on scalp potential as a spatial filter (Srinivasan et al., 1996; 1998). *One important implication of Figure 3.4 is that spatial filtering by volume conduction can lead to temporal filtering of source activity in the scalp EEG.* If synchronous source activity in different frequency bands takes place in dipole layers of different sizes, frequency bands that are synchronized broadly over the cortical surface can easily generate higher power in the scalp potentials than a stronger but smaller dipole layer. The power at any frequency in the spectrum of scalp EEG is determined not only by the source strength but also by spatial properties of the source such as its size and synchrony. Thus, we anticipate that EEG recorded within the brain can have quite different spectra than EEG recorded on the scalp, a prediction well-supported by experimental studies. Moreover, strong correlations between EEG data recorded on the scalp and cognitive processes or clinical disease states may have no obvious correlation in EEG recorded within the brain.

In summary, these simulations demonstrate that relative EEG power in different frequency bands and power changes between brain states can easily result from changes in source synchrony, source region size, and meso-source strength. Furthermore, source strength $\mathbf{P}(\mathbf{r},t)$, measured as dipole moment per unit volume, is itself a measure of source synchrony at smaller scales because synaptic (microsource) synchrony influences effective pole separation as shown in Chapter 4. Thus, the relative power level measured by an EEG electrode at any one frequency is closely related to the degree of synchronization of synaptic currents at that frequency (with no phase lag) over tangential cortical distances roughly in the range of 5–10 cm.

3.5 Spatial Statistics of EEG

In this section, we introduce *spatial analysis* of the EEG by means of the analysis of a joint observation of time series $\{V_{mk}(t)\}$ consisting of $k = 1, K$ observations in $m = 1, M$ data channels. These joint observations of time series are the realization of a stochastic process distributed in space and time over the cortical surface and recorded on the scalp with EEG electrodes. The *coherence* between pairs of EEG channels provides an entry point to examine the spatial properties of the stochastic source activity. As in the case of other statistical measures, we can never know the coherence of a stochastic process, we can only obtain estimates. In this section, we define *coherence as a linear correlation coefficient* that primarily estimates the amount of phase synchronization between any two data channels. Coherence of a random process is a statistical measure of the relationship between two time series (or data channels) *across observations*. As we shall see, coherence is a measure very similar to a squared correlation coefficient, which measures the proportion of variance in one data channel that can be explained by a linear transformation of another data channel.

To calculate coherence we first define a *cross spectrum* (Bendat and Piersol, 2001), which is a measure of the joint spectral properties of two channels. The cross spectrum $C_{uv}(f_n)$ of two channels u and v at frequency f_n can be estimated from pairs of Fourier coefficients as an average over K epochs, that is

$$C_{uv}(f_n) = A_{uv}e^{j\phi_{uv}} = \frac{2}{K}\sum_{k=1}^{K} F_{uk}(f_n)F_{vk}^{*}(f_n) \quad n = 0,1,2,\ldots(N-1)/2 \tag{3.5}$$

When $u = v$ the cross spectrum reduces to the power spectrum (2.3), and the factor of two again reflects the fact that our spectra are restricted to positive frequencies.

Unlike the power spectrum, which is real valued, the cross spectrum is complex valued, and can be expressed as magnitude (or cross-power) A_{uv} and phase φ_{uv}. The phase of the cross spectrum is the average phase difference between the two channels which we also label the *relative phase*. The cross spectrum is a measure of the covariance between two signals at one frequency across observations analogous to the ordinary *covariance* between two time series. In fact, similar to the relationship between the power spectrum and the autocorrelation function, the cross spectrum is the Fourier transform of the crosscorrelation function R_{uv}:

$$R_{uv}(\tau) = E\left[V_u(t)V_v(t+\tau)\right] \tag{3.6}$$

If t spans the interval $[-T/2, T/2]$ the crosscorrelation function contains the same information as the crossspectrum. The crosscorrelation function is at the heart of the multivariate spectral analysis methods discussed at the end of the chapter.

If we normalize the squared magnitude of the cross spectrum by the power spectrum of each channel, we obtain the coherence $\gamma_{uv}^2(f_n)$ between the two channels

$$\gamma_{uv}^2(f_n) = \frac{\left|C_{uv}(f_n)\right|^2}{P_u(f_n)P_v(f_n)} \quad n = 0,1,2,\ldots(N-1)/2 \tag{3.7}$$

The form of Equation 3.7 follows closely from the equation for a Pearson correlation coefficient (squared). The numerator is the squared magnitude of the cross spectrum (or squared cross power), analogous to squared covariance. The power spectrum is analogous to the variance of the signal. Thus, Equation 3.7 is analogous to dividing squared covariance by the variance of each channel, which is a squared correlation coefficient. Like the usual r^2 statistic, coherence $\gamma_{uv}^2(f_n)$ measures the fraction of variance of channel u at frequency f_n that can be explained by a constant linear transformation of the Fourier coefficients at frequency f_n obtained at channel v. *In the frequency domain, a constant linear transformation means both constant gain (relative amplitude) and constant relative phase.*

The form of Equation 3.7 indicates that the coherence measure is quite sensitive to the relative phases between two channels. If the relative phase is constant over epochs, the average of the product on the right-hand side of Equation 3.5 is equal to the average product of the magnitude of the Fourier coefficients and coherence is equal to one. If the relative phase varies across the K epochs, then some cancellation will take place and coherence (Equation 3.7) will be less than one. If the phase difference is purely random from epoch to epoch, the coherence estimate will approach zero as the number of epochs (K) is increased. A coherence of 0.5 in one frequency band indicates that at that frequency 50% of the variance at one channel can be explained by a linear transformation of the other channel. *This interpretation does not imply that there is a linear relationship between possible dynamic processes linking the data channels.* A coherence of 0.5 only indicates that we can only partly account for the data by a linear model. If the relationship was purely linear, the coherence estimate would be close to one if enough epochs were averaged to remove noise effects. Coherence can be less than one because the linear relationship between channels is *stochastic* as there is some randomness in the phase differences between channels but restricted to a narrow range. Another possibility is that the relationship between the channels is deterministic but nonlinear, in which case coherence provides a measure of the degree of linearity.

In describing coherence effects in EEG, we emphasize that coherence is a measure of phase synchronization. But, coherence depends both on relative amplitude and on relative phase between the two channels. If the phases at two channels are identical (phase difference = 0), coherence is still less than one if the amplitudes fluctuate independently at each channel. If our main goal is to estimate phase synchronization independent of amplitude fluctuations, we can measure coherence by normalizing each Fourier coefficient by its amplitude (phase-only coherence) or use entropy measures on the relative phase distribution across epochs to measure synchronization (Tass et al., 1998). One reason to use coherence measures rather than directly measuring phase correlation is that coherence measures are weighted in favor of epochs with large amplitudes. This makes good practical sense because phase estimates are likely to be more reliable when amplitudes are large if large amplitudes indicate large signal to noise ratio as is usually the case in EEG after obvious artifact has been removed. If only epoch phase information is used (independent of epoch amplitudes), equal emphasis is placed on low- and high-amplitude epochs in estimates of phase synchronization potentially reducing signal-to-noise ratio.

To summarize, coherence estimates provide a measure of phase synchronization between EEG channel pairs. Fluctuations in EEG amplitude are expected to produce relatively small changes in coherence, when used with epochs containing minimal artifact (Nunez, 1995). Coherence can be greater than zero or less than one for several reasons: (i) the presence of additive noise at each channel; the effects of additive noise can be minimized by averaging over a larger number of epochs; (ii) the system that gives rise to the amplitude and phase relationship between the two channels is stochastic and fluctuates across the observations; (iii) the system that gives rise to the relationship between the two channels is nonlinear; and (iv) a mutual influence between the two channels is present in the same frequency band.

3.6 Effects of Volume Conduction on EEG Coherence

Our goal in obtaining EEG coherence estimates is to estimate statistical properties of random source processes distributed in space and time over the cortical surface. In order to develop a theoretical model relating scalp potential statistics to source statistics, it is useful to think of source statistics in terms of continuous variables of time and space rather than discrete sets of sources. EEG sources are most likely dipole layers of varying size and shape which are described in terms of continuous functions of cortical location; discrete sources are simply special cases of this picture. Thus, the so-called "EEG generators" can be expressed generally in terms of the field $\mathbf{P}(\mathbf{r}, t)$ defined over the three dimensional volume of the brain, which generates a scalp potential field $V(\mathbf{r}, t)$. If the field $\mathbf{P}(\mathbf{r}, t)$ represents a random process, we can characterize it by its mean $\mu_B(\mathbf{r}, t)$ and cross-spectral density function $C_B(\mathbf{r}_1, \mathbf{r}_2, f)$. The cross-spectral density function is a spatial correlation function that depends on temporal frequency. The mean depends on brain location $\mathbf{r}$, and the cross-spectral density function depends on pairs of locations $(\mathbf{r}_1, \mathbf{r}_2)$. The mean $\mu_V(\mathbf{r}, t)$ and cross-spectral density function $C_V(\mathbf{r}_1, \mathbf{r}_2, f)$ of the scalp potential field $V(\mathbf{r}, t)$ are similarly defined, but are now continuous functions of position rather than being defined only at discrete EEG electrode locations.

For the purpose of this discussion, we assume the random process is weakly stationary, so that we can assume zero mean without loss of generality. The cross-spectral density function of the scalp potential is related to the cross-spectral density function of the source distribution by

$$C_V(\mathbf{r}_1,\mathbf{r}_2,f) = \int_{B_1'}\int_{B_2'} G_H^*(\mathbf{r}_1,\mathbf{r}_1')C_B(\mathbf{r}_1',\mathbf{r}_2')G_H(\mathbf{r}_2,\mathbf{r}_2')\,dV(\mathbf{r}_1')\,dV(\mathbf{r}_2') \tag{3.8}$$

where $G_H(\mathbf{r},\mathbf{r}')$ is the Green's function that gives the potential at location $\mathbf{r}$ due to a dipole source of unit strength located at $\mathbf{r}'$ and the integration is over the entire source distribution. In general, Equation 3.8 is an integral over the volume of the brain, but practically this volume is constrained to conform to the geometry of the cortical surface. The Green's function depends on the volume conduction properties of the head, source locations, and measurement locations.

Equation 3.8 defines a spatial filtering of the brain cross-spectral density function to obtain the scalp cross-spectral density function. Although, the exact details depend on the volume conduction model, the Green's function for scalp potentials in both spherical and realistic (BEM) volume conduction models appears to be a low pass filter (Srinivasan et al., 1998, 2007). To examine the effects of spatial filtering on the cross spectrum or coherence estimates, we consider a simple case where the source activity is a spatially uncorrelated stationary random process defined on a sphere of radius r_z in a spherical model of the head:

$$C_B(\theta_1,\varphi_1,\theta_2,\varphi_2,f) = p^2(f)\delta(\cos\theta_1 - \cos\theta_2)\delta(\varphi_1 - \varphi_2) \tag{3.9}$$

Here φ and θ are the azimuth and elevation coordinates on a spherical surface, $p(f)$ is the source variance as a function of frequency, in other words the power spectrum of the sources. If we place the source in a concentric spheres models of the head, the cross-spectral density function of the scalp potentials can be calculated substituting the Green's function using the Green's function for a concentric sphere model to obtain (Srinivasan et al., 1998)

$$C_V(\theta_1,\varphi_1,\theta_2,\varphi_2,f) = p^2(f)\sum_{n=1}^{\infty}\frac{4\pi H_n(r_z)}{2n+1}P_n(\cos\chi_{12}) \tag{3.10}$$

where χ_{12} is the angle between two electrodes positioned at (θ_1, φ_1) and (θ_2, φ_2), the $P_n(x)$ are the Legendre polynomials (Morse and Feshbach, 1953), and the H_n are the coefficients of the Legendre Polynomial expansion of the Green's function G_H for a concentric sphere model. The power spectral density function can be obtained from Equation 3.10 for the case of identical electrode positions, that is, $\chi_{12} = 0$. The coherence function γ_V^2 for the scalp potential can then be derived by substituting cross-spectral density function given in Equation 3.10 and the corresponding power spectral density function into Equation 3.7 to obtain:

$$\gamma_V^2(\chi_{12}) = \left[\frac{\sum_{n=1}^{\infty}(H_n(r_z)/2n+1)P_n(\cos\chi_{12})}{\sum_{n=1}^{\infty}(H_n(r_z)/2n+1)}\right]^2 \tag{3.11}$$

The coherence function given by Equation 3.11 is the scalp potential coherence predicted by the concentric spheres model if the source distribution is a spatially uncorrelated Gaussian random process. Thus, when coherence in the brain sphere is zero between all possible source locations, we can predict the scalp potential coherence that is due only to volume conduction.

We note immediately that the coherence function given by Equation 3.11 is independent of frequency, which does not appear as a parameter on the right-hand side of the equation. Second, we note that this theoretical coherence does not depend on the position of the electrodes but only on the angular distance between electrodes χ_{12}. Figure 3.5 shows the coherence function plotted as a function of the separation distance between electrodes measured in centimeters along the spherical scalp surface. The sources consist of a superficial spherical dipole layer placed in concentric spheres models with different assumed ratios of brain to skull conductivity. Coherence introduced by volume conduction falls off with distance, reaching a minimum at a surface distance of about 10 cm. At very large distances, there is a small rise in

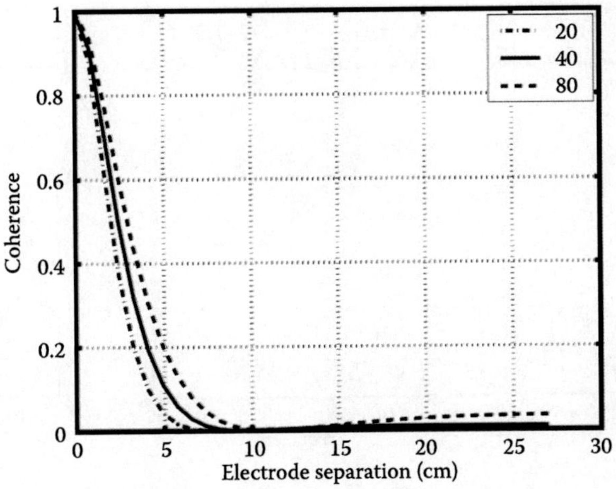

FIGURE 3.5 Theoretical predictions of coherence between scalp potentials due to volume conduction alone with an assumed spatial white-noise source distribution in the concentric spheres model of the head given by Equation 3.11. The source is a spherical dipole layer at a radial location $r_z = 7.8$ cm. The model parameters are radii $(r_1, r_2, r_3, r_4) = (8, 8.1, 8.6, 9.2)$ and conductivity ratios $(\sigma_1/\sigma_2, \sigma_1/\sigma_3, \sigma_1/\sigma_4) = (0.2, 40, 1)$. Source coherence is zero and scalp potential coherence depends only on distance.

the coherence. The implication is that over short to moderate inter-electrode distances (<10 cm in the spherical model) we may expect a significant contribution of volume conduction to coherence. This effect is similar at the three values of brain to skull conductivity ratio that spans the range of most estimates of the conductivity ratio. The same picture emerges from numerical simulations using concentric spheres and realistic models derived from MRI (Srinivasan et al., 2007).

This theoretical prediction of coherence due to volume conduction suggests that *the main effect of volume conduction is to artificially inflate coherences at short to moderate distances, and that this effect is independent of frequency.* This prediction may be evaluated with genuine EEG data. Figure 3.6 shows the coherences between an electrode labeled x and a ring of electrodes at progressively greater distances from x labeled 1–9. The subject is at rest with eyes closed, a state in which coherence is usually high in the alpha band (Nunez, 1995). The estimated coherence between electrode X and electrode n is labeled x:n. The electrode positions are indicated and the typical distance between adjacent electrodes is 2.7 cm. At the closest electrode pair x:1, coherence is very high (above 0.75) at all frequencies; coherence is

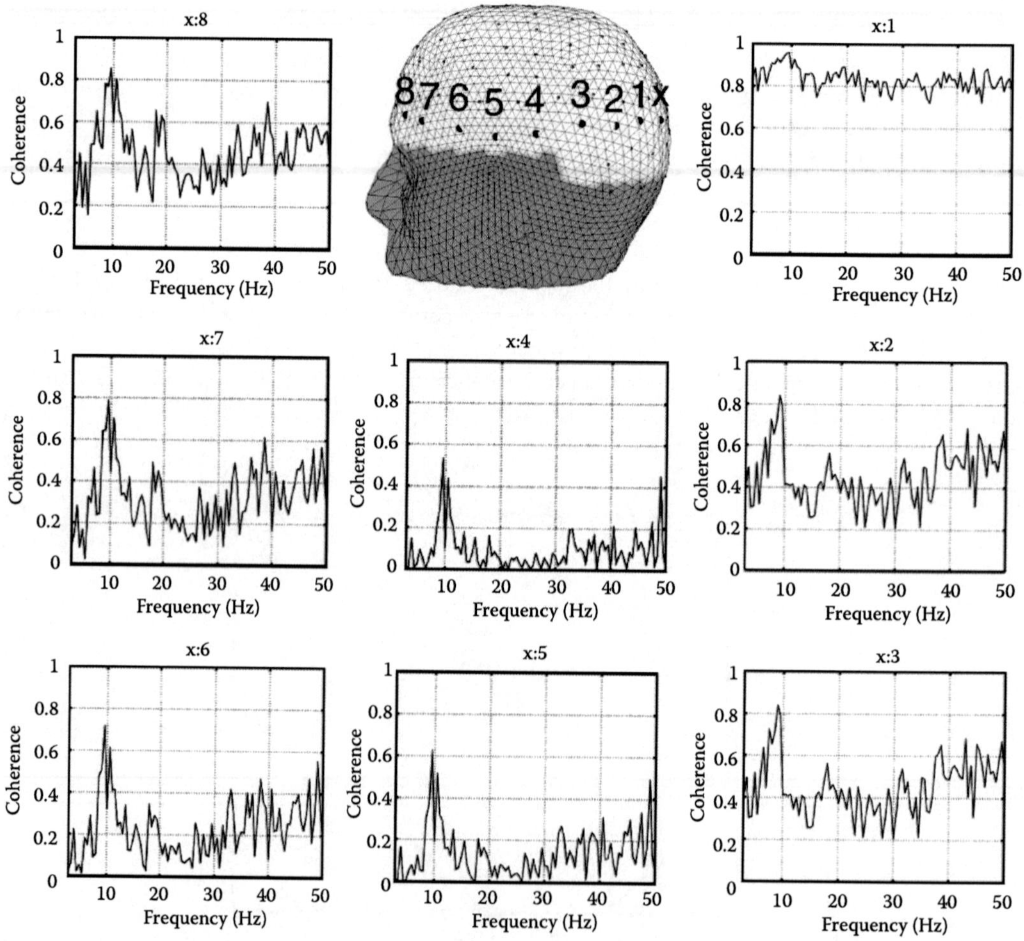

FIGURE 3.6 Scalp potential coherence spectra from a 22-year-old female subject at rest with eyes closed (to maximize alpha coherence). Coherence was estimated with $T = 2$ s ($\Delta f = 0.5$ Hz) in a 60 s record. The head plot shows the location of 9 electrodes, labeled x and 1 through 8. Coherence spectra between electrode x and each of the other electrodes 1–8 are shown, with increasing separations along the scalp. Note that very close electrodes have higher coherence independent of frequency as predicted by the theoretical model. Alpha band coherence is high for large electrode separations, apparently reflecting the large cortical source coherence. Power spectra for this subject are shown in Figure 3.2.

generally independent of temporal frequency. As the electrode separation is increased, the pair x:2 shows lower coherences, but at most frequencies coherence is still above 0.4 suggesting a strong component of coherence that is independent of frequency. A peak is visible in the alpha band at 9.5 Hz, but it is difficult to evaluate this peak, since there is also a broad elevation of coherence. As the sensor separation is further increased (x:3), the floor of the coherences reduces further to about 0.2, and a peak becomes more evident in the 18 Hz range. For pairs of electrodes involving temporal electrodes (x:4 and x:5) the floor of the coherences approaches zero at most frequencies except for the alpha band where a second peak at 10.5 Hz is visible. At very long distance, a pair with a prefrontal electrode (x:8) the coherences are again elevated across all frequencies, suggesting a very small volume conduction effect at long distances as also observed with the model shown in Figure 3.5.

The coherence spectra shown in Figure 3.6 have strong qualitative similarity to the coherence effects predicted by volume conduction of uncorrelated source activity. At short distances coherence is high across all frequencies. The level of coherence independent of frequency systematically decreases as distance increases. This suggests that it is difficult to interpret coherence between closely spaced electrodes. The electrode pair x:3 shows a clear coherence peak of about 0.4 at 18 Hz, while the pair x:2 shows many peaks of about the same size. Clearly we cannot easily determine if the source coherence of the pair x:3 is genuinely higher than x:2, since we observe a strong contribution by volume conduction that is independent of frequency. In addition, there is even a small rise in coherence at very large distances as predicted by the theoretical model (due to the head's closed surface). Many experimental papers on EEG coherence have ignored this volume conduction effect by reasoning (incorrectly) that volume conduction effects are *additive* and can be ignored in the comparison of two or more conditions in the same subject or between groups of subjects. It is important to appreciate the underlying process in filtering as expressed by Equation 3.10. *The implication of the curves shown in Figure 3.5 is that the EEG electrodes separated by less than 10 cm are averaging over many of the same sources.* Thus, if two closely spaced electrodes record from the same source region and the power of the source region increases, coherence between these electrodes will also increase. If there are two source regions, one close to each electrode, changes in source power and changes in source coherence will both cause increases in coherence when the distance between electrode pairs is small to moderate.

The implication of these results is that coherence (or any measure of correlation) between EEG electrodes can only be easily interpreted as increased coherence (or correlation) between two distinct source regions, if the electrodes are at least 10 cm apart in surface tangential directions along the scalp, but are also partly compromised at longer distances (>20 cm). This provided only a limited view of the spatial statistics of the underlying sources. Figure 3.7 shows coherence between all pairs of electrodes for the same data as Figure 3.6, but at six selected frequencies. Coherence is plotted as a function of electrode separation distance, where each point represents one pair of electrodes. Not surprisingly, at frequencies in the alpha band (9.5–12.5 Hz), coherences are very high at both short and long distances, and theta coherence (7.5 Hz) is lower than alpha coherence at long distances, but still higher than the coherence expected due to volume conduction (see Figure 3.5). At 14.5 Hz coherences are reduced and more closely resemble the characteristics of coherence due only to volume conduction. A similar pattern is observed at most higher frequencies.

High-resolution EEG methods such as the surface Laplacian (Srinivasan et al., 1996) can reduce the impact of volume conduction on coherence or correlation estimates but will also remove a substation amount of source coherence that is broadly distributed, or involves deeper sources, for instance in the sulcal walls (Srinivasan et al., 1998), also providing a limited view of the source dynamics. Despite these limitations, both conventional and high-resolution EEG coherence estimates have been used in cognitive and clinical studies to extract correlates of cognitive functions or brain disease. However, the interpretation of these coherences in terms of brain networks remains problematic and there are practical statistical problems with coherence estimates. For instance, using 128 electrodes, there are more than 8000 unique pairs of electrodes to evaluate coherence at each frequency. This is a daunting visualization problem and poses an even greater multiple comparisons problem for statistical contrasts. In the next section, we introduce a multivariate signal

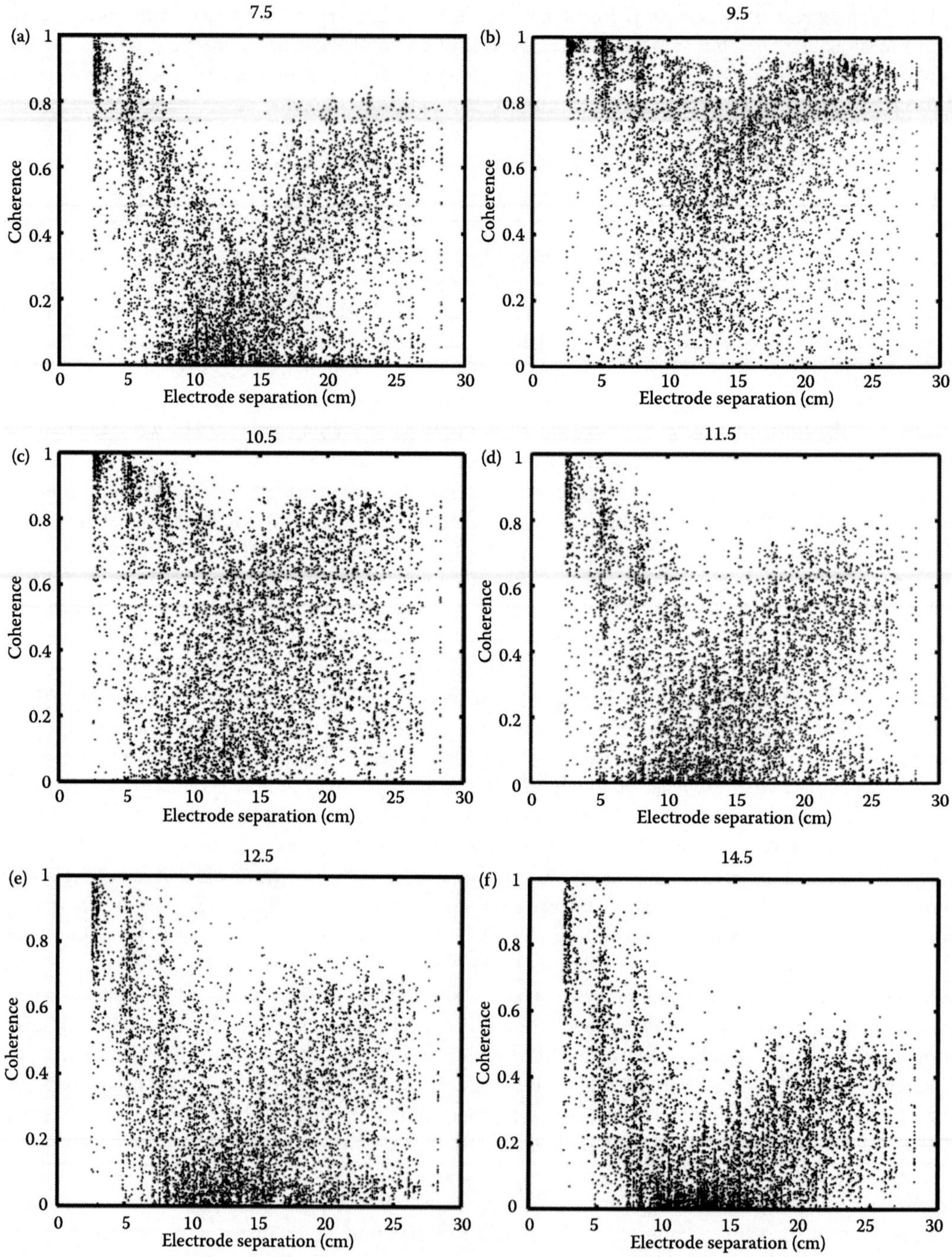

FIGURE 3.7 Scalp potential coherence at different frequencies as a function of electrode separation for the female subject at rest with eyes closed. Detailed coherence spectra for this subject are shown in Figure 3.6. (a) 7.5 Hz coherence versus electrode separation distance, (b) 9.5 Hz coherence, (c) 10.5 Hz coherence, (d) 11.5 Hz coherence, (e) 12.5 Hz, and (f) 14.5 Hz coherence. In Part (f) power is low and coherence follows electrode separation consistent with the effects of volume conduction. At the other frequencies, coherence is elevated at long distances.

processing method that has been developed for BSS using second-order statistics (correlation). In the following section, we adapt this method for multivariate spectral analysis to identify the coherent sources of EEG oscillations.

3.7 Second-Order Blind Identification

EEG signals are mixtures of potentials generated by sources distributed throughout the brain. Although we have some knowledge of the nature of the mixing process for volume conduction models (which is the Green's function G_H), the problem is more complicated because the time series of the dipole sources are not statistically independent, and have structure that reflects the dynamic functional connectivity of brain networks. Thus, EEG signals are mixtures of signals generated by multiple source distributions, each likely composed of synchronous sources distributed over the brain. Thus, there has been considerable interest in using BSS techniques to separate the source on the basis of statistical criterion. In the section we will detail the SOBI algorithm, and in the next section make use of it to obtain multivariate spectral analysis of EEG records.

The SOBI algorithm (Belchourani et al., 1997) can be described as follows. Consider an multichannel-channel time series $\{V_m,\ m = 1{:}M\}$, with mean zero. Each sample is assumed to be an instantaneous linear mixture of up to m unknown sources s, where the mixing occurs through some unknown linear mixing matrix **A**:

$$\mathbf{V} = \mathbf{AS} \tag{3.12}$$

The goal of BSS analysis is to determine a separation matrix, **B** such that

$$\mathbf{S} = \mathbf{BV} \tag{3.13}$$

Each source is described by a distribution of loadings across the electrodes (the component) and the source time series. The SOBI algorithm is closely related to spectral analysis because of the criteria used to estimate **B**. We will present the method in a manner to highlight the relationship between SOBI and spectral analysis, which is less compact and elegant than other discussions (Belchourani et al., 1997; Tang et al., 2004).

From the multichannel time series V, we can construct the crosscorrelation function $R_{mn}(\tau)$ for any pair of electrodes m and n following Equation 3.6. When $m = n$, the crosscorrelation function reduces to the autocorrelation function given by Equation 3.4. For each value of τ, we define the matrix $\mathbf{R}_{V,\tau}$ whose elements are $R_{mn}(\tau)$. We note that $R_{mn}(-\tau) = R_{nm}(\tau)$, so the upper and lower triangles of this matrix correspond to channel m leading n by τ and channel n leading m by τ, respectively. For a range of values of positive τ up to the period the Nyquist frequency, an ensemble of correlation matrices can be constructed $\{\mathbf{R}_{V,\tau}\}$. This ensemble of matrices contains the auto- and crosscorrelations between channels for a range of lags including both the positive and negative lags in the upper and lower triangles of each matrix.

In the SOBI algorithm, the first step is to find the eigenvalues and eigenvectors of the correlation matrix at lag $\tau = 0$ (the ordinary correlation matrix):

$$\mathbf{R}_{V,0} = \mathbf{PDP}^{T} \tag{3.14}$$

Here, **P** is a matrix whose columns are the eigenvectors of the correlation matrix and **D** is a diagonal matrix whose diagonal entries are the eigenvalues. The eigenvalues and eigenvectors of the correlation can be used to "prewhiten" the data, that is, to remove all correlation between channels at lag $\tau = 0$. A whitening matrix **W** is defined as

$$\mathbf{W} = \mathbf{D}^{-1/2}\mathbf{P}^{T} \tag{3.15}$$

The whitening step can be recognized as a principal components analysis (PCA), with the projection onto each component normalized by the eigenvalues to define new variables **Z**:

$$\mathbf{Z} = \mathbf{WV} \tag{3.16}$$

that have a correlation matrix that is the identity matrix:

$$\mathbf{R}_{Z,0} = \mathbf{W}\mathbf{R}_{V,0}\mathbf{W}^{T} = \mathbf{I} \tag{3.17}$$

Thus the effect of the PCA is to diagonalize the correlation matrix at lag $\tau = 0$.

The entire set of correlation matrices (for all lags) can each be similarly transformed:

$$\mathbf{R}_{Z,\tau} = \mathbf{W}\mathbf{R}_{V,\tau}\mathbf{W}^{T} \tag{3.18}$$

The key procedure of SOBI is to find a unitary transformation **U** that jointly diagonalizes the set of correlation matrices $\{\mathbf{R}_{Z,\tau}\}$ by minimizing a diagonality measure M:

$$\mathbf{U} = \arg\min \sum_{\tau} M(\mathbf{U}^{T}\mathbf{R}_{Z,\tau}\mathbf{U}) \tag{3.19}$$

For example, Cardoso (1998) uses the following measure:

$$M(A) = \sum_{i \neq j} A^2 \tag{3.20}$$

that is, minimizing the sum of squares of the off-diagonal terms. These off-diagonal terms are the correlations between the PCA components with nonzero lag τ. U can be obtained via various matrix diagonalization techniques, including classical eigenanalysis methods such as the Jacobi method (Cardoso, 1998) or the Levenberg–Marquardt algorithm (Ziehe et al., 2003). In a typical implementation the algorithm proceeds until a very small amount of correlation remains with the tolerance determined by the user (Cardoso, 1998).

After the joint-diagonalization of crosscorrelations, the estimate of the separation matrix **B** is thus obtained as

$$\mathbf{B} = \mathbf{UW} \tag{3.21}$$

After estimating the separation matrix, the source time series can be reconstructed and the statistical properties (e.g., power and coherence) of the source time series can be estimated.

3.8 Multivariate Spectral Analysis Using SOBI

The definition of the SOBI algorithm provided above was developed in the context of a single time series observed with multiple channels. We can easily generalize the above approach to account for multiple observations by extending the expectations across multiple observations (Deng et al., 2010), which is entirely consistent with the definitions of the autocorrelation and crosscorrelations.

Previous studies using SOBI (Tang et al., 2004) have typically made use of time delays that span a wide range on a logarithmic scale. The motivation for this choice is to capture the correlation structure over a wide range of time scales while minimizing the number of correlation matrices that must be diagonalized. We will consider an entirely different basis of selection of τ, which will closely tie the results of SOBI analysis to spectral analysis. Consider the analysis of 1 s of data sampled at 1000 Hz. With the second of data we can easily calculate correlations matrices with lags (in ms) from the domain {0,1,. . ..,999}. However for very long lags, we do not have as many observations to obtain a robust estimate of the crosscorrelations. Moreover, the correlation matrices for lag τ and $\tau + 1$ ms are also not expected to vary greatly, except for the contributions of very small oscillations that are close to the Nyquist frequency. We can reasonably expect that the EEG has been sampled at a frequency at least 2.5 the highest frequency with any power present in the recording (the Engineer's Nyquist), and that analog filters in the EEG amplifier have been used to remove any power at frequencies above the Nyquist.

Consider instead the crosscorrelation matrices $\{\mathbf{R}_{V,\tau}\}$ obtained for a set of lags $\tau = \{0, 10, 20,\ldots,500 \text{ ms}\}$ using a 1 s record sampled at 1000 Hz. Here we have defined a uniform step in the lags of 10 ms. These crosscorrelation matrices can accurately represent the spectral content of the signal up to 50 Hz (Nyquist criterion) or more practically 40 Hz (Engineer's Nyquist). The maximum lag chosen here is 500 ms, which can be used to capture the correlation at frequencies down to 1 Hz. Thus, between 1 Hz and 50 Hz all of the spectral information in the record has been preserved by the set of crosscorrelation matrices, and this information can always be recovered by applying a Fourier transform. Thus, applying the SOBI algorithm to this set of matrices has the goal of minimizing the crosscorrelation function between these channels over a bandwidth of 1–50 Hz.

We have applied the SOBI algorithm to the data whose power and coherence are shown in Figures 3.2, 3.3, 3.6, and 3.7 using the set of lags $\tau = \{0, 10, 20,\ldots, 500 \text{ ms}\}$. In these data we have 30 epochs of duration 2 s, sampled at 1000 Hz. Figure 3.8 shows the power spectra of all the EEG channels (upper left), and the power spectra of all the SOBI components (upper right). The SOBI components have been sorted by the total variance explained by the component. The EEG channels all show highest power in the alpha band, which is also shown in the peak frequency histogram (lower left) where almost every channel is shown to peak in the alpha band, with most channels showing the peak at 9.5 Hz. The SOBI components show the largest components having power in the alpha band, with a total of 16 components showing the highest

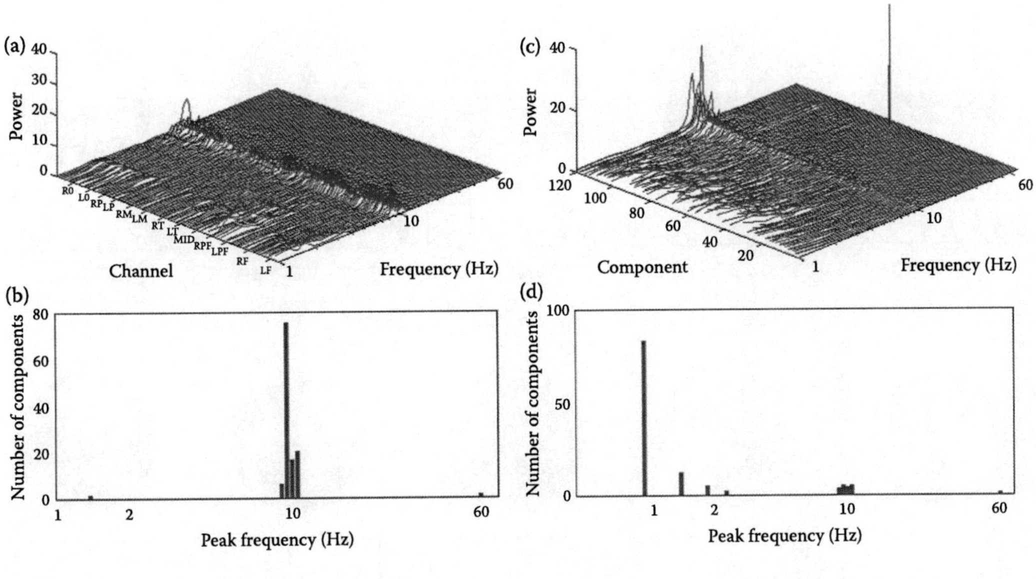

FIGURE 3.8 **(See color insert.)** Average power spectra and peak histogram of the raw EEG and SOBI components. (a) The raw EEG power spectra of all 120 channels, averaged across all 30 2-s epochs. The frequency axis is in log-scale. (b) Average peak power histogram of raw EEG spectra, which shows the frequency distribution of peak power for each channel. (c) Average SOBI component spectra, ordered by power in alpha band (8–12 Hz). (d) Average peak power histogram of the 120 SOBI components.

power in the alpha band. Of these 16 components, 6 had negligible power and were discarded leaving 10 components. All of the other components had much less power and peaked at very low frequencies except for one component which contains all the 60 Hz line noise picked up by the EEG electrodes.

Figure 3.9 shows the spatial distribution of the component loading and the corresponding source power spectrum for each of the 10 components that contribute all the power in the alpha band. Each of these "alpha" components has a distinct spatial distribution. The components have been labeled C1–C10 by the total power contributed to the alpha band. Component C1 captures the main features of the broadly distributed signal which peaks at 9.5 Hz. Components C2 and C3 capture the main features of the signal that peaks at 10.5 Hz prominently at occipital and temporal channels which is less prominent at dorsal frontal channels (see Figures 3.2 and 3.3). Component C4 also peaks at 9.5 Hz and is focused on parietal channels. The other components shown correspond to independent sources of alpha rhythm power with distinct spatial distribution.

Since the SOBI analysis performed a multivariate analysis of the crosscorrelation between channels over a range of lags, we might reasonably have expected that different SOBI components would correspond to oscillations of different frequencies. However, our analysis of this simple eyes closed resting EEG record, reveals multiple components with identical peak frequency. For example, components C1, C4, C7, and C10 all have time series with peak power at 9.5 Hz. To understand why these time series are indicative of separate sources, we calculated the coherence between the source time series corresponding to the components C1–C10. We found that at all frequencies, including the alpha band, coherence between the source time series is negligible. Figure 3.10 shows the coherences between components at four frequencies in the alpha band including the dominant frequencies of 9.5 and 10.5 Hz. In all cases the highest coherences observed are <0.3. In comparison, Figure 3.7 shows that even at long electrode separations (>10 cm) very high coherences (>0.8) are observed between many electrode pairs at 9.5 Hz, but at other pairs coherence is much lower. When the SOBI decompositions separate components that oscillate centered on the same frequency, they indicate the oscillations in this frequency

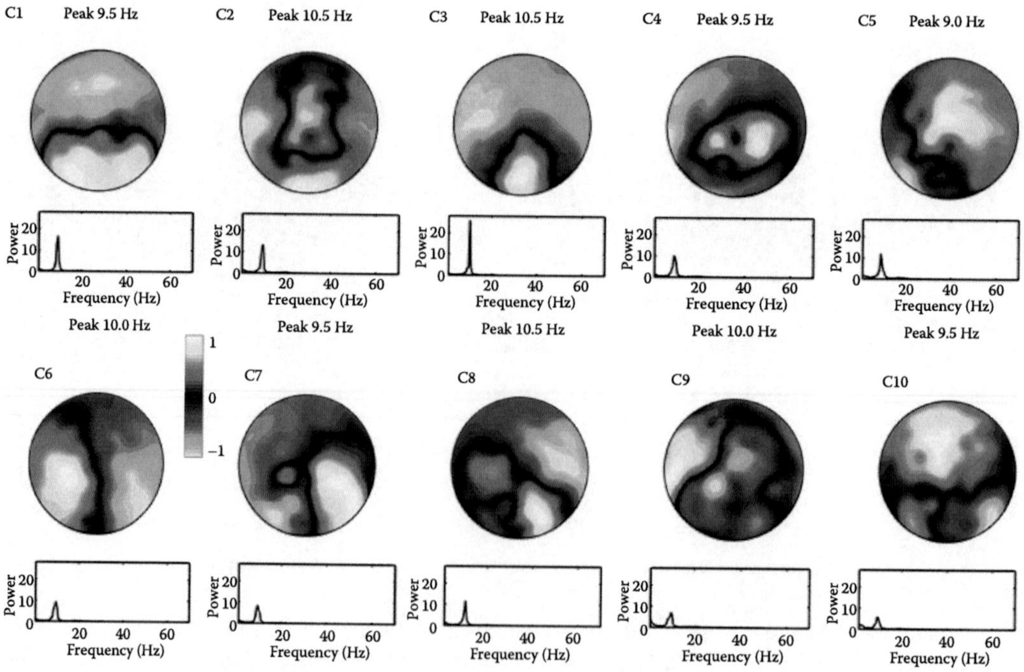

FIGURE 3.9 **(See color insert.)** Spatial loading topography of first 10 SOBI components and average spectra. The SOBI components are ordered by the total power within alpha band (8–12 Hz).

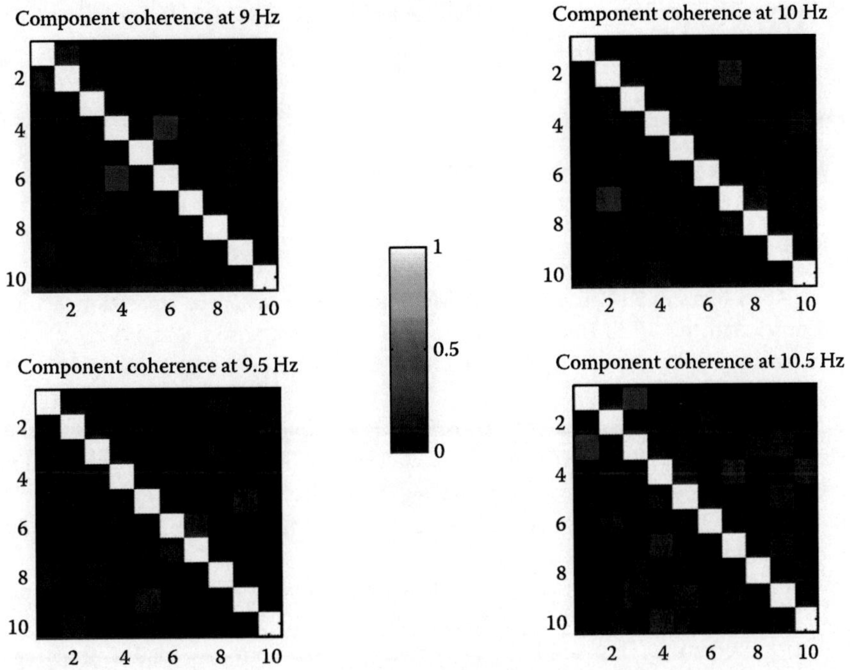

FIGURE 3.10 **(See color insert.)** Coherence of the first 10 SOBI components in the alpha band. These are the same group of components as shown in Figure 3.2. Coherence was calculated between the source time series for each component. Coherence at 9, 9.5, 10, and 10.5 Hz are shown. Coherence between components is negligible, even when they peak at the same frequency.

band generated by distinct source distributions that are relatively incoherent. This picture is consistent with our understanding of alpha rhythms; there are multiple independent alpha rhythms generated by networks spanning different regions of cortex, which are selectively manipulated by different tasks. This picture is also consistent with the observation the coherence between channels in the alpha band reveals a complex pattern of high and low coherence between pairs of electrode all of whom show significant power in the alpha band (see Figure 3.8). Thus, the SOBI components identified here are a multivariate decomposition of the EEG spectra to identify the underlying coherent sources whose time series are incoherent in the sense of second-order statistics.

3.9 Summary

We view source dynamics as a stochastic (random) process having statistical properties that change with changes in behavior and cognition. This general framework has an important advantage over viewpoints that may prejudge the nature of EEG dynamics, thereby biasing experimental design. Spectral analysis is the obvious entry point for studying EEG dynamics, but the physics of volume conduction places constraints on the interpretation of the EEG spectrum. The EEG power spectrum is straightforward to estimate using Fourier methods and should be interpreted in terms of synchronization of the underlying sources, including spatial synchronization. The effects of volume conduction on EEG coherence are severe for closely spaced electrode, and limit the use of coherence to estimate spatial properties of brain networks. SOBI algorithm is a BSS method that operates on the crosscorrelation between channels over a range of lags. We show that in effect the SOBI algorithm isolates "sources" (brain networks) that oscillate at different frequencies, or within the same frequency oscillate incoherently. This provides a direct method for multivariate spectral analysis to decompose the spatio-temporal statistics of EEG signals into independent source signals.

Acknowledgment

This work was supported by a grant from NIH 2R01-MH68004.

References

Belouchrani A, Abed-Meriam K, Cardoso JF, and Moulines E, A blind source separation technique using second-order statistics. *IEEE Transactions on Signal Processing*, 45:434–444, 1997.

Bendat JS and Piersol AG, *Random Data. Analysis and Measurement Procedures*, Third Edition. New York: Wiley, 2001.

Cardoso JF, Blind signal separation: Statistical principles. *Proceedings of the IEEE*, 9:2009–2025, 1998.

Deng S, Srinivasan R, Lappas T, and D'Zmura M, EEG classification of imagined speech using Hilbert Spectrum methods. *Journal of Neural Engineering*, 7, 046006, 2010.

Deng S and Srinivasan R, Semantic and acoustic analysis of speech by functional networks with distinct time scales. *Brain Research*, 1346:132–144, 2010.

Ding JD, Sperling G, and Srinivasan R, Attentional modulation of SSVEP power depends on network tagged by flicker frequency. *Cerebral Cortex*, 16:1016–1029, 2006.

Lachaux JP, Lutz A, Rudrauf D, Cosmelli D, Le Van Quyen M, Martinerie J, Varela F, Estimating the time-course of coherence between single-trial brain signals: An introduction to wavelet coherence. *Electroencephalography and Clinical Neurophysiology*, 32(3):157–174, 2002.

Le Van Quyen M, Foucher J, Lachaux J, Rodriguez E, Lutz A, Martinerie J, and Varela FJ, Comparison of Hilbert transform and wavelet methods for the analysis of neuronal synchrony. *Journal of Neuroscience Methods*, 111(2):83–98, 2001.

Lopes da Silva FH, and Storm van Leeuwen W, The cortical alpha rhythm in dog: The depth and surface profile of phase. In: MAB Brazier MAB and H Petsche (eds) *Architectonics of the Cerebral Cortex*. New York: Raven Press, pp. 319–333, 1978.

Lopes da Silva FH, Dynamics of EEGs as signals of neuronal populations: Models and theoretical considerations. In: E Niedermeyer and FH Lopes da Silva (eds) *Electroencephalography. Basic Principals, Clinical Applications, and Related Fields. Forth Edition*. London: Williams & Wilkins, pp. 76–92, 1999.

Makeig S, Debener S, Onton J, and Delorme A, Mining event-related brain dynamics. *Trends in Cognitive Science*, 8(5):204–210, 2004.

Morse PM and Feshbach M, *Methods of Theoretical Physics*. McGraw-Hill Interamericana, 1953.

Murias M, Swanson JM, and Srinivasan R, Functional connectivity of frontal cortex in healthy and ADHD children reflected in EEG coherence. *Cerebral Cortex*, 17:1788–1799, 2007.

Nunez PL and Srinivasan R, *Electric Fields of the Brain: The Neurophysics of EEG*, 2nd Edition. New York: Oxford University Press, 2006.

Nunez PL, *Neocortical Dynamics and Human EEG Rhythms*. New York: Oxford University Press, 1995.

Nunez PL, *Electric Fields of the Brain: The Neurophysics of EEG*. Oxford University, New York, 1981.

Nunez PL, Toward a quantitative description of large scale neocortical dynamic function and EEG. *Behavioral and Brain Sciences*, 23:371–398 (target article), 2000a.

Nunez PL, Neocortical dynamic theory should be as simple as possible, but not simpler. *Behavioral and Brain Sciences*, 23:415–437 (response to commentary by 18 neuroscientists), 2000b.

Percival DB and Walden AT, *Spectral Analysis for Physical Applications: Multitaper and Conventional Univariate Techniques*. Cambridge, UK: Cambridge University Press, 1993.

Petsche H and Etlinger SC, *EEG and Thinking. Power and Coherence Analysis of Cognitive Processes*. Vienna: Austrian Academy of Sciences, 1998.

Pfurtscheller G and Lopes da Silva FH, Event-related EEG/MEG synchronization and desynchronization: Basic principles. *Electroencephalography and Clinical Neurophysiology*, 110:1842–1857, 1999.

Srinivasan R, Nunez PL., Tucker DM, Silberstein RB, and Cadusch PJ, Spatial sampling and filtering of EEG with spline Laplacians to estimate cortical potentials. *Brain Topography*, 8:355–366, 1996.

Srinivasan R, Nunez PL, and Silberstein RB, Spatial filtering and neocortical dynamics: Estimates of EEG coherence. *IEEE Transactions on Biomedical Engineering*, 45:814–826, 1998.

Srinivasan R, Anatomical constraints on source models for high-resolution EEG and MEG derived from MRI. *TCRT*, 5:389–399, 2006.

Srinivasan R, Winter WR, Ding J, and Nunez PL, EEG and MEG coherence: Measures of functional connectivity at distinct spatial scales of neocortical dynamics. *Journal of Neuroscience Methods*, 166:41–52, 2007.

Tang AC, Sutherland MT, and McKinney CJ, Validation of SOBI components from high-density EEG. *NeuroImage*, 25:539–553, 2004.

Tass P, Rosenblum MG, Weule J, Kurths J, Pikovsky A, Volkmann J, Schnitzler A, and Freund HJ, Detection of n:m phase locking from noisy data: Application to magnetoencephalography. *Physical Review Letters* 81:3291–3294, 1998.

Ziehe A, Laskov P, Muller KR, and Nolte G, A linear least-squares algorithm for joint diagonalization. *Proc. 4th Intern. Symp. on ICA and BSS 2003 (ICA2003)*, 469–474, 2003.

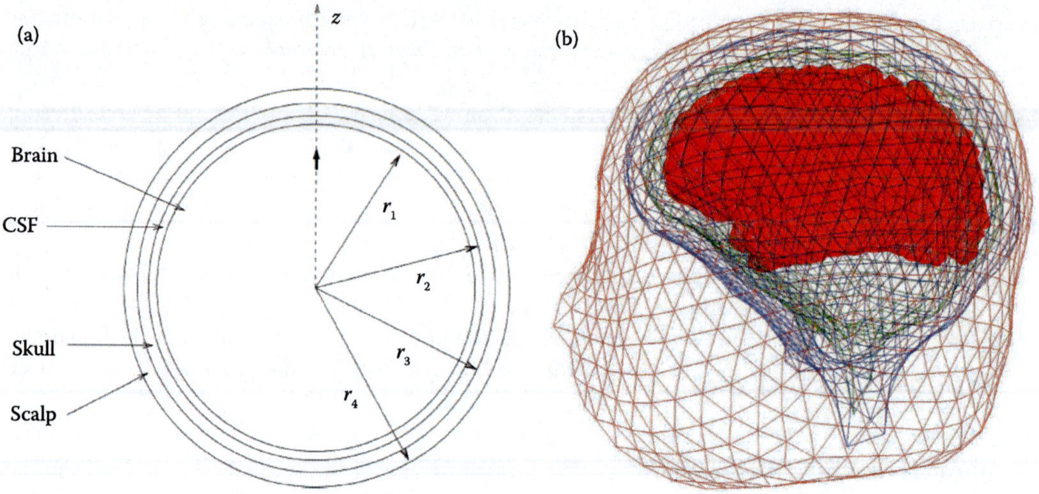

FIGURE 3.1 Volume conduction models for EEG. (a) A dipole is shown in the inner sphere of a *4-concentric spheres head model* consisting of the inner sphere (brain) and three spherical shells representing CSF (cerebrospinal fluid), skull and scalp. The parameters of model are the radii (r_1, r_2, r_3, r_4) of each shell and the conductivity ratios (σ_1/σ_2, σ_1/σ_3, σ_1/σ_4). Typical values are: radii (8, 8.1, 8.6, 9.2 cm) and conductivity ratios (0.2, 40, 1). (b) A realistic shaped BEM of the head. The brain and scalp boundaries were found by segmenting the images with a threshold, and opening and closing operation, respectively, while the outer skull boundary was obtained by dilation of the brain boundary (ASA, Netherlands). Although geometrically more accurate that the spherical model, the (geometrically) realistic BEM is potentially a less accurate model than concentric spheres because tissue resistivity is poorly known.

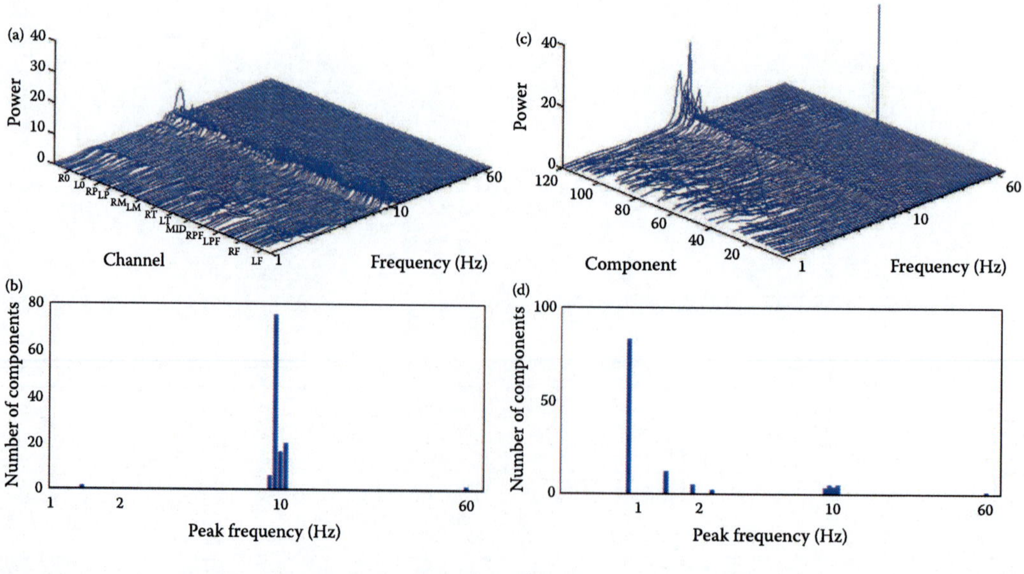

FIGURE 3.8 Average power spectra and peak histogram of the raw EEG and SOBI components. (a) The raw EEG power spectra of all 120 channels, averaged across all 30 2-s epochs. The frequency axis is in log-scale. (b) Average peak power histogram of raw EEG spectra, which shows the frequency distribution of peak power for each channel. (c) Average SOBI component spectra, ordered by power in alpha band (8–12 Hz). (d) Average peak power histogram of the 120 SOBI components.

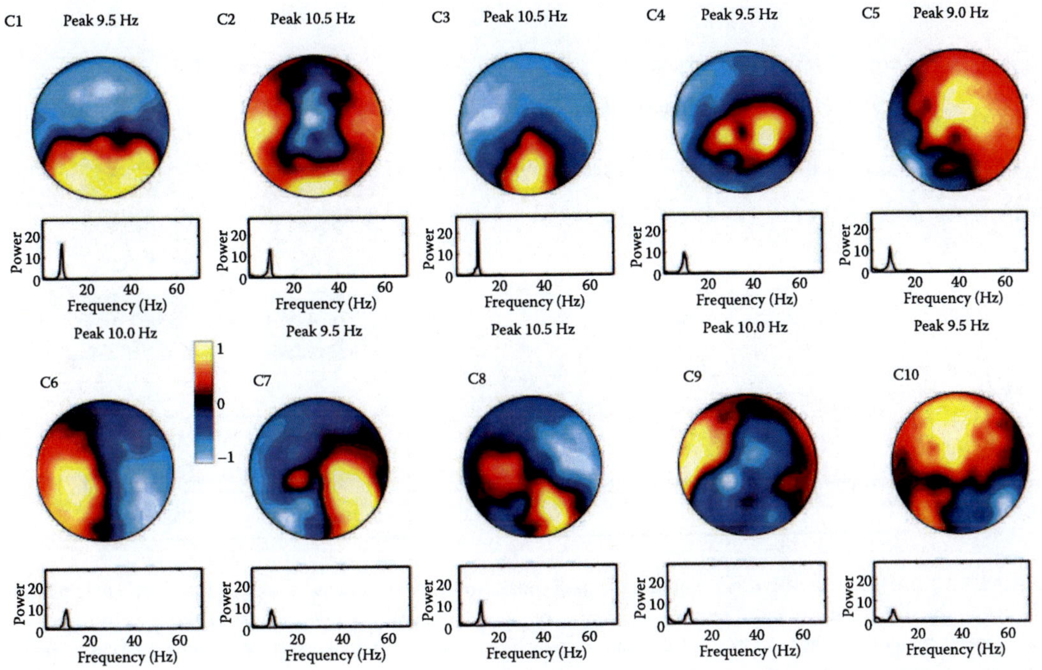

FIGURE 3.9 Spatial loading topography of first 10 SOBI components and average spectra. The SOBI components are ordered by the total power within alpha band (8–12 Hz).

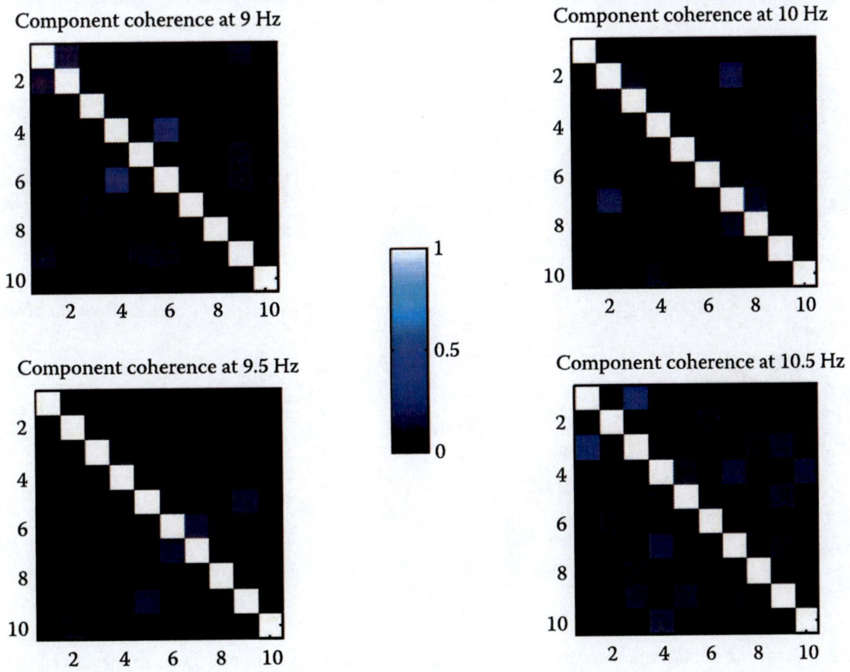

FIGURE 3.10 Coherence of the first 10 SOBI components in the alpha band. These are the same group of components as shown in Figure 3.2. Coherence was calculated between the source time series for each component. Coherence at 9, 9.5, 10, and 10.5 Hz are shown. Coherence between components is negligible, even when they peak at the same frequency.

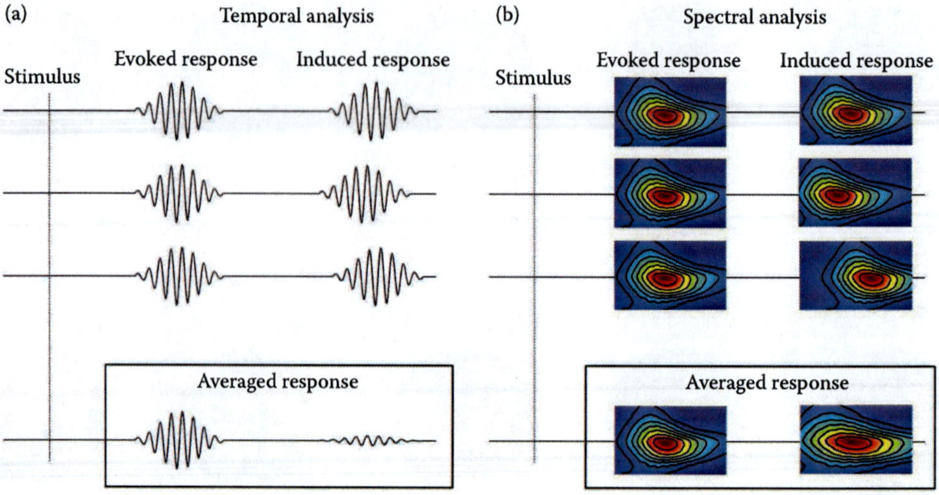

FIGURE 4.1 MEG brain activity in response to a task consists of two components: evoked responses that are phase-locked to the stimuli, and induced responses that are not. (a) Averaging the MEG time-series over epochs preserves the evoked components, but suppresses the induced (nonphase-locked) components. (b) Averaging the power time–frequency decompositions of the time-series preserves both evoked and induced components.

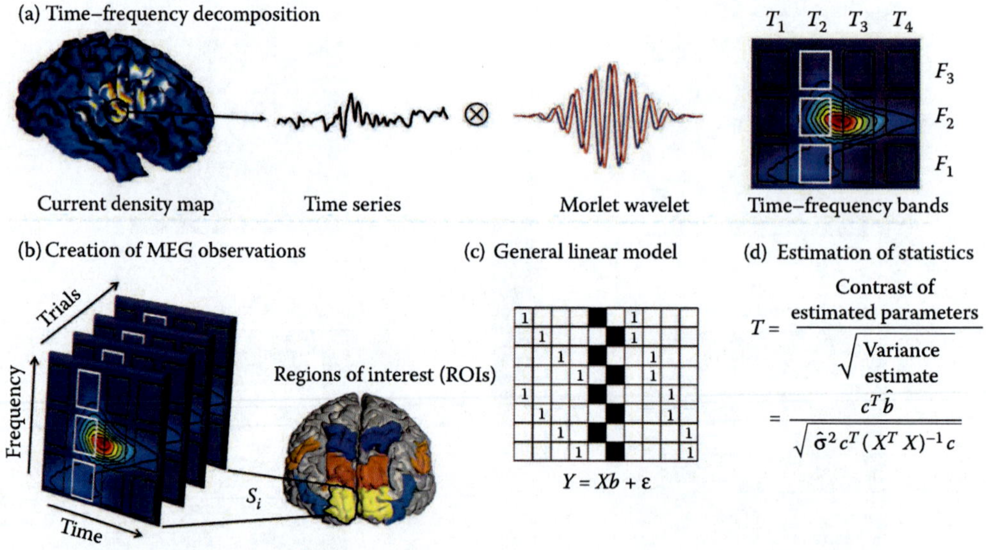

FIGURE 4.2 Creation of statistical maps of brain activation: (a) inverse methods produce distributed cortical activation maps which are expanded to time–frequency components using, for example, Morlet wavelets; (b) MEG data observations are created over several spatial-temporal-spectral bands. Alternative data reduction techniques can be used, such as singular value decomposition; (c) observations are fitted into GLMs following a mass-univariate approach or a multivariate approach; (d) a contrast of interest is defined and the statistic is normalized by its standard deviation.

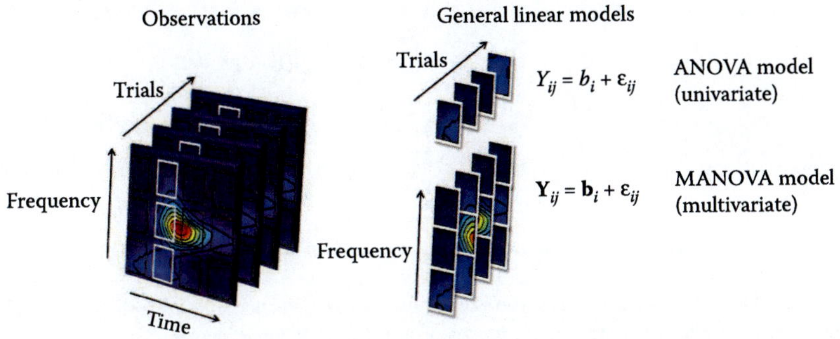

FIGURE 4.3 Power observations are fitted into GLMs using either a univariate or a multivariate approach. In the latter case, observations at multiple frequency bands are grouped together into vectors and fitted into MANOVA models.

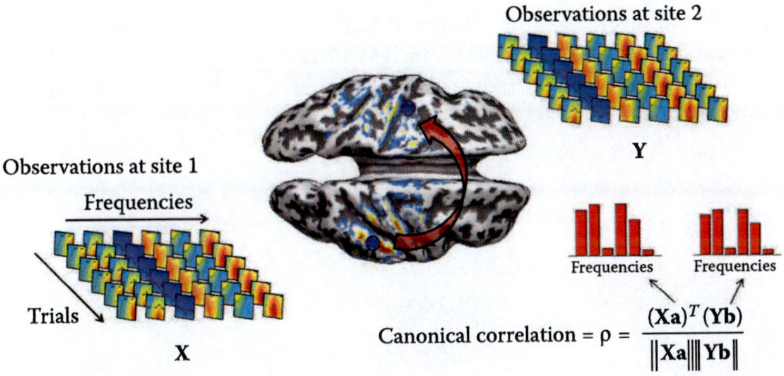

FIGURE 4.4 Observation matrices ($n_{trials} \times n_{frequencies}$) are estimated in each cortical site for a specific time band. Canonical correlation then produces the optimal combination of frequencies in one cortical site that best explains the frequencies in another site.

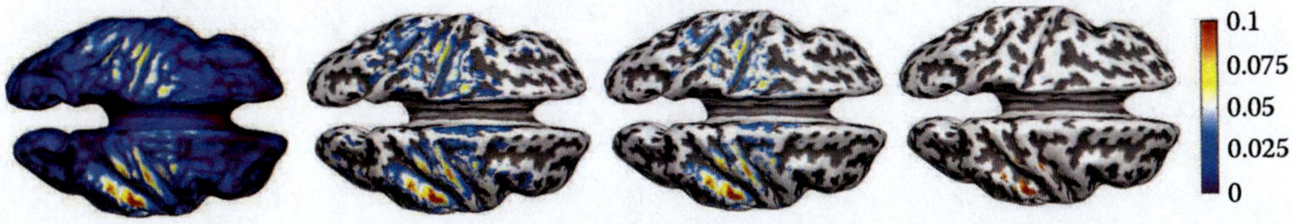

FIGURE 4.6 A statistic map thresholded at several arbitrary levels. Do both hemispheres show experimental effects, or just the right one? Interpretation of these activation results clearly depends on principled selection of the threshold for significance.

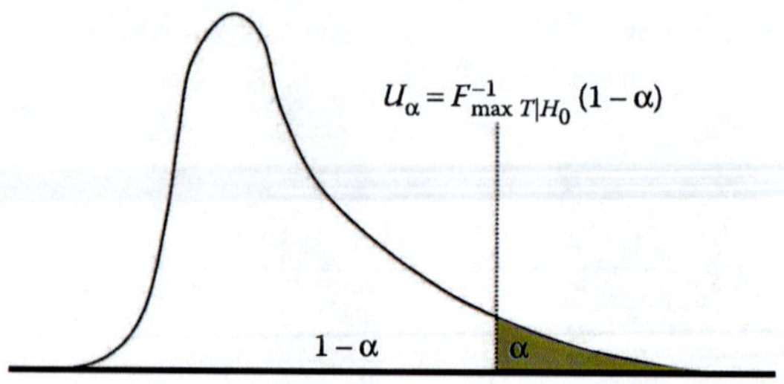

FIGURE 4.8 Probability density function of the maximum statistic. By choosing a threshold u_α which leaves only α (typically 5%) of the distribution to the right of u_α, we control the FWER at level α.

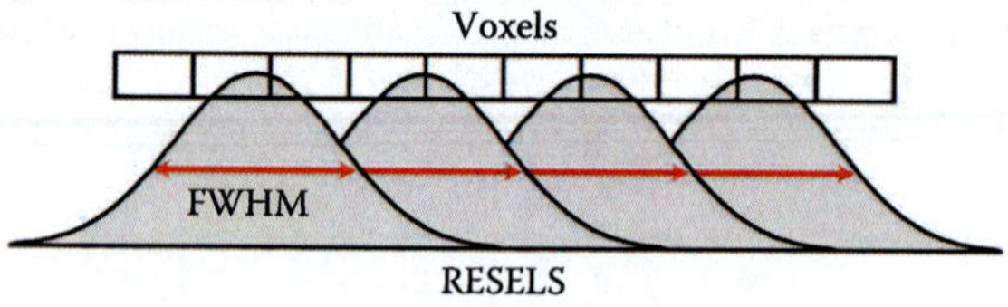

FIGURE 4.9 Random field theory uses the topological features of a statistical map to convert the voxels into RESELS, a dimensionless quantity that represents the image with interpretable units of smoothness. Under the null hypothesis of no experimental effects, it is the degree of spatial correlation in the noise in the statistical maps that determines the RESEL count.

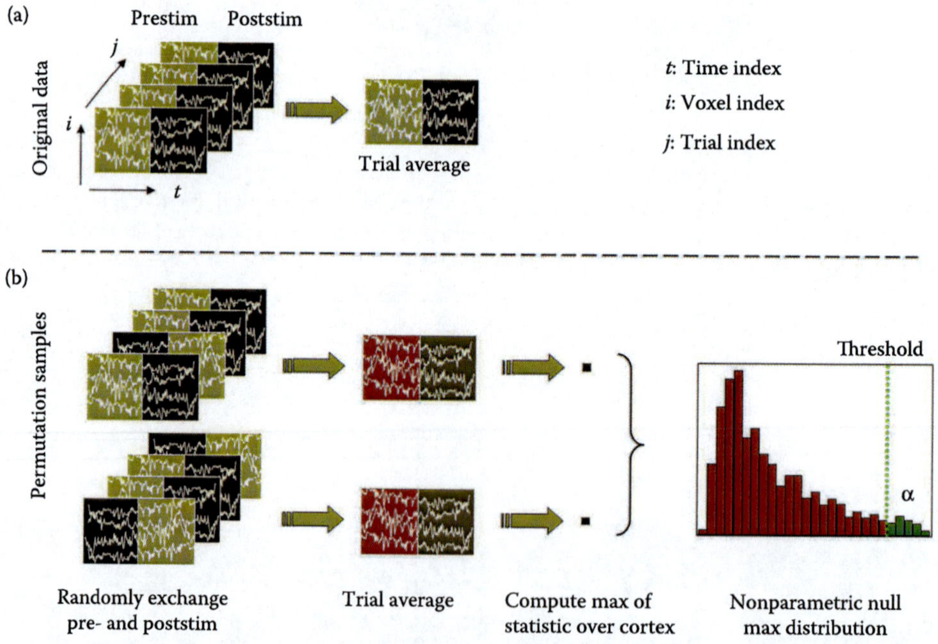

FIGURE 4.10 Permutation scheme on a single-subject multitrial MEG study. (a) Averaging of original statistical maps. (b) Generation of permutation samples by randomly exchanging pre- and poststimulus conditions within each trial. An empirical distribution of the maximum statistic is generated by averaging the permuted trials and computing the max over the cortex. The α level threshold at the upper tail of the empirical distribution is applied to the original averaged data to control the FWER.

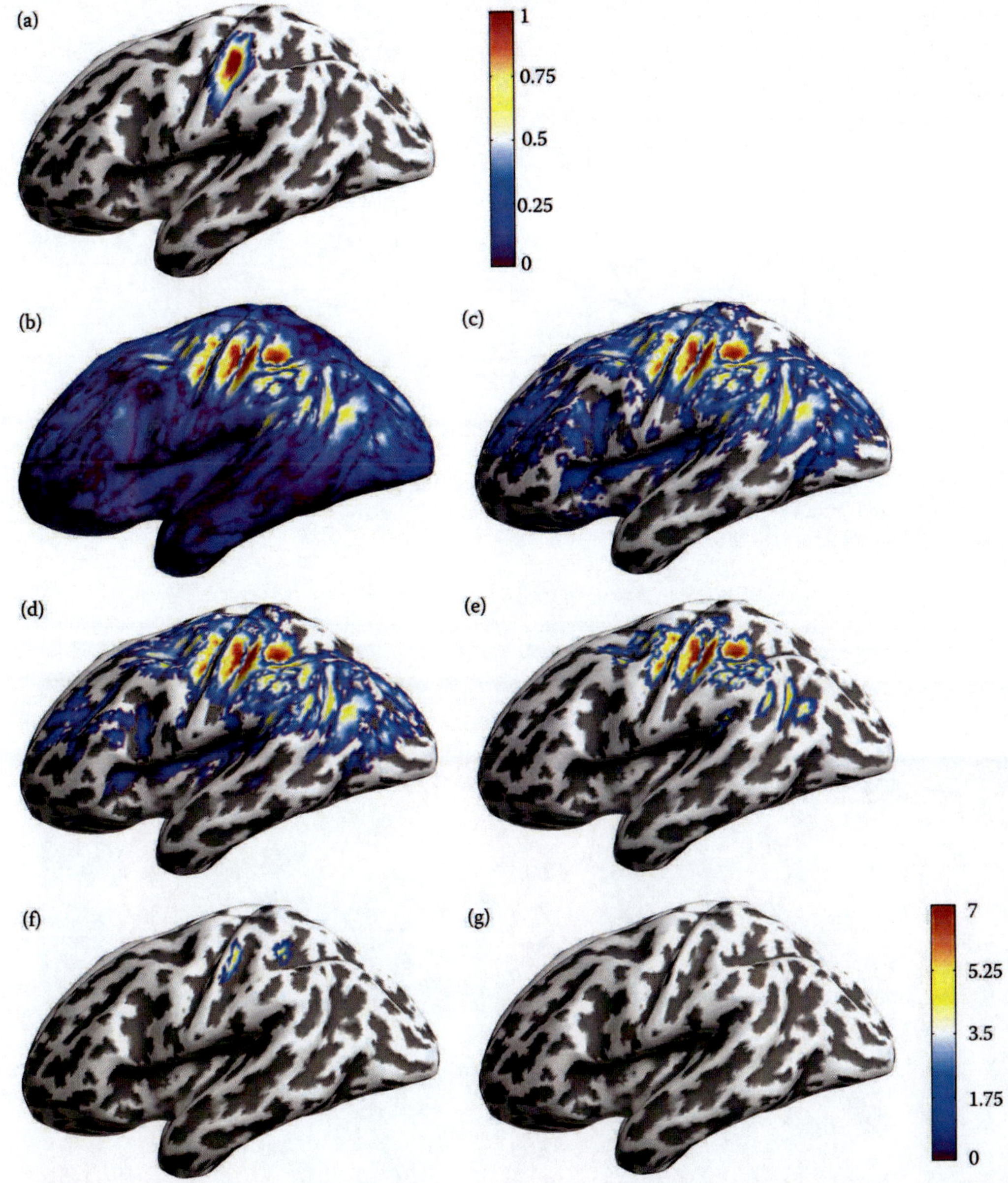

FIGURE 4.11 Simulated MEG source on the left hemisphere and reconstructed dSPM statistical map, thresholded using several methods to control false-positives. (a) Simulated sources, (b) statistical map, (c) uncorrected, (d) FDR, (e) permutations, (f) random field, and (g) Bonferroni. Uncorrected thresholding (p-value = 0.05) and FDR (p-value = 0.0065) produced many false-positives. Permutations and random field theory gave 5% FWER thresholds $t = 3.99$ and $t = 4.12$, respectively. The Bonferroni approach was very conservative (p-value $0.05/7501 = 6.6610^{-6}$) and did not identify the source.

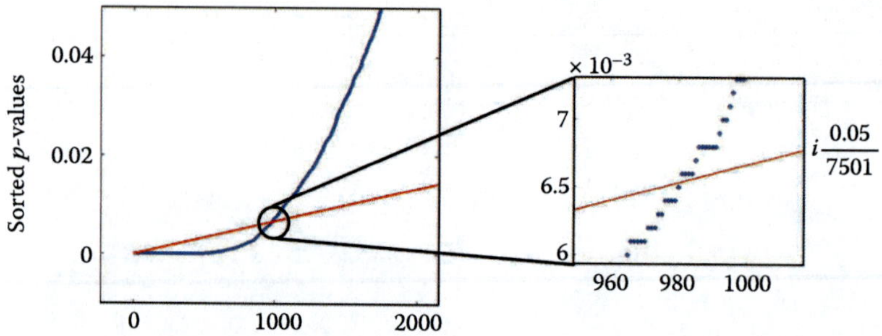

FIGURE 4.12 Graphical representation of the FDR procedure. The blue line represents the sorted p-values of the statistical map in Figure 4.11, and the red line is $i\,\alpha/V = i\,0.05/7501$. The largest p-value below the line is 0.0065 and corresponds to a 5% level FDR threshold.

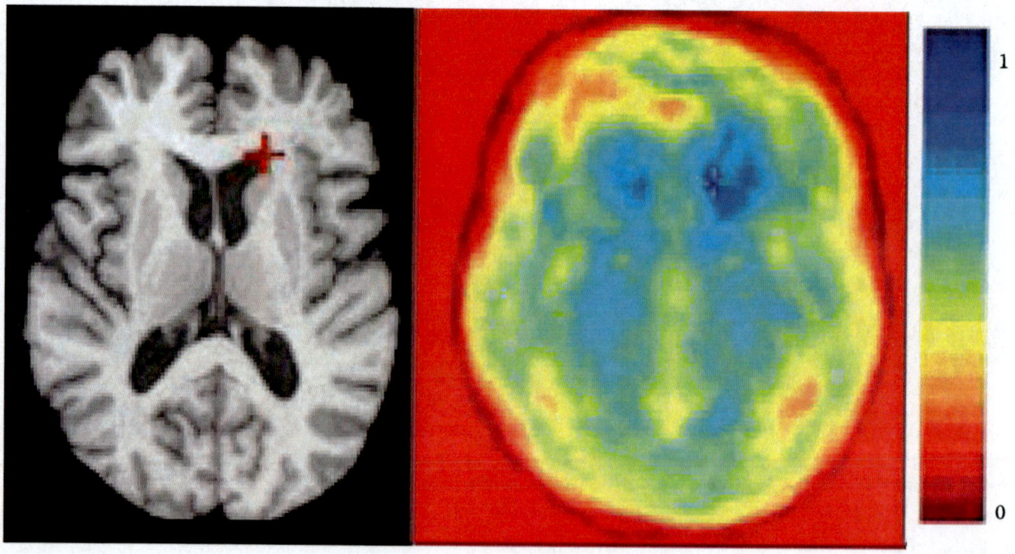

FIGURE 5.1 Color-coded map (right) of the degree of similarity between the attribute vectors of the marked point (the red cross in the left image) and every other point in the brain. Blue denotes for high similarity and red for low similarity. (Adapted from D. Shen and C. Davatzikos, *Medical Imaging, IEEE Transactions on*, 21, 1421–1439, © 2002 IEEE.)

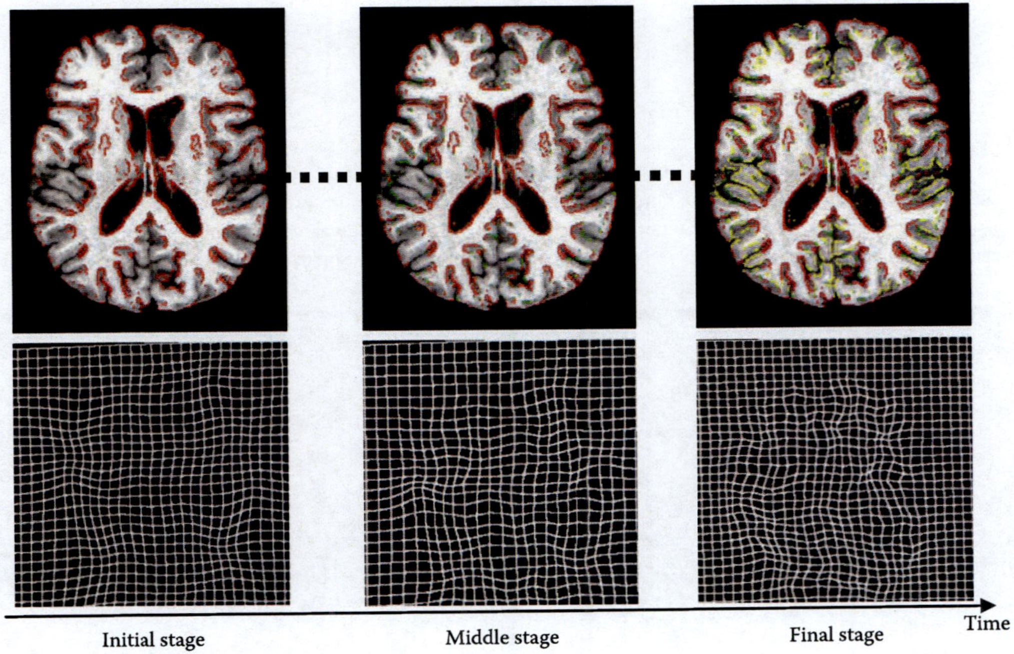

FIGURE 5.2 Hierarchical selection of the driving voxels, and evolution of deformation fields in different registration stages. In the initial stage, only a small number (around approximately 2% of total voxels) of voxels with distinctive attribute vectors (displayed in red), located at sulcal roots, gyral crowns, and ventricular boundaries, are selected to steer the registration of other less distinctive voxels. As registration progresses, more and more voxels are selected as the driving voxels, as shown in green and yellow, respectively. The bottom row shows the corresponding deformation fields estimated at three different stages. It can be observed that, as the number of the driving voxels increases, the deformation field is gradually refined. (Adapted from G. Wu et al., *NeuroImage*, 49, 2225–2233, 2010.)

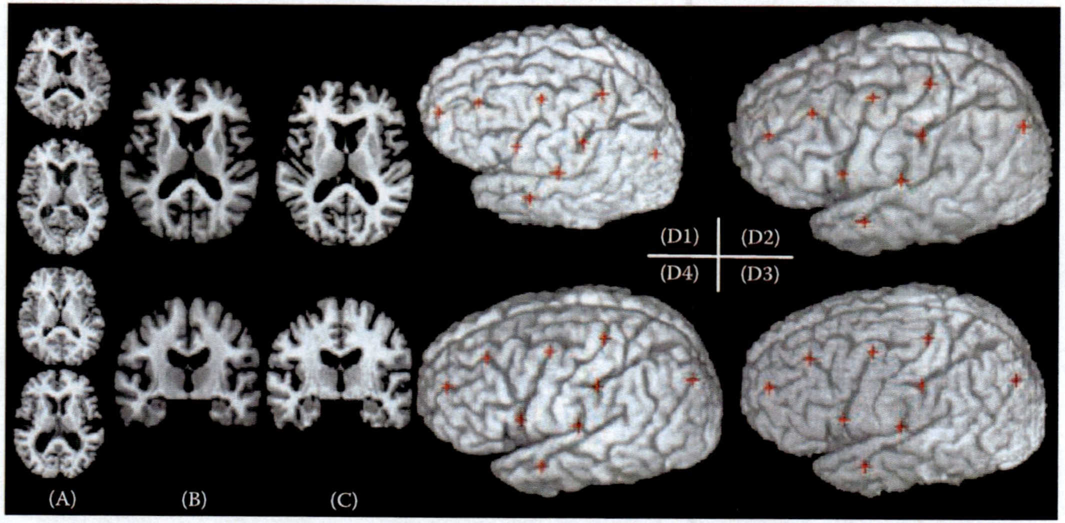

FIGURE 5.3 Results from HAMMER algorithm. (A) Four representative cross sections from BLSA dataset; (B) Representative views from the average of the 18 images after normalization onto the template in (C) by HAMMER; (D1–D4) The 3D rendering of a representative case, its warped configuration using HAMMER, the template and the average of 18 warped brains, respectively. The anatomical details seen in (B) and (D4) are the evidences of the registration accuracy. The red crosses in (D1–D4) are identically placed to allow for visual inspection of point correspondences. (Adapted from Z. Lao et al., *NeuroImage*, 21, 46–57, 2004.)

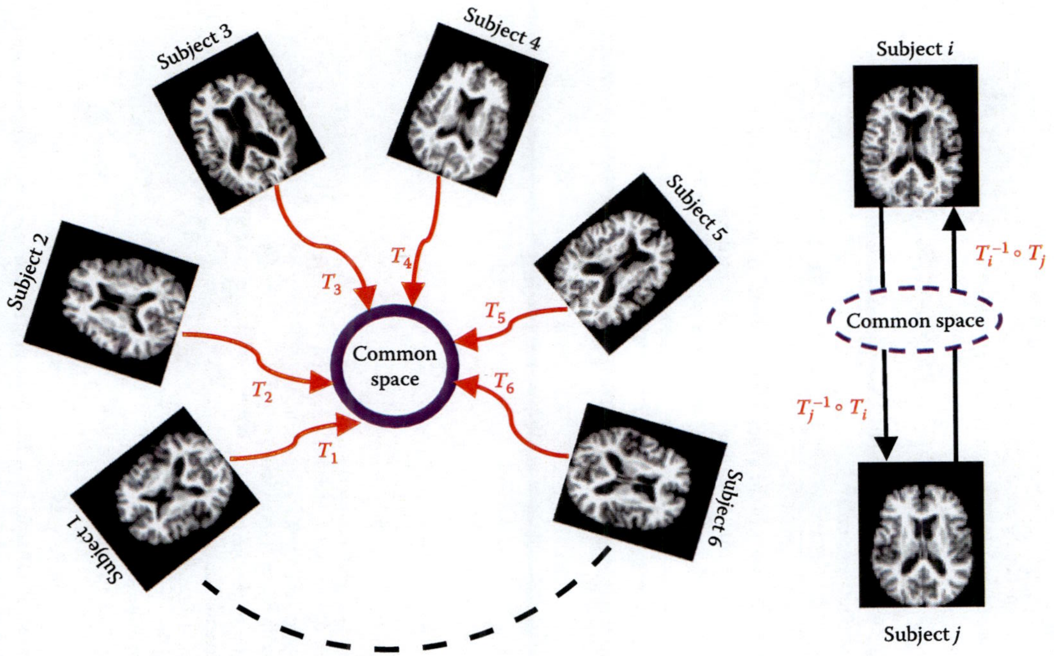

FIGURE 5.4 In groupwise registration, all subjects are warped onto a common space by following their individual deformations (as indicated by red arrows). Also, any subject I_i is connected to another subject I_j via the common space by a composed transformation, that is, $T_j^{-1} \circ T_i$, as shown in the right panel.

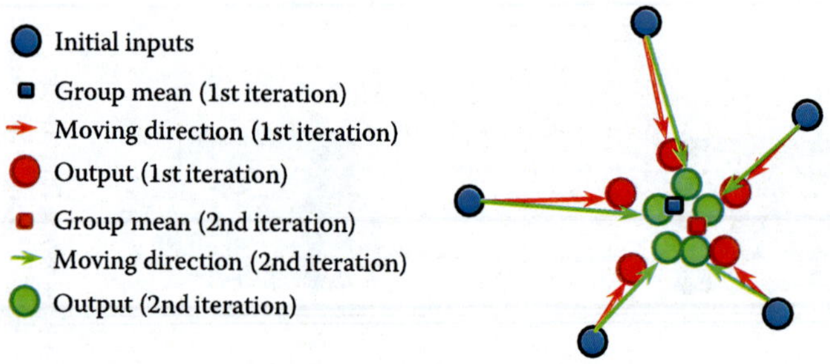

FIGURE 5.5 Illustration of the framework of the group mean method. In each iteration, the subjects are warped toward the tentatively estimated group mean. And the group mean is refined based on newly warped subjects.

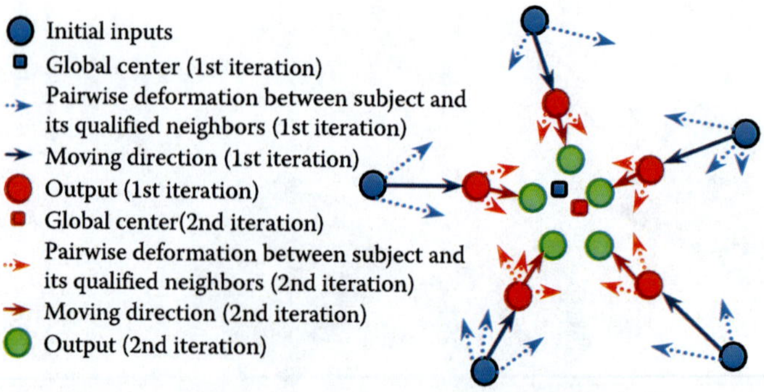

FIGURE 5.6 Illustration of the ABSORB framework. In each iteration, each subject is deformed toward its selected neighbors, which are closer to the population center. The estimated population center is updated iteratively based on the tentatively warped images. (Adapted from H. Jia et al., *NeuroImage*, 51(3), 1057–1070, 2010.)

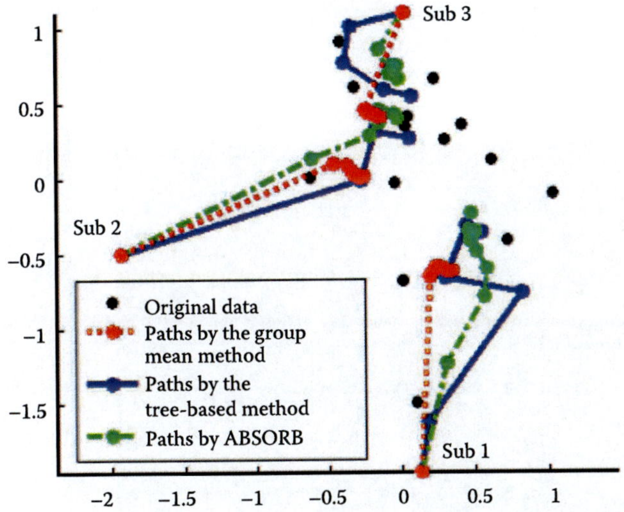

FIGURE 5.7 The registration paths produced by three different methods. The paths generated by ABSORB (with green dashed curves) are much smoother than the tree-based method (with blue solid curves), and the paths given by the group mean method (with red dotted curves) show that there is not much progress after the first iteration of registration. (Adapted from H. Jia et al., *NeuroImage*, 51(3), 1057–1070, 2010.)

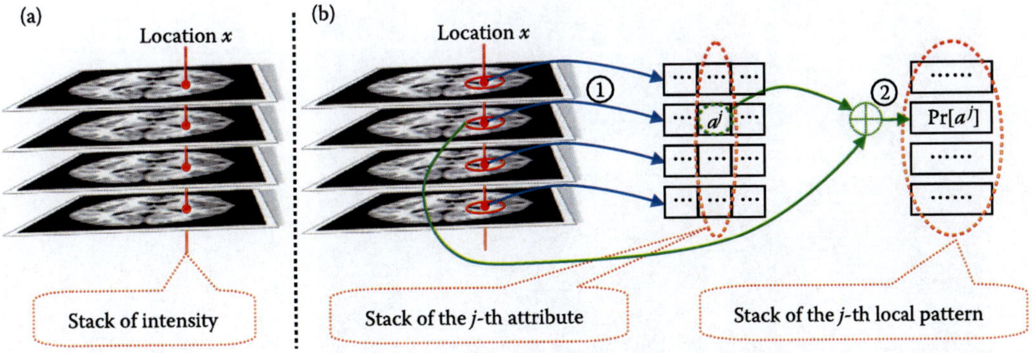

FIGURE 5.8 In (a), a stack of intensities is sampled from the identical locations of different images. (Adapted from Q. Wang et al., *NeuroImage*, 50, 1485–1496, 2010.) In (b), not only the single intensity but also more attributes are sampled to form an attribute vector as a morphological signature of each voxel. Moreover, the neighborhood of each voxel is considered as a local pattern, described by the local probability density function, to construct a robust objective function.

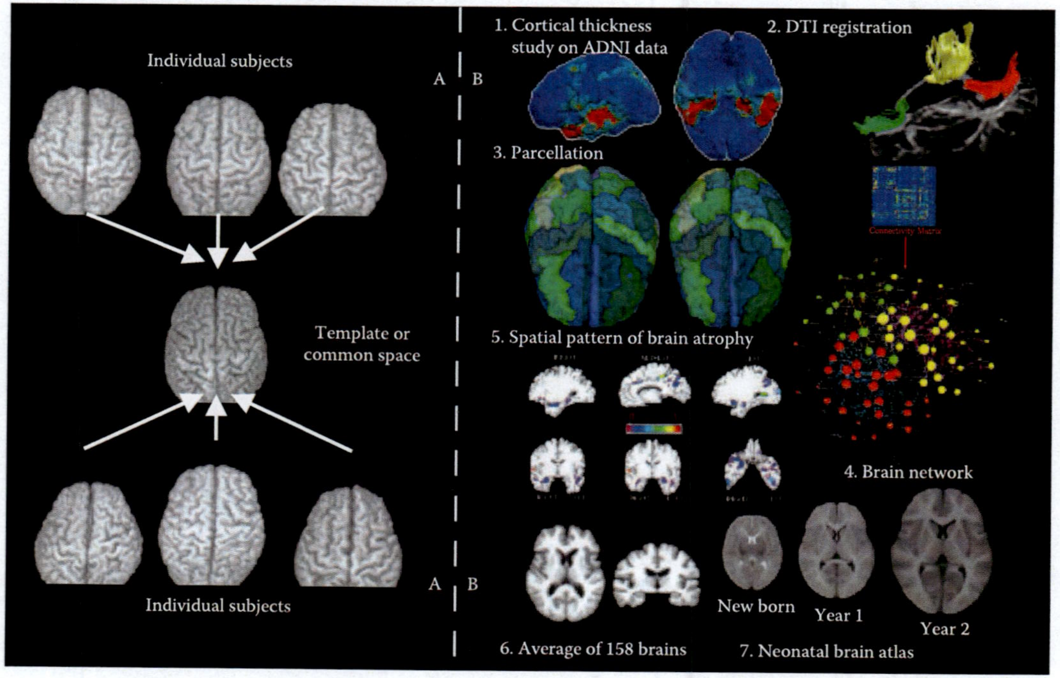

FIGURE 5.9 Illustration of various applications of image registration. Panel (A) shows the procedure of warping individuals subjects (top and bottom rows) to the template (in a pairwise scenario) or common space (in a group-wise scenario). After spatial normalization, numerous clinical applications can be performed, with some typical ones shown in the right panel (B). From (B1) to (B7), we show the illustrative results of (B1) cortical thickness study on ADNI data, (B2) DTI registration, (B3) image parcellation, (B4) brain network discovery on structural images, (B5) spatial pattern of brain atrophy with respect to MCI, (B6) normalization of elderly brains, and (B7) study on infant brain development, respectively.

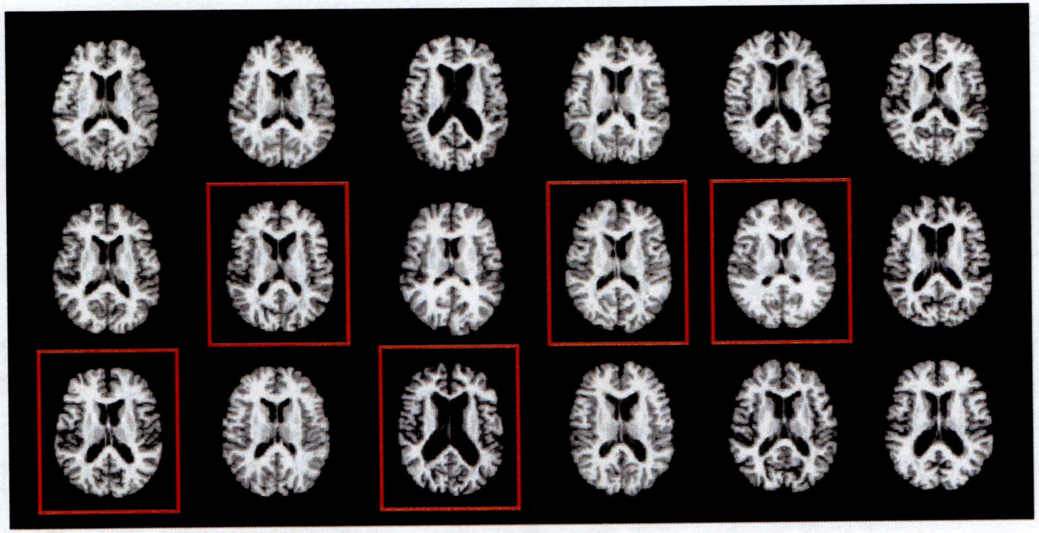

FIGURE 5.10 Eighteen elderly brain images used in evaluation of three registration methods. The five subjects with red rectangles are selected as template images in the pairwise registration algorithm for a fair performance evaluation of the pairwise registration algorithms.

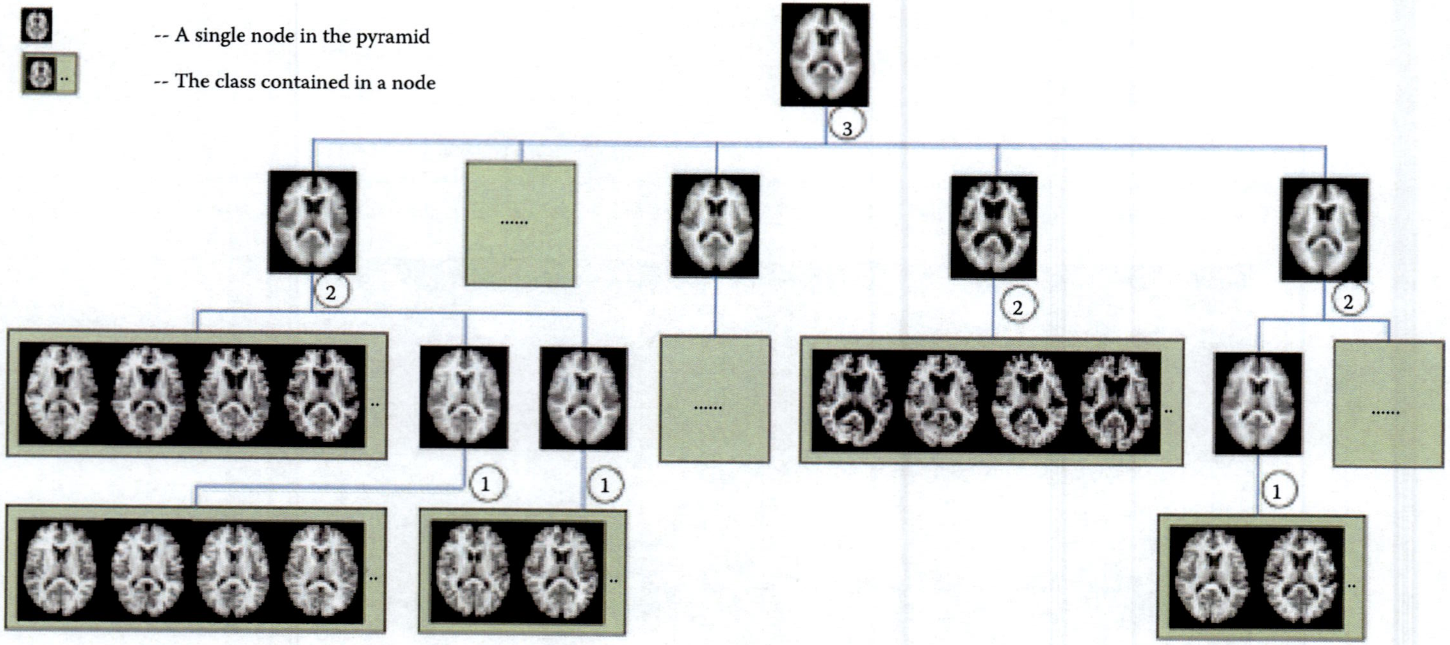

FIGURE 5.11 An image population of 150 brain MR images is hierarchically clustered into a pyramid, based on the similarity definition between any two images. Groupwise registration is performed in each class, producing the representative image for the class (label ϕ). The representative images participate into intraclass registrations in the higher level (label κ). Finally, a single representative is estimated (label λ), as the whole registration process reaches the top of the pyramid. Each input image then can be warped to the common space by following its respective deformation path. (Adapted from Q. Wang et al., *Human Brain Mapping*, 31(8), 1128–1140, 2010.)

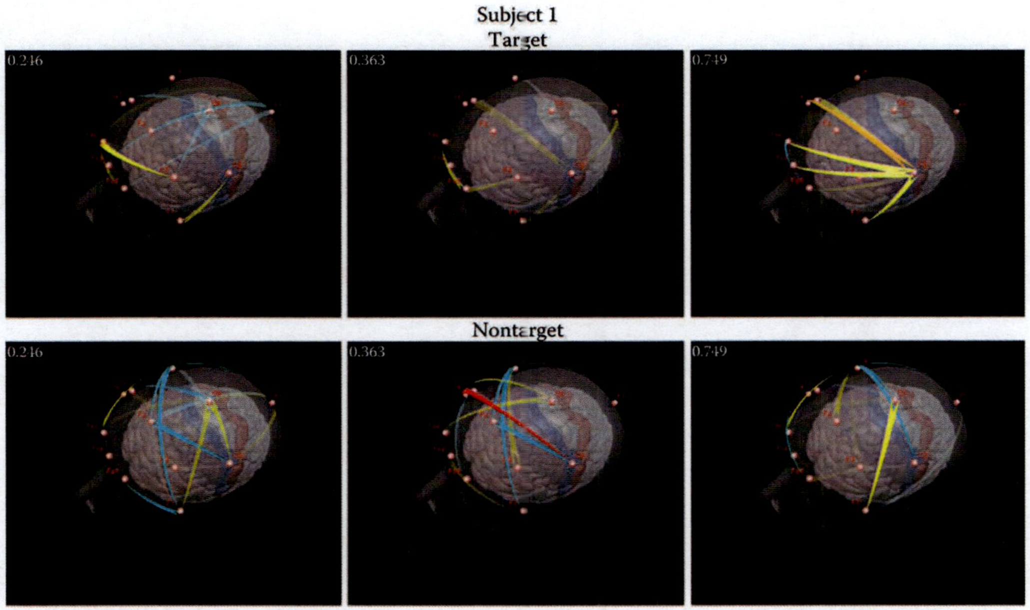

FIGURE 7.10 Snapshots from the movie presenting significant changes in transmissions in one subject, for target (upper) and nontarget (lower part). Intensity of flow changes for increase: from pale yellow to red, for decrease: from light to dark blue. In the right upper corner the time after cue presentation (in seconds). (Reprinted from Blinowska K et al. *Brain Topogr* 2010; 23:205–213.)

4

General Linear Modeling of Magnetoencephalography Data

Dimitrios Pantazis
University of Southern California

Juan Luis Poletti Soto
University of Southern California

Richard M. Leahy
University of Southern California

4.1 Introduction

Magnetoencephalography (MEG) has become increasingly popular in clinical and cognitive neuroscience as an imaging tool for studying human brain function. As more whole head systems and novel experimental paradigms become available, researchers are using MEG to explore many aspects of the workings of the human brain. To assure an objective scientific interpretation of these studies, it is important that experimental findings be accompanied by appropriate statistical analysis that effectively controls for false-positives.

This chapter reviews the statistical tools available for the analysis of distributed activation maps defined either on the 2D cortical surface or throughout the 3D brain volume. Statistical analysis of MEG data bears a great resemblance to the analysis of functional magnetic resonance imaging (fMRI) or positron emission tomography (PET) activation maps, therefore much of the methodology can be borrowed or adapted from the functional neuroimaging literature. In particular, we describe the general linear modeling (GLM) approach, where the MEG data are first mapped into brain space, and then fit to a univariate or multivariate model at each surface or volume element. A desired contrast of the estimated parameters produces a statistical map, which is then thresholded for evidence of an experimental effect.

We review several methods for generating statistical maps of brain activation based on the distributed source imaging. They all consist of these steps: process the MEG measurements to create a collection of observations, use a GLM to fit the observations at each location, and finally generate a contrast of the estimated parameters and normalize with its variance to create a map of pivotal statistics (t-maps, F-maps, etc.). This methodology is a standard approach in fMRI and PET data analysis, and together with subsequent statistical inference, is generally referred to as statistical parametric mapping (SPM) (Friston et al., 1995b).

We describe GLM formulations for the analysis of induced and evoked response in MEG. These methods include both univariate and multivariate analysis. We also extend these models to the problem of investigating large-scale cortical interactions. Finally, we describe different approaches to thresholding statistical maps to control for false-positives when testing multiple hypotheses, a problem that arises when analyzing spatial maps of cortical activity.

4.2 Special Considerations in MEG General Linear Modeling

Statistical inference in MEG distributed activation maps typically uses the GLM framework (Kiebel, 2003), which has been widely successful and is considered a standard in fMRI and PET neuroimaging studies. However, there are important differences from the other neuroimaging modalities related to how observations are created and fitted in GLM models, as well as how subsequent statistical inference is performed.

The temporal resolution of MEG is on the order of milliseconds, much higher than fMRI and PET. Standard analysis of MEG data involves the use of stimulus locked averaging over epochs to produce the evoked response. Recently there has also been a great deal of interest in analysis of the induced response, which corresponds to stimulus-related variations in power in different oscillatory bands as a function of time. This allows us to detect experimental oscillatory effects corresponding to modulations in power in specific frequency bands, even though the oscillations themselves are not phase-locked to the stimulus or response. Induced effects are typically investigated using time–frequency decomposition such as the Morlet wavelet transform (Teolis, 1998). Averaging over epochs of the power in the time–frequency maps gives us an estimate of induced components which can then be tested for experimental effects. These two forms of processing, stimulus-locked averaging and averaging of time–frequency powermaps, are the two basic approaches that are used for analyzing, respectively, evoked and induced components in the MEG data (Figure 4.1).

The fact that we often want to identify and localize experimental effects not only over space, as traditionally done in fMRI with the notion of voxels, but also in time and possibly frequency, introduces challenges that differentiate MEG analysis from that of PET and fMRI. The high dimensionality of the data (space × time × frequency × experimental design) presents challenges, in terms of the high computational costs, but also possibilities, in terms of the greater flexibility that this affords us in the design of the linear models.

Another important difference relative to fMRI is that MEG offers only limited spatial resolution. Distributed cortical imaging involves the reconstruction of thousands of elemental current sources from a few hundred measurements. The problem is highly underdetermined and requires regularization to produce a stable solution. The resulting images are typically of low resolution so that reconstructions of focal sources are blurred with extended point spread functions (PSFs). The shape of the PSF will depend on the reconstruction space, cortical or volumetric, and whether the orientations of the sources are constrained to be normal to the cortical surface. Unlike in fMRI, the PSFs for MEG are highly asymmetric and can extend over mutiple gyri or sulci. As a result, even after thresholding to control for false-positives, one can still observe false-positives at locations within the point spread of truly active regions and, therefore, care must be taken in interpreting these results. Figure 4.11, shown later in this chapter,

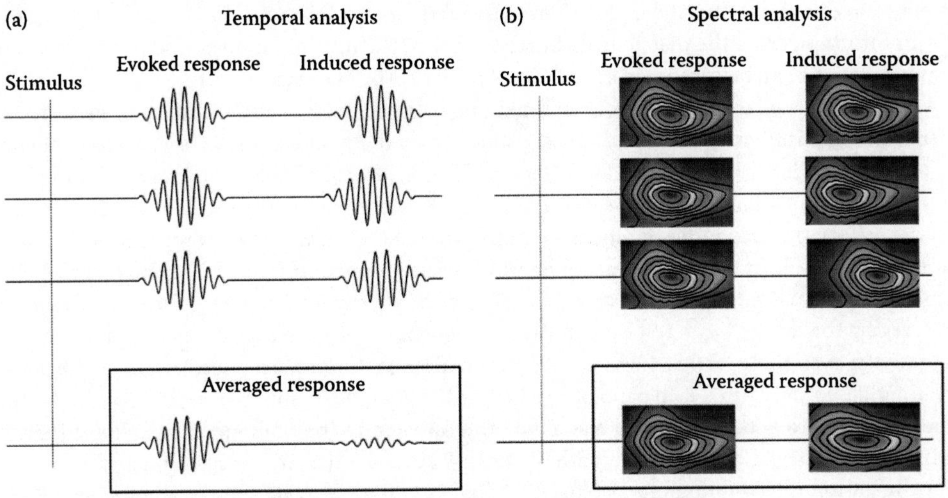

FIGURE 4.1 **(See color insert.)** MEG brain activity in response to a task consists of two components: evoked responses that are phase-locked to the stimuli, and induced responses that are not. (a) Averaging the MEG time-series over epochs preserves the evoked components, but suppresses the induced (nonphase-locked) components. (b) Averaging the power time–frequency decompositions of the time-series preserves both evoked and induced components.

illustrates this issue; the reconstructed statistical map has much greater spatial extent than the single simulated cortical patch, and subsequent thresholding procedures identify significant activity in broad cortical areas.

fMRI analysis is typically performed in the 3D volumetric space while in MEG the 2D cortical surface is often chosen as the source space. Cortically constrained maps can complicate the analysis in several ways. For example, isotropic smoothing on the cortical surface when applying random field methods requires the use of the Laplace–Beltrami operator (Chung, 2001). In group analysis, the data should be brought into a common coordinate system, which requires cortical surface alignment rather than volumetric registration (Fischl et al., 1999; Joshi et al., 2007b), and the resulting areas of activation should be reported with respect to cortical anatomy rather than the standard Talairach coordinates. Orientation-free MEG reconstructions produce vector rather than scalar fields (three elemental dipoles at each location), which can also complicate analysis.

In addition to producing a nonuniform PSF, the MEG inverse operator also introduces a highly nonstationary spatial covariance structure in reconstructed images. Contributions to the covariance can include trial-to-trial variations in induced and evoked responses as well as physiological and environmental noise. Furthermore, the covariance can also vary substantially over the course of an experiment so that we can often not assume temporal stationarity. In comparison, variations in fMRI data can often reasonably be approximated as spatially and temporally stationary. As a result, statistical inference for MEG with random field theory requires the use of special formulas that correct for nonstationarity (Worsley et al., 1999).

4.3 Observations

Using source imaging methods, MEG channel measurements are converted into 2D cortical or 3D volumetric maps of brain activation. Examples of these methods include the regularized minimum-norm (Hamalainen and Ilmoniemi, 1984) and its variants depth-weighted (Fuchs et al., 1999), Tikhonov-regularized (Tikhonov and Arsenin, 1977) and noise-normalized (Dale et al., 2000), beamformers (van Veen et al., 1997), MUSIC maps (Mosher and Leahy, 1998), and sLORETA (Pascual-Marqui, 2002).

Different source assumptions underlie each of these methods, for example, the dipole model in MUSIC and beamforming versus the distributed source model in the minimum norm methods. However, in each case a statistic can be computed at each voxel in the 2D or 3D space.

To explore the spectral components of induced brain activation, it is also common to perform time–frequency decompositions of the image maps, using, for example, short-time Fourier transform (Bruns, 2004) or complex Morlet wavelet transform (Figure 4.2a). As described before, the resulting inverse solutions are of high dimension: (2D or 3D) space, time, frequency, and experimental condition for each subject. There is, therefore, tremendous flexibility in processing the MEG data; we can create observations using any of these dimensions, treat them as univariate or multivariate observations, and fit them to different GLMs.

Some form of data reduction is desirable. For example, we can summarize information by forming discrete regions or "bands" with respect to the time, frequency, and/or spatial dimensions and integrating brain activity over these bands (Figure 4.2b). Even though this reduces resolution, as we have no discrimination power within each band, it can benefit the analysis in multiple ways: reduce data storage requirements, improve the signal-to-noise ratio, and ameliorate the multiple comparison problem by reducing the number of concurrent hypothesis tests. Data reduction in the spatial, temporal, and frequency dimension is a common practice in MEG studies and we provide a few examples here: Pantazis et al. (2007) defined 10 temporal bands (100 ms each), a single α-frequency band (8–14 Hz), and 6 spatial bands (or equivalently, cortical regions of interest) and integrated power over these bands in each trial. Brooks et al. (2004) analyzed the data only in a couple of frequency bands. Kilner et al. (2005) completely collapsed the spatial information by performing time–frequency analysis on a single channel, or equivalently, a single source. Finally, Singh et al. (2003) filtered the data into four frequency bands and averaged out the temporal dimension using a spatial power map computed from an LCMV beamformer output.

If oscillatory analysis is not required, a time–frequency decomposition is not necessary and the frequency dimension is ignored (Barnes and Hillbrand, 2003; Carbonell et al., 2004b; Pantazis et al., 2005b; Sekihara et al., 2005). An alternative form of data reduction is the application of principal

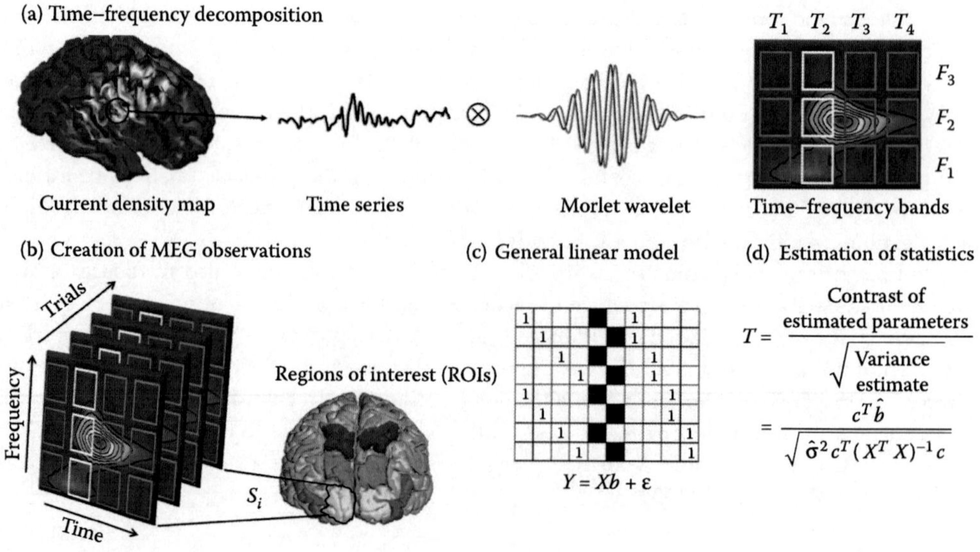

FIGURE 4.2 **(See color insert.)** Creation of statistical maps of brain activation: (a) inverse methods produce distributed cortical activation maps which are expanded to time–frequency components using, for example, Morlet wavelets; (b) MEG data observations are created over several spatial-temporal-spectral bands. Alternative data reduction techniques can be used, such as singular value decomposition; (c) observations are fitted into GLMs following a mass-univariate approach or a multivariate approach; (d) a contrast of interest is defined and the statistic is normalized by its standard deviation.

components analysis (PCA) or independent component analysis (ICA) to the MEG data. For example, Friston et al. (1996) used singular value decomposition (SVD) in the spatiotemporal dimension to reduce the set of components for each multivariate observation.

4.4 Simple General Linear Modeling Example

After the construction of observations, a GLM approach is used to model the data at each location (Figure 4.2d). The MEG observations, as described before, can be current density estimates, time–frequency power maps, or others. GLM theory assumes normal distributions, which is reasonable for averaged evoked responses due to the central limit theorem. However, power time–frequency decompositions of single trial data have a χ^2-distribution. Fortunately, Kiebel et al. (2005b) has shown that, under most circumstances, one can appeal to the central limit theorem or transform the MEG power estimates with a log or square-root transform to make the error terms normal, and thus GLM theory is still appropriate.

Under the GLM framework, the MEG observations Y are predicted from the parameters b:

$$Y = Xb + \varepsilon \tag{4.1}$$

where ε is the modeling error. X is the design matrix whose elements model an experimental paradigm and consist of qualitative (0s or 1s) and/or quantitative variables.

To provide intuition on using the GLM theory for MEG data modeling, consider the following example. In an MEG visual attention study, we acquire multitrial data for two conditions: subject attends to the right (condition 1), or to the left (condition 2). By combining an inverse method with time–frequency analysis of individual trials, we produce dynamic images of brain activity in the α-frequency band. The α-power observations for a single voxel, $y_{11}, \ldots, y_{1N}$ for N trials under condition 1 and $y_{21}, \ldots, y_{2M}$ for M trials under condition 2, are fitted into a one-way analysis of variance (ANOVA) GLM model with two predictor variables, b_1 and b_2, for the two conditions:

$$y_{ij} = b_i + \varepsilon_{ij} \tag{4.2}$$

where $i = \{0,1\}$ denotes the condition, j the trial index for each condition, and ε_{ij} is the model error.

The same ANOVA model can be written in matrix notation. If the observations y_{ij} are arranged as a single observation vector Y, and the rows of the design matrix X have 0s and 1s to indicate the condition for each MEG observation, the ANOVA model becomes $Y = Xb + \varepsilon$, explicitly written as

$$\begin{bmatrix} y_{11} \\ y_{12} \\ \vdots \\ y_{1N} \\ y_{21} \\ y_{22} \\ \vdots \\ y_{2M} \end{bmatrix} = \begin{bmatrix} 1 & 0 \\ 1 & 0 \\ \vdots & \vdots \\ 1 & 0 \\ 0 & 1 \\ 0 & 1 \\ \vdots & \vdots \\ 0 & 1 \end{bmatrix} \begin{bmatrix} b_1 \\ b_2 \end{bmatrix} + \begin{bmatrix} \varepsilon_{11} \\ \varepsilon_{12} \\ \vdots \\ \varepsilon_{1N} \\ \varepsilon_{21} \\ \varepsilon_{22} \\ \vdots \\ \varepsilon_{2M} \end{bmatrix} \tag{4.3}$$

By assuming independent error distributions with equal variance for both conditions, $N(0, \sigma^2)$, we can solve the GLM using ordinary least squares:

$$\hat{b} = (X^T X)^{-1} X^T Y = \begin{bmatrix} \bar{y}_{1\cdot} \\ \bar{y}_{2\cdot} \end{bmatrix} \tag{4.4}$$

where the bar denotes the mean over the dotted subscript. The estimated error variance $\hat{\sigma}^2$ has $N+M-2$ degrees of freedom, because two of them were used to estimate the model predictors. The error and error variance are estimated as

$$\hat{\varepsilon} = Y - X\hat{b} = (I - X(X^TX)^{-1}X^T)Y = \mathrm{P}Y \tag{4.5}$$

$$\hat{\sigma}^2 = \frac{\hat{\varepsilon}^T\hat{\varepsilon}}{\mathrm{trace}\{P\}} = \frac{\sum_i (y_{1i} - \bar{y}_{1\cdot})^2 + \sum_i (y_{2i} - \bar{y}_{2\cdot})^2}{N + M - 2} \tag{4.6}$$

where P is a projection operator onto the left null space of X. Suppose we want to test whether there is a difference between the two conditions, or equivalently whether the difference $b_1 - b_2$ is significantly different from zero. The statistic of interest is, therefore, the contrast of the two parameters, $c^T\hat{b} = \begin{bmatrix} 1 \\ -1 \end{bmatrix}^T \hat{b} = b_1 - b_2$, which is then normalized with an estimate of its standard deviation. The resulting statistic T is a two-sample t-test between the two conditions.

$$T = \frac{c^T\hat{b}}{\sqrt{\hat{\sigma}^2 c^T (X^TX)^{-1} c}} = \frac{\bar{y}_{1\cdot} - \bar{y}_{2\cdot}}{\sqrt{\hat{\sigma}^2(1/N + 1/M)}} \tag{4.7}$$

Even though we could have derived the T statistic directly, it is useful to see how it is estimated in the GLM framework and gain intuition for more complex designs where the theory becomes important. The design matrix X can have multiple columns with indicator variables, as above, but also quantitative variables that correspond to covariates. The observations can be arranged in multiple ways and several contrasts can capture the experimental effect of interest.

4.5 Contrast Statistic and Normalization

After selection of a GLM approach, the MEG observations are fitted to the models and a contrast (or linear combination) of the parameters is computed (Figure 4.2d). This contrast statistic captures the effect of interest, for example, the difference between two experimental conditions or the correlation of a response variable with brain activation. It is then preferable to normalize the statistics into known parametric distributions (pivotal statistics). This allows the application of random field theory, which as we will see, requires a Gaussian distribution or one derived from Gaussian data (e.g., a t or F statistic). The normalization also helps when using nonparametric permutation methods, because it makes the variance at all voxels homogeneous under the null hypothesis, which should produce approximately uniform specificity, that is, false-positives are equally likely at all locations.

We conclude by showing that the GLM framework is parsimonious in MEG analysis. Consider, for example, the simple case where the MEG data are used to create dSPM maps (Dale et al., 2000), that is, minimum-norm inverse maps normalized with an estimate of the noise standard deviation at each location. As we will show, this corresponds to the simplest case of GLM analysis following a mass-univariate approach: the one-way ANOVA model $y_j^{it} = b^{it} + \varepsilon_j^{it}$ is fitted to the current density data y_j^{it} data separately at each spatial location i and temporal location t, where j is the trial repetition index and b^{it} is the main effect (brain response) (Pantazis et al., 2005b). We use superscripts for i and t to denote that the same model is fit separately in each spatial-temporal location. The contrast of interest is the parameter itself, which is equal to the trial average according to the minimum-norm solution: $c^T\hat{b}^{it} = [1]\hat{b}^{it} = \hat{b}^{it} = \bar{y}_{\cdot}^{it}$, where the bar indicates an average over the dotted subscript. Since the error terms ε_j^{it} are assumed to be

Gaussian, the estimated contrast is also a Gaussian statistic. Finally, to create a map of *t*-distribution statistics, we normalize with the standard deviation at each location $T^{it} = \hat{b}^{it}/\hat{\sigma}^{it}/\sqrt{J}$, where $\hat{\sigma}^{it}$ is the estimated standard deviation and J is the total number of trials. This is equivalent to the noise normalization performed in dSPM for orientation-constrained linear inverses. For the unconstrained case, the dSPM output is an *F*-map computed as the ratio of the magnitude squared of the vector current density to the noise variance at each spatial location. The sLORETA solution (Pascual-Marqui, 2002) is similar to dSPM, but with a different normalization coefficient. In this case, we normalize by the standard deviation computed from the data covariance rather than the noise only covariance. Under the null hypothesis of noise only (or equivalently a zero experimental effect), sLORETA and dSPM are identical. Similarly, the beamformer neural activity index (van Veen et al., 1997) corresponds to a *t*-map for the orientation-constrained case or an *F*-map for the orientation-free case, which can be again cast in a GLM framework (Kucukaltun-Yildirim et al., 2006).

4.6 Multisubject Studies

In multisubject studies, the measurement variance has two sources: the within-subject variance and the between-subject variance. Depending on how we model the error variance, two types of statistical analysis can be used: fixed-effect and mixed (or random) effect. Fixed-effect analysis considers only the within-subject variance and; therefore, all measurements are fitted to the same GLM in the same manner as for a single subject. Statistical inferences apply only to the particular subjects participating in the experiment. To generalize to the whole population, mixed-effect analysis is required, where both within- and between-subject variances are considered in making statistical inferences.

Mixed-effect analysis typically involves fitting hierarchical models (Friston et al., 2002; Mumford and Nichols, 2006), where we specify the complete model in stages: a first or lower level model fits the data for each subject separately, and a second level combines the different subjects. Estimation of the parameters in the two-stage analysis is a challenge since it involves iterative optimization and is generally not practical, unless we follow the summary statistics approach. This approach is computationally efficient because it dissociates estimation of the parameters of the two-stage models, and can be implemented with algorithms such as Markov chain Monte Carlo (Beckmann et al., 2003), or restricted maximum likelihood (Verbeke and Molenberghs, 2000).

Under specific assumptions, the summary statistic approach simplifies and the parameters can be estimated without the need for an iterative procedure (Holmes and Friston, 1998; Mumford and Nicholas, 2006). We describe this method here because it has become the most popular approach for multisubject analysis in MEG. The first stage model fits the data from each subject $k = 1,\ldots,K$ separately*:

$$Y_k = X_k b_k + \varepsilon_k \tag{4.8}$$

where Y_k is the MEG observations and b_k is the model parameters for subject k. While each design matrix X_k can have a different number of rows (e.g., different number of MEG trials per subject), all the design matrices must have the same number of columns, each column expressing the same effect among subjects. The subject parameters are estimated using a generalized least squares solution, which normally requires the estimation of the error covariance matrix C_k:

$$\hat{b}_k = (X_k^T C_k^{-1} X_k)^{-1} X_k^T C_k^{-1} \tag{4.9}$$

* To ease notation, we now use subscripts rather than superscripts, for indices where we follow a mass-univariate approach.

The second stage model takes only one contrast $c^T \hat{b}_k$ from each subject and fits it to the group GLM:

$$\begin{bmatrix} c^T \hat{b}_1 \\ c^T \hat{b}_2 \\ \vdots \\ c^T \hat{b}_K \end{bmatrix} = X_g b_g + \varepsilon_g \tag{4.10}$$

where X_g and b_g are the group design matrix and group level parameters, respectively. The summary statistic model error ε_g has two variance components, the intrasubject and intersubject variance. Under the assumption of homogeneous intrasubject variance (i.e., $c^T \hat{b}_k$ has the same variance for all subjects), the intrasubject variance is a scaled identity matrix. Similarly, under the assumption of independent subjects, the intersubject variance is a scaled identity matrix. Therefore, the covariance of ε_g is also a scaled identity matrix and the generalized least squares solution of the second stage model (which normally requires estimation of the error covariance matrix) becomes equivalent to an ordinary least squares solution that does not require the covariance matrix:

$$\hat{b}_g = (X_g^T X_g)^{-1} X_g \hat{b} \tag{4.11}$$

The key assumption here is the homogeneity of the intrasubject variances; without it the ordinary least squares solution could not have been used and iterations would be necessary to estimate both the intrasubject and the intersubject components of the variance.

With multisubject studies, we first coregister all subjects to a common coordinate system using either volumetric brain coregistration (Christensen and Johnson, 2001; Hellier et al., 2002; Shen and Davatzikos, 2002) or cortical surface alignment methods (Fischl et al., 1999; Thompson et al., 2001; Joshi et al., 2007a). Then the first stage model, which can be a mass-univariate approach, a multivariate approach, or a general univariate framework, estimates subject specific parameters. These parameters are then fitted to a second stage model and finally a statistic map is computed on the common coordinate system using a contrast of the group parameters b_g at each voxel. This statistic map can then be thresholded for significant activity at the group level using any of the methods described later in this chapter.

Consider the following example. In Pantazis et al. (2007), the first stage model consisted of fitting a univariate model for each subject in the α band for each of several cortically defined regions of interest and time bands. A contrast statistic was then estimated that captured an attention effect: ipsilateral minus contralateral alpha power in each spatiotemporal band. The contrast for all subjects was then fitted to a second stage GLM (Equation 4.10), whose design matrix X_g is a column of 1s. This simply leads to averaging the responses from all subjects (Equation 4.11), since the assumption of homogeneous intrasubject variance allows application of the simple summary statistic approach described above. Finally, the false discovery rate (FDR) approach, as described below, was used to threshold the resulting statistic map. Other examples of multisubject MEG studies can be found in Singh et al. (2003).

Besides the summary statistic approach, other methods for multisubject analysis have been proposed in functional neuroimaging. They consist of two steps: first, the statistic map from each subject is converted into a p-value map; then, the p-value maps from all subjects are combined into a single statistic map, which can finally be thresholded for significance with any of the error control methods described below. One important factor in determining how the individual p-value maps will be combined is the null hypothesis to be tested: one may consider, for instance, that there is a group effect if at least one subject has an effect (global null) (Friston et al., 1999), or that all subjects must have an effect for a group effect to be considered (conjunction null) (Friston et al., 2005; Nichols et al., 2005), or even that, for a group effect to be present, a predefined number of subjects having the effect is sufficient (partial conjunction null) (Benjamini and Heller, 2007; Heller et al., 2007). Once the null hypothesis is defined, we can choose between a variety of expressions for pooling individual p-values; some of these are due to Fisher (1950); Stouffer et al. (1949) and Worsley and Friston (2000), among others. The properties of each of these expressions are discussed elsewhere (Lazar et al., 2002; McNamee and Lazar, 2004).

4.7 Univariate versus Multivariate GLMs

We can analyze MEG data using either mass-univariate or multivariate approaches (Kiebel and Friston, 2004). The mass-univariate approach considers the data at each location in isolation. Therefore, a separate but identical GLM is fitted at each spatial-temporal-spectral location and analyzed using an ANOVA or ANCOVA approach. The data correlations in the respective dimensions are ignored at this stage, and accommodated at the inference stage through adjusting the p-values associated with the statistical maps. For example, even though the activation of nearby voxels is correlated, the mass-univariate approach ignores the spatial correlation, but corrects for it when random field theory or permutation tests define a threshold for significant activation. The mass-univariate approach can identify regionally specific effects, since it can test for rejection of the null hypothesis independently at each location. This property, together with its ease of implementation, has made it the most popular approach in functional neuroimaging.

In fMRI, univariate GLMs are typically fit in each cortical location to produce statistical maps that are then thresholded for significance (Friston et al., 1995a). Even though MEG does not have comparable spatial resolution, it affords high temporal resolution on the order of milliseconds (Barnes and Hillbrand, 2003; Brookes et al., 2004). This allows time–frequency decompositions of the recorded time series, which are then used as observations in mass-univariate GLMs in the spatial, temporal, and spectral dimensions (Durka et al., 2004; Kiebel et al., 2005a; Pantazis et al., 2009).

We have recently seen an increased interest in multivariate fMRI studies (Carlson et al., 2003; Cox and Savoy, 2003; Haynes and Rees, 2006; Norman et al., 2006; Pereira et al., 2009). Multivariate observations are formed across neighboring voxel locations, for example, following the searchlight approach (Kriegeskorte et al., 2006). These are then analyzed using pattern recognition techniques. Multivariate approaches offer increased sensitivity in detecting spatially distributed effects and can reveal the spatial encoding of mental states as well as assess the amount of information encoded in a particular brain region (Norman et al., 2006). Multivariate approaches should offer similar benefits for MEG data analysis. While fMRI has better spatial resolution, and multivariate observations are formed across neighboring voxels, MEG has excellent temporal resolution, allowing us to form multivariate observations across multiple frequencies. These observations are formed by first creating dynamic maps of cortical activity (regularized minimum-norm maps) through inverse mapping of MEG data (Baillet et al., 2001), and then applying time–frequency decompositions, such as the complex Morlet wavelet transform (Teolis, 1998).

In the multivariate approach we use the multivariate analysis of variance (MANOVA) or multivariate analysis of covariance (MANCOVA) framework. In this case, the MEG observations are organized into vectors and stacked as rows in an observation matrix Y (Figure 4.3). Classical analysis of this model proceeds by computing sample covariance matrices of the data and the residuals, and then estimating test statistics such as Roy's maximum root, Wilk's lambda, Pillai's trace, or Hotelling's trace (Seber, 2004).

An example of multivariate analysis in MEG is given in Soto et al. (2009). In this chapter, vectors of observations were formed by concatenating the power in six frequency bands and fit into separate multivariate linear models for each time band and cortical location with experimental conditions as predictor variables. The resulting Roy's maximum root statistic maps were thresholded for significance using permutation tests and the maximum statistic approach (described later in this chapter). Their results indicated that the multivariate method is more powerful than the univariate approach in detecting experimental effects when correlations exist between power across frequency bands.

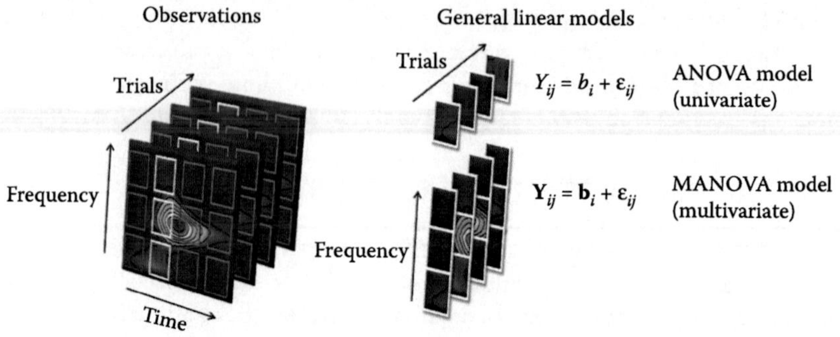

FIGURE 4.3 **(See color insert.)** Power observations are fitted into GLMs using either a univariate or a multivariate approach. In the latter case, observations at multiple frequency bands are grouped together into vectors and fitted into MANOVA models.

4.8 Canonical Correlation Analysis

Until now, we have focused on investigating experimental effects by contrasting conditions between locations in space, time, and frequency. However, one may also be interested in exploring how the brain forms cortical functional networks. Given the excellent temporal resolution of MEG, we can explore functional interactions between cortical sites and even resolve these interactions at individual frequency bands.

Cortical interactions often involve several frequency bands, indicating that a multivariate (multifrequency) approach would have better sensitivity in detecting neural effects than univariate ones. Recent findings include theta–gamma coupling in visual memory (Schack et al., 2002; Bruns and Eckhorn, 2004; Schack and Weiss, 2005; Penny et al., 2008), word recognition (Mormann et al., 2005), and behavioral tasks (Canolty et al., 2006; Jensen and Colgin, 2007); delta–gamma in visual attention (Lakatos et al., 2008); alpha–gamma in mental arithmetic tasks (Palva et al., 2005) and rest (Osipova et al., 2008); beta–gamma in hand movement simulation (De Lange et al., 2008; Jerbi and Bertrand, 2009); and coupling of ultraslow rhythms with frequencies between 1 and 40 Hz during somatosensory tasks (Monto et al., 2008). Within-frequency interactions have also been reported recently (Lachaux et al., 1999; Fries, 2005; Hummel and Gerloff, 2006; Jerbi et al., 2007a; Pantazis et al., 2009).

Despite the importance of interactions across frequencies, most popular connectivity measures in MEG, such as coherence (Nunez et al., 1997; Gross et al., 2001; Le Van Quyen et al., 2001), phase synchrony (Tass et al., 1998; Lachaux et al., 1999; Lin et al., 2004), and Granger's causality (Kaminski et al., 2001; Brovelli et al., 2004; Kus et al., 2004), typically consider only interactions in amplitude or phase at the same frequency. Given the wealth of information in MEG data, analysis using a single-frequency approach requires either prior knowledge of the frequencies at which interactions will occur or, conversely, a large number of tests, one for each possible type of interaction.

Interpretation of interaction measures is further confounded by the ill-posed nature of the inverse problem in MEG, producing images of low resolution with blurred cortical sources resulting in linear mixing or crosstalk between regions, which may be mistaken as neural interactions between these regions. Approaches to reduce linear mixing when computing interactions include eliminating zero-lag correlations (Nolte et al., 2004; Gomez-Herrero et al., 2008; Marzetti et al., 2008), reconstructing current density maps that cancel interfering signals (Dalal et al., 2006; Hui and Leahy, 2006; Hui et al., 2010), and simply excluding *a priori* a number of spatial locations from the analysis (Carbonell et al., 2004a). However, all these approaches suffer from limitations and are not ideal solutions to the linear mixing problem. Because most interaction measures are sensitive to the linear mixing of sources, even small crosstalk can produce spurious interactions (Nunez et al., 1997). Here we describe a new alternative approach dealing with linear mixing: we accept as true interactions only those whose spectral profile cannot be explained by crosstalk between regions (which is equivalent to requiring canonical correlation vectors a and b to be nonparallel, as described below).

Our multivariate analysis of cortical interactions is based on canonical correlation analysis (Seber, 2004). Canonical correlation (or subspace correlation) extends the idea of simple correlation to multivariate signals; given two sets of signals, it finds the best way to linearly combine the two sets to achieve the maximum correlation. Multivariate observations are formed using the power or phase at multiple frequency bands, thus allowing us to automatically find the optimal set of frequencies contributing to neural interactions.

Time–frequency representations of brain activity are computed from MEG as described earlier in this chapter. Observations can then be formed by integrating the power of the wavelet coefficients over the frequency bands of interest, for example theta (4–7 Hz), alpha (8–14 Hz), beta (15–30 Hz), and gamma (31–50 Hz). The resulting observation matrices at each spatial location have dimension $n_{\text{trials}} \times n_{\text{bands}}$ and are normalized to have a zero mean and unit variance at each band.

Given two observation matrices **X** and **Y** from distinct voxel locations, the maximum canonical correlation seeks linear combinations of the columns of these matrices that maximize the correlation between them (Figure 4.4). In other words, we want to find vectors **a** and **b** such that ρ is maximized:

$$\rho = \frac{(\mathbf{Xa})^T(\mathbf{Yb})}{\|\mathbf{Xa}\|\|\mathbf{Yb}\|} \tag{4.12}$$

The maximum value of ρ, called the maximum canonical correlation, is given by the largest singular value of the matrix $\mathbf{M} = (\mathbf{X}^T\mathbf{X})^{1/2}(\mathbf{X}^T\mathbf{Y})(\mathbf{Y}^T\mathbf{Y})^{1/2}$ and the vectors **a** and **b** associated with the maximum ρ are $\mathbf{a} = (\mathbf{X}^T\mathbf{X})^{1/2}\mathbf{u}$ and $\mathbf{b} = (\mathbf{Y}^T\mathbf{Y})^{1/2}\mathbf{v}$, **u** and **v** being the left and right singular vectors of the largest singular value of **M**, respectively. We can use the canonical vectors **a** and **b** to find the relative contribution of each frequency to the correlation between **X** and **Y** (Rencher, 1992).

To create canonical correlation statistical maps, we can either choose a seed voxel and compute the maximum canonical correlations between the seed and all other voxels on the cortical surface, or compute the canonical correlations between all possible pairs of cortical locations.

Apart from amplitude/amplitude coupling, we can also detect other forms of coupling by extending each observation vector to also include the phase of the wavelet coefficients in each band of interest. This will allow automatic detection of all possible relations: amplitude–amplitude (Bruns and Eckhorn, 2004), amplitude–phase (Canolty et al., 2006), and phase–phase (Lachaux et al., 1999).

We can use canonical vectors **a** and **b** to find the relative contribution of each frequency to the correlation between two cortical regions. However, low-resolution inverse solutions in EEG cause linear

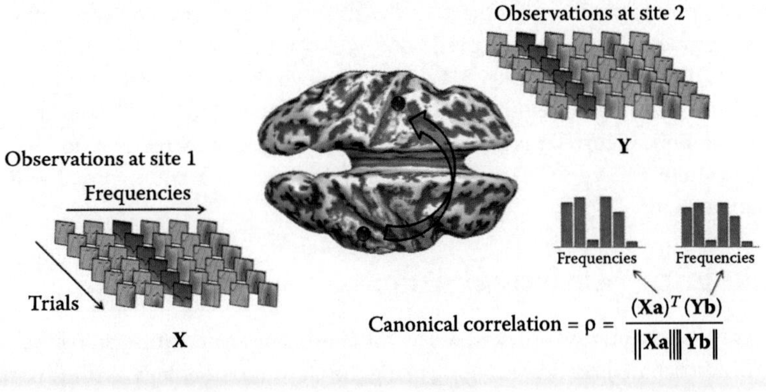

FIGURE 4.4 **(See color insert.)** Observation matrices ($n_{\text{trials}} \times n_{\text{frequencies}}$) are estimated in each cortical site for a specific time band. Canonical correlation then produces the optimal combination of frequencies in one cortical site that best explains the frequencies in another site.

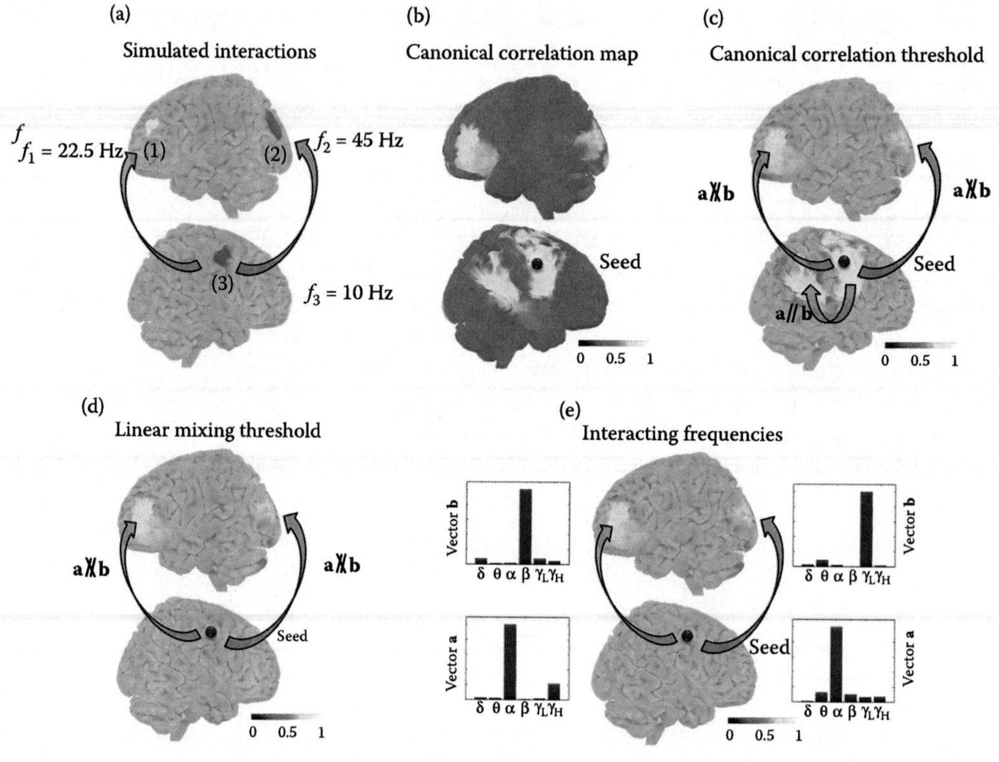

FIGURE 4.5 Identifying cortical networks with canonical correlation. (a) Simulated interactions between sources 1–3 and 2–3. Even though sources have different frequency content, their power is correlated with each other; (b) a canonical correlation map is estimated between the seed and all other cortical locations; (c) test for symmetry in cross correlation matrix to detect linear mixing; (d) interactions after controlling for linear mixing; (e) individual frequencies contributing to canonical correlation.

mixing of activation sources, causing large values in canonical correlation, even when true interaction does not exist (the same is true for simple correlations and phase synchrony). We can separate such spurious results from true cortical interactions by testing whether the cross correlation matrix between each pair of locations is symmetric. Specifically, we can show that in case of pure linear mixing, the cross correlation is symmetric. Therefore asymmetry implies true cortical interaction. Consequently the canonical correlation maps should be subjected to a statistical test, with correction for multiple comparisons, against symmetry of the cross correlation.

This procedure is illustrated in Figure 4.5. We simulate two cortical interactions and then estimate a map of canonical correlation between the seed and all other cortical locations. We successively threshold for significant canonical correlation and for asymmetry of cross correlation, to identify significant interactions that are not caused by linear mixing. Finally, vectors **a** and **b** reveal which frequencies contribute to the interaction.

4.9 Thresholding Statistical Maps

In the first half of this chapter, we reviewed several approaches to creating statistical maps of brain activation in MEG distributed cortical imaging using the GLM methodology. Arbitrary thresholding of these maps can lead to different interpretations of brain activation (Figure 4.6) and undermine the validity of a functional neuroimaging study. Objective assessment of the statistic maps requires a principled approach to identifying regions of activation. This involves testing thousands of hypotheses

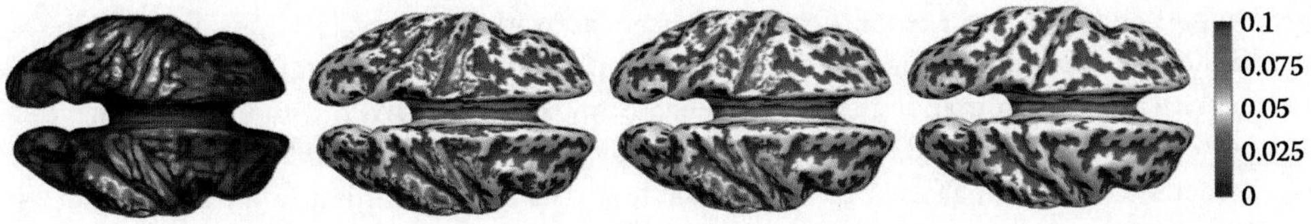

FIGURE 4.6 **(See color insert.)** A statistic map thresholded at several arbitrary levels. Do both hemispheres show experimental effects, or just the right one? Interpretation of these activation results clearly depends on principled selection of the threshold for significance.

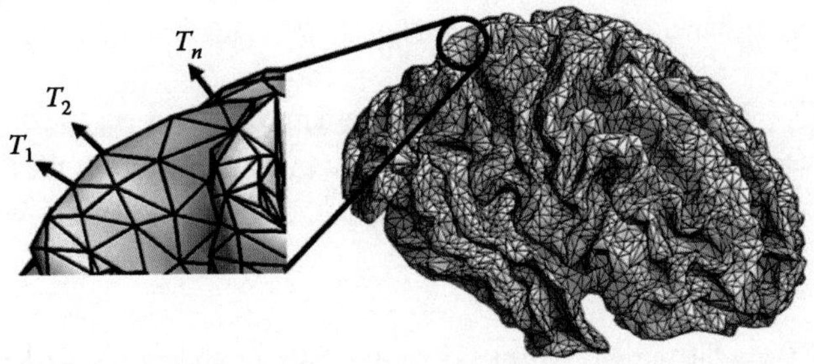

FIGURE 4.7 A statistical map typically consists of activation measures at thousands of voxels T_i on the brain surface. In the case of multidimensional statistical maps, we acquire activation measures for multiple time points and frequencies at each voxel.

(one for each spatial/temporal/frequency band or region of interest) for statistically significant experimental effects (Figure 4.7), and raises the possibility of large numbers of false-positives simply as a result of multiple hypothesis testing.

In the following, we first define measures of false-positives and show the important role that the maximum statistic plays in statistical inference. We then describe the Bonferroni correction, random field theory (RFT), permutation methods, and false discovery error rate (FDR), which provide corrected thresholds for statistical maps.

4.9.1 False-Positive Measures

Thresholding statistical maps should control some measure of the false-positive rate that takes into account the multiple hypothesis tests. Several measures of false-positives have been proposed, the most popular of which is the familywise error rate (FWER), that is, the probability of making at least one false-positive under the null hypothesis that there is no experimental effect. The Bonferroni method and two approaches based on the maximum statistic distribution, RFT and permutation tests, control the FWER. Another measure that is becoming increasingly popular is FDR, which controls the expected proportion of errors among the rejected hypotheses. Other measures of false-positives exist, such as positive false discovery rate, false discovery rate confidence, and per-family error rate confidence (Nichols and Hayasaka, 2003), but they are not as common and not covered in this chapter.

There are two types of FWER control: weak and strong. In *weak FWER control*, false-positives are controlled only when the complete null hypothesis holds, that is, when there is no experimental effect at any location in the brain. If a cortical site (or a temporal/spectral band) is truly active, control of false-positives is not guaranteed anywhere in the brain. Effectively, this implies that with weak FWER control we cannot achieve any localization of an experimental effect, but rather only reject the complete null hypothesis. Conversely, in *strong FWER control*, the false-positives are controlled for any subset where the null hypothesis holds. So, even if there is true brain activation at some locations, false-positives are still controlled at the other locations, and therefore we can localize experimental effects. Fortunately, the Bonferroni, RFT, and permutation methods achieve strong control of FWER, and therefore have localization power. On the other hand, the FDR method only has weak control of FWER.

FWER methods control the false-positives at an α level, typically 5%. This means that with 100 repetitions of the entire experiment only 5 of them will have one or more false-positives, or type I errors, at any location in the brain. We now investigate how the FWER is related to the maximum statistic.

4.9.2 Maximum Statistic

The FWER is directly related to the maximum value in the statistical image; one or more voxels T_i will exceed the threshold u_α under the null hypothesis H_0 only if the maximum exceeds that threshold:

$$\begin{aligned} P(\text{FWER}) &= P(\cup_i \{T_i \geq u_\alpha\} \mid H_0) \quad \text{(Probability that any voxel exceeds the threshold)} \\ &= P(\max_i T_i \geq u_\alpha \mid H_0) \quad \text{(Probability that max voxel exceeds the threshold)} \\ &= 1 - F_{\max T|H_0}(u_\alpha) \quad \text{(1 – cumulative density function of max voxel)} \\ &= 1 - (1 - \alpha) = \alpha \end{aligned} \tag{4.13}$$

where $F_{\max} T|H_0$ is the cumulative density function of the maximum statistic under the null. Therefore, we can control the FWER if we choose the threshold u_α to be in the $(1 - \alpha)$100th percentile of the maximum distribution (Figure 4.8).

To control FWER, random field theory estimates the right tail of the maximum statistic distribution using a topological measure called the Euler Characteristic. Permutation tests, on the other hand, resample the data to estimate the empirical distribution of the maximum statistic. The Bonferroni method relies on the Bonferroni inequality and makes no use of the maximum distribution described here.

Rather than use the statistic value directly, these can first be converted to p-values by either assuming a parametric distribution or estimating an empirical distribution at each location (Pantazis et al., 2005b). In cases where the distribution of the statistic is spatially variant, p-values can improve control of FWER. We then use the distribution of the minimum p-value for control of FWER. As we see below, p-values are also used when controlling the FDR.

4.9.3 Bonferroni Correction

The simplest approach to controlling the FWER is the Bonferroni correction method (Hochberg and Tamhane, 1987; Nichols and Hayasaka, 2003). It is based on the Bonferroni inequality and assumes independence of each of the multiple hypothesis tests; under dependency Bonferroni is still valid but can be very conservative. To control false-positives at an α level, we threshold each voxel separately at the $\alpha_b = \alpha/V$ level, where V is the total number of voxels.

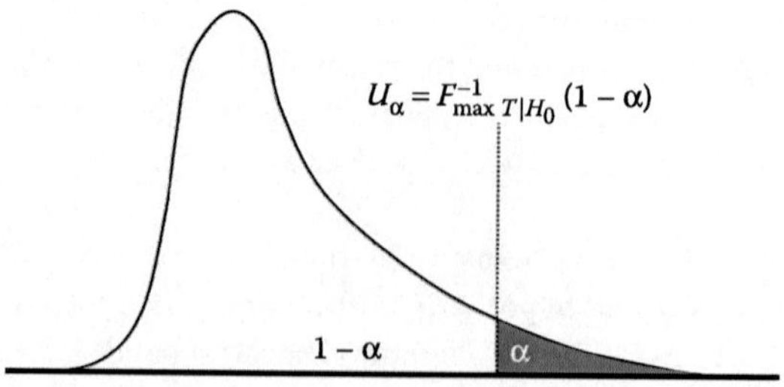

FIGURE 4.8 **(See color insert.)** Probability density function of the maximum statistic. By choosing a threshold u_α which leaves only α (typically 5%) of the distribution to the right of u_α, we control the FWER at level α.

$$
\begin{aligned}
P(\text{FWER}) &= P(\cup_i \{T_i \geq u_{\alpha_b}\} \mid H_0) \\
&\leq \sum_i P(T_i \geq u_{\alpha_b}\} \mid H_0) \quad \text{(Bonferroni in equality)} \\
&= \sum_i \alpha_b \\
&= \sum_i \alpha / V = \alpha
\end{aligned}
\tag{4.14}
$$

The Bonferroni method requires the estimation of the marginal distribution at each location in the statistical map, or equivalently, its conversion into a p-value map. We can do this either parametrically, by assuming, for example, a Gaussian t, or F distribution at each voxel, or nonparametrically, by resampling the data using a permutation scheme and estimating the empirical distribution separately at each voxel. In Figure 4.11, we estimated the distributions using the later approach. Since the cortical surface was defined using 7501 nodes, the Bonferroni adjusted 5% level threshold was $\alpha_b = 0.05/7501 = 6.66 \cdot 10^{-6}$ and no voxel exceeded this very small threshold.

This is not surprising as the Bonferroni method produces very conservative thresholds unless the tests are independent or has weak dependency (Nichols and Hayasaka, 2003). This is rarely if ever the case in MEG since the number of MEG sensors rarely exceeds a few hundred, while the number of voxels in a statistical map may number several thousand. The inverse procedure that maps from sensors into brain space will inevitably introduce correlation among voxels. Many Bonferroni variants have been proposed, such as the Kounias inequality and step-up or step-down procedures (Hochberg and Tamhane, 1987). However, they offer little improvement over the original Bonferroni method.

4.9.4 Random Field Methods

As shown in Equation 4.13, the FWER can be determined directly from the probability distribution of the maximum statistic. Adler (1981) demonstrated that the expected value of the Euler Characteristic (EC), a topological measure of the suprathreshold region of a statistical map, is a good approximation of this probability when the threshold is large. Therefore, random field theory (RFT) approximates the upper tail of the maximum distribution $F_{\max}T$ using the expected value of the EC of the thresholded image (Worsley et al., 1996). Computational procedures for calculating this value are implemented in several software packages for analysis of functional imaging data (SPM—http://www.fil.ion.ucl.ac.uk, VoxBo—http://www.voxbo.org, and FSL—http://www.fmrib.ox.ac.uk/fsl among others), and are widely used in fMRI and PET functional neuroimaging studies.

Worsley et al. (1996) provides a formula for the expected value of the EC that unifies the results for all types of random fields:

$$
\begin{aligned}
P(\text{FWER}) &= P(\cup_i \{T_i \geq u\} \mid H_0) \\
&\approx \sum_{d=0}^{D} R_d(S)\rho_d(u)
\end{aligned}
\tag{4.15}
$$

This equation gives the probability of an FWER for threshold u in a D-dimensional random field T_i in a search region S, which can be the cortical surface ($D = 2$) or the brain volume ($D = 3$). The term $R_d(S)$ is the d-dimensional RESEL (RESolution Element) count, a unitless quantity that depends on the smoothness of the statistical map in the search region S under the null hypothesis (Figure 4.9). The term $\rho_d(u)$ is the EC density that depends only on the threshold u and the type of statistical field (such as z, t, χ^2, and Hotelling's T^2). In Equation 4.15, the lower dimensional terms ($d < D$) compensate for the case when the excursion set, that is, the regions of voxels in a field above a threshold u, touches the boundary. They can usually be omitted because they have only a small impact on the RESEL count.

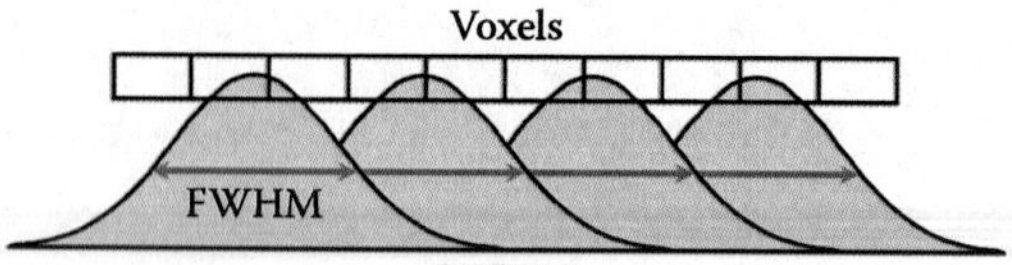

FIGURE 4.9 **(See color insert.)** Random field theory uses the topological features of a statistical map to convert the voxels into RESELS, a dimensionless quantity that represents the image with interpretable units of smoothness. Under the null hypothesis of no experimental effects, it is the degree of spatial correlation in the noise in the statistical maps that determines the RESEL count.

While in fMRI and PET the random fields can be assumed to be statistically stationary, in MEG we need to compensate for nonstationarity in the spatial, temporal, and spectral dimensions (Worsley et al., 1999), both for maximum statistic inference and cluster size tests (Hayasaka et al., 2004). Such corrections in the spatial dimension were applied by Pantazis et al. (2005b) and Barnes and Hillbrand (2003) to threshold 2D cortical maps and 3D volumetric maps, respectively. Singh et al. (2003) and Park et al. (2002) used RFT as implemented in the SPM software to threshold beamformer and LORETA (Pascual-Marqui et al., 1994) volumetric maps from a multisubject MEG/EEG study. Kilner et al. (2005) used single channel EEG data to create time–frequency maps that were thresholded with SPM under the assumption of stationarity. Finally, Carbonell et al. (2004b) applied RFT on a 1D Hotelling T^2 statistical map created from multichannel EEG data in the temporal dimension.

To derive corrected thresholds for statistical maps, RFT relies on several assumptions including the following: the image has the same parametric distribution at each spatial location, the point spread function has two derivatives at the origin, the field has sufficient smoothness to justify application of continuous RFT, and the threshold is sufficiently high for the asymptotic results to be accurate. When these assumptions hold, RFT is a very powerful method; when this is not possible, for example with statistical maps of nonstandard distributions, nonparametric alternatives should be considered.

To apply RFT in Figure 4.11, the statistical map was first smoothed with the Laplace–Beltrami operator (Chung, 2001), a generalization of Gaussian smoothing on an arbitrary Riemannian manifold. The spatial filtering corresponded to a 16.7 mm full-width half-maximum (FWHM). Since the mean distance between the vertices in the tessellated cortical surface was 5.7 mm, the spatial filtering was equivalent to 2.93 vertices FWHM, which is considered sufficient when smoothing 3D Gaussian images (Hayasaka and Nichols, 2003). On the smoothed statistical map, RFT produced 334.91 RESELS from 7501 cortical vertices or voxels. Using Equation 4.15, the adjusted 5% level threshold was 4.12.

RFT results are available not only for the maximum statistic (peak statistic height), but also for the size of a cluster, the number of clusters, and joint inference on peak height and cluster size (Poline et al., 1997; Hayasaka and Nichols, 2004; Hayasaka et al., 2004). Furthermore, the theory is applicable to the multivariate analog of the F-statistic, Roy's maximum root, and therefore multivariate GLM modeling can also be used in conjunction with RFT (Worsley et al., 2004).

4.9.5 Permutation Methods

The standard approach to permutation tests is to find units exchangeable under the null hypothesis. Units are exchangeable if by randomly rearranging these units we can create permutation samples that are statistically equivalent under the null hypothesis to the original data. The simplest example involves a study in which we want to detect differences between two experimental conditions. Under the null hypothesis that there is no difference, epochs from the two conditions can be exchanged, provided that equal numbers of samples (in time, space, and frequency) are collected under each condition.

A test statistic is computed from each permutation sample that, including the statistic representing the original data, constitute the reference set for determining significance. The proportion of data permutations in the reference set that have test statistic values greater than or equal to the value for the experimentally obtained results are the *p*-value (significance or probability value). An excellent treatment of permutation tests can be found in Edgington (1995) and Nichols and Holmes (2001).

For FWER control, the test statistic is the maximum in the statistical map. Therefore, unlike the RFT approach, which estimates the upper tail of the maximum distribution based on geometrical features of a parametric statistical map, permutation methods resample the data and create an empirical maximum distribution. By setting a threshold at the α100th percentile of the upper tail of the empirical distribution, we have exact control of the FWER.

Since the permutation samples must be statistically equivalent to the original data, permutations that destroy the inherent correlation structure of the MEG data are not allowed. For example, we cannot exchange channel labels or randomize time-series because the spatial or temporal structure would be altered. Therefore, it is important to apply valid permutation schemes for both single-subject and multisubject studies.

In single-subject studies, permutations are feasible between experimental conditions (Maris and Oostenveld, 2007). The MEG data are assigned to conditions either beforehand, with respect to the baseline and types of stimuli provided, or on-the-fly based on the subject's responses, such as fast/slow button presses. In between-trials design, every trial is assigned to one experimental condition; in within-trials design every trial is assigned to multiple experimental conditions in different time segments. The latter is far more common, as a baseline is typically included before the presentation of a stimulus, and therefore a single trial has two conditions. Most researchers are willing to assume statistical independence between MEG trials or between nonoverlapping time segments within trials, especially if they are separated by some minimum time interval, and thus satisfy the exchangeability requirement. Figure 4.10 shows an example permutation scheme used in Pantazis et al. (2005b) to threshold minimum-norm cortical maps while controlling for false-positives.

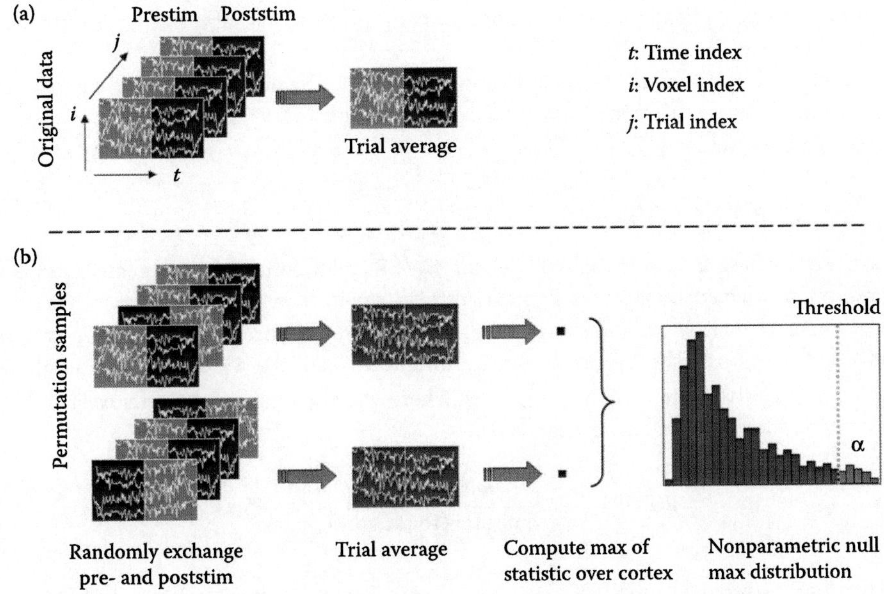

FIGURE 4.10 **(See color insert.)** Permutation scheme on a single-subject multitrial MEG study. (a) Averaging of original statistical maps. (b) Generation of permutation samples by randomly exchanging pre- and poststimulus conditions within each trial. An empirical distribution of the maximum statistic is generated by averaging the permuted trials and computing the max over the cortex. The α level threshold at the upper tail of the empirical distribution is applied to the original averaged data to control the FWER.

In multisubject studies, permutations are only performed on the second-level GLM for random effect statistical inference (see Section 4.6). In the simple summary statistic approach in Equation 4.10, each subject's estimated contrast $c^T \hat{b}_k$ is assumed to have a symmetric distribution around zero under the null hypothesis. Therefore, randomly multiplying it by 1 or −1 does not change its distribution under the null hypothesis. With K subjects (and thus K contrasts), a total of 2^K permutation samples can be created, which can then each be fitted to the second-level GLM to estimate permuted group parameters that are used in turn to estimate the empirical distribution of the group-averaged map. Such an approach was followed for example by Singh et al. (2003); Pantazis et al. (2007). Unfortunately, with small K the empirical distribution may be coarsely quantized and more subjects may be necessary to achieve a desired FWER control.

Permutation tests have many advantages. They are exact, that is, give precise control of FWER, they do not assume parametric distributions, they adapt to underlying correlation patterns in the data, and they are very flexible as any test statistic can be used. The only assumptions required are those to justify permuting the labels of the conditions, such as that the distributions under the null hypothesis have the same shape or are symmetric. Even though we are free to consider any statistic summarizing evidence for the effect of interest at each location, it is usually best to use the same statistics for a nonparametric approach as we would for a comparable parametric approach. The reason is that parametric statistics often have optimal power; for example, a t-statistic is the most powerful in detecting differences between populations in many circumstances. Furthermore, to achieve uniform specificity, that is, equal chances of false-positives at any location in the statistical map, we should use statistics that have approximately homogeneous null permutation distributions.

On account of their flexibility, permutation tests are more commonly used in MEG than the parametric RFT. Permutation tests have been proposed to control false-positives in the channel domain: (Blair and Karnisky, 1993, 1994; Karnisky et al., 1994; Galan et al., 1997; Achim, 2001; Maris, 2004) and in the source domain: (Park et al., 2002; Pantazis et al., 2003, 2005b; Singh et al., 2003; Chau et al., 2004; Sekihara et al., 2005). These methods have been applied in multiple MEG studies: (Kaiser et al., 2000; Lutzenberger et al., 2002; Pantazis et al., 2005a, 2007; Bayless et al., 2006; Cheyne et al., 2006; Itier et al., 2006). Reviews on the application of permutation tests in MEG are available in Maris and Oostenveld (2007), Maris et al. (2007).

Various thresholding methods are illustrated in Figure 4.11. The permutation method was based on that described in Pantazis et al. (2005b) and produced a threshold of 3.99, which controls FWER over the whole cortex at a 5% level.

4.9.6 Control of False Discovery Rate

In contrast to the above methods that control the FWER, FDR controls the expected proportion of errors among the rejected hypotheses Pantazis et al. (2005b). For example, if we set $\alpha = 5\%$ FDR threshold, then on average we should expect 5% of our suprathreshold voxels to be false-positives.

The standard FDR method proposed by (Benjamini and Hochberg, 1995; Genovese et al., 2002) is conservative, as it controls the FDR at a $\frac{V_0}{V}\alpha$ level, where V is the total number of voxels and V_0 is the number of voxels where the null hypothesis is true:

$$E(\text{FDR}) = E\left(\frac{\text{False positives}}{\text{Suprathreshold voxels}}\right) \leq \frac{V_0}{V}\alpha \tag{4.16}$$

When the true brain activation extends over broad areas, V_0 may become small and the FDR procedure too conservative. Thus, a number of adaptive procedures improve on the original FDR approach by first estimating V_0, and then using this estimate to tighten the threshold (Benjamini et al., 2006).

The FDR methods adapt to the properties of the data; when a large number of voxels are truly active, the threshold will adjust to allow for more false-positives; when no truly activated voxels exist, FDR controls the FWER, but in a weak sense (see Section 4.9.1). They are more powerful than Bonferroni,

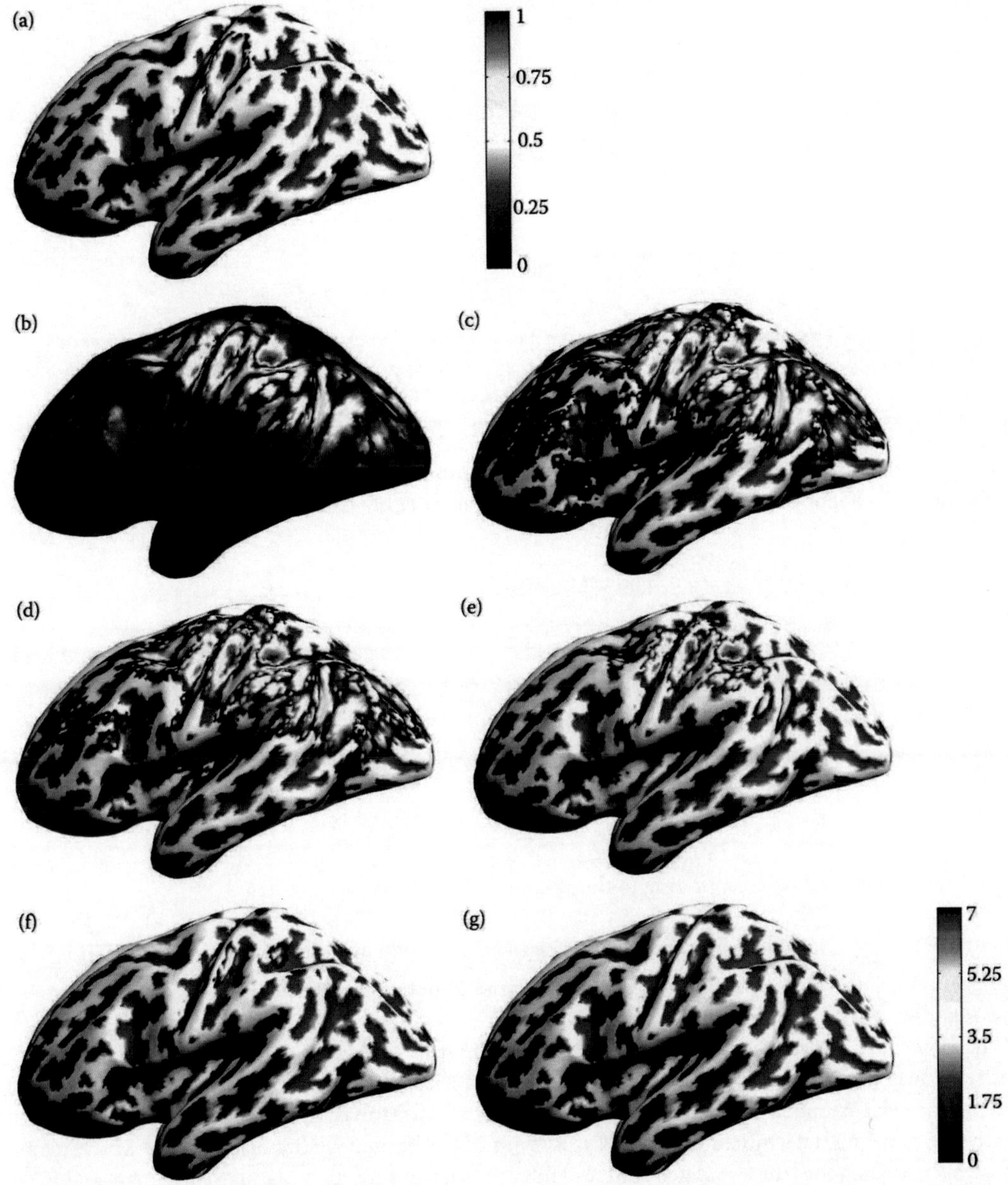

FIGURE 4.11 **(See color insert.)** Simulated MEG source on the left hemisphere and reconstructed dSPM statistical map, thresholded using several methods to control false-positives. (a) Simulated sources, (b) statistical map, (c) uncorrected, (d) FDR, (e) permutations, (f) random field, and (g) Bonferroni. Uncorrected thresholding (p-value = 0.05) and FDR (p-value = 0.0065) produced many false-positives. Permutations and random field theory gave 5% FWER thresholds $t = 3.99$ and $t = 4.12$, respectively. The Bonferroni approach was very conservative (p-value 0.05/7501 = 6.6610^{-6}) and did not identify the source.

random field, and permutation control of FWER, and for this reason may become popular for thresholding MEG maps.

The FDR approach requires the estimation of the marginal distribution at each location in the statistical map, or equivalently, conversion of the statistic value at each location into an equivalent p-value. We can do this parametrically or nonparametrically, as described for the Bonferroni approach.

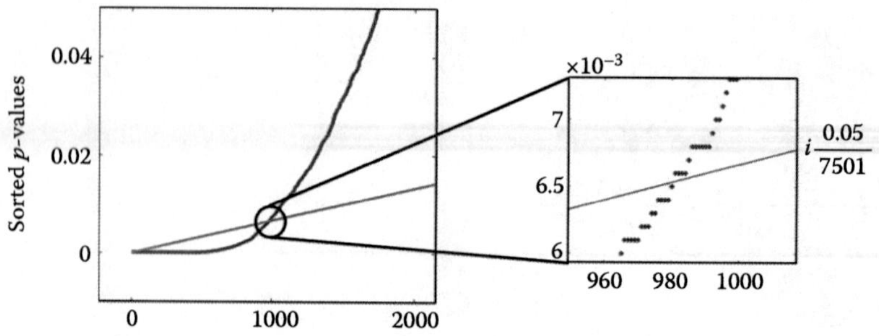

FIGURE 4.12 **(See color insert.)** Graphical representation of the FDR procedure. The blue line represents the sorted p-values of the statistical map in Figure 4.11, and the red line is $i\ \alpha/V = i\ 0.05/7501$. The largest p-value below the line is 0.0065 and corresponds to a 5% level FDR threshold.

Once the maps are converted to p-values, implementation of the standard FDR method is relatively straightforward (Genovese et al., 2002). If V is the total number of voxels being tested, the procedure is as follows:

1. Order the voxel p-values from smallest to largest:

$$P_{(1)} \leq P_{(2)} \leq \cdots \leq P_{(V)} \tag{4.17}$$

2. Let r be the largest i for which

$$P_{(i)} \leq \frac{i}{V} \frac{\alpha}{c(V)} \tag{4.18}$$

3. Declare all voxels corresponding to the p-values $P_{(1)}, \ldots P_{(r)}$ active.

where $c(V) = \sum_{i=1}^{V} 1/i$ if no assumptions on the joint distribution of the p-values across voxels is made, and $c(V) = 1$ if the p-values in different voxels are independent or they have positive dependence (Benjamini and Yekutieli, 2001).

The procedure is demonstrated graphically in Figure 4.12 for the FDR procedure applied to the statistical map in Figure 4.11. The estimated threshold for 7501 cortical voxels at the 5% level was 0.065, and produced an extended region of suprathreshold voxels. Unfortunately, the large extent of the significantly active region determined using FDR is a result of the limited spatial resolution of MEG; many voxels surrounding the true simulated source exhibit significant activity in the statistical map, and FDR is sensitive enough to identify them. Conversely, the more conservative thresholds from FWER control tend to reduce the size of activated regions as also shown in Figure 4.11. Other examples of the application of FDR in MEG maps include Edwards et al. (2005); Jacobs et al. (2006); Pantazis et al. (2007); Jacques and Rossion (2007).

4.10 Discussion

We have presented a GLM framework to produce statistical maps from MEG distributed cortical imaging, and subsequently threshold them while controlling for false-positives. Choosing a thresholding method depends on the data available: Bonferroni is simple and efficient for a small number of tests with minimal dependence; random fields are robust when their parametric assumptions are satisfied and strong correlation exists in the data; permutation tests are very general, adapt to the underlying data correlations, can use any statistic, and are more powerful than random fields for data with low degrees of freedom (e.g., studies with a few subjects); FDR is more powerful, works well with sparse signals, and recommended when we can afford a few false-positives. However as we have shown in our simulations, FDR can produce large regions of significant activation as a result of the limited resolution of MEG inverses.

A number of important statistical issues are beyond the scope of this chapter such as conjunction analysis (Nichols et al., 2005), that is, the identification of brain areas that are simultaneously active in multiple tasks, extraction of confidence intervals for distributed solutions using the bootstrap (DiNocera and Ferlazzo, 2000; Gross et al., 2003; Darvas et al., 2005), and thresholding using cluster size tests (Hayasaka et al., 2004). Also, the theory was developed for distributed inverse methods in MEG. However, discrete solutions are also popular in MEG, especially with well-localized activation when a few equivalent current dipoles can represent most cortical activity. In this case alternative approaches can be used to establish significance, for example the bootstrap resampling approach or Monte Carlo simulations to find localization accuracy and confidence intervals for current dipoles (Braun et al., 1997; Darvas et al., 2005).

A related problem in MEG data analysis is testing for the statistical significance of cortical interactions (Gross et al., 2001; Varela et al., 2001; Hui and Leahy, 2006; Jerbi et al., 2007b; Maris et al., 2007). In some cases, a few cortical locations are investigated and corrections for multiple comparisons are generally not employed. In the case where tests are made for interactions between multiple pairs of locations, the theory described in this chapter can be applied. The DICS algorithm, for example, can be used to investigate cortical coherence at all locations in the cortex relative to a reference, which may be a single cortical location or an electromyograph reference signal (Gross et al., 2001). The resulting maps are a measure of coherence at each cortical location for a single frequency band but can be easily extended to multiple frequency bands. The methods described in this chapter for analysis of time–frequency representations of brain activity can be adapted to testing for significant activation in these coherence maps.

References

Achim, A., 2001. Statistical detection of between-group differences in event-related potentials. *Clinical Neurophysiology* 112, 1023–1034.

Adler, R. J. (ed.), 1981. *The Geometry of Random Fields*. New York: Wiley.

Baillet, S., Mosher, J. C., Leahy, R. M., 2001. Electromagnetic brain mapping. *IEEE Signal Processing Magazine* 18, 14–30.

Barnes, G. R., Hillbrand, A., 2003. Statistical flattening of MEG beamformer images. *Human Brain Mapping* 18, 1–12.

Bayless, S. J., Gaetz, W. C., Cheyne, D. O., Taylor, M. J., 2006. Spatiotemporal analysis of feedback processing during a card sorting task using spatially filtered MEG. *Neuroscience Letters* 410, 31–36.

Beckmann, C. F., Jenkinson, M., Smith, S. M., 2003. General multilevel linear modeling for group analysis in fMRI. *NeuroImage* 20(2), 1052–1063.

Benjamini, Y., Heller, R., 2007. Screening for partial conjunction hypotheses. Technical Report RP-SOR-06-06, http://www.math.tau.ac.il/departments/st/.

Benjamini, Y., Hochberg, Y., 1995. Controlling the false discovery rate: A practical and powerful approach to multiple testing. *Journal of the Royal Statistical Society* 57, 289–300.

Benjamini, Y., Krieger, A. M., Yekutieli, D., 2006. Adaptive linear step-up procedures that control the false discovery rate. *Biometrica* 93(3), 491–507.

Benjamini, Y., Yekutieli, D., 2001. The control of the false discovery rate in multiple testing under dependency. *The Annals of Statistics* 29(4), 1165–1188.

Blair, R. C., Karnisky, W., 1993. An alternative method for significance testing of waveform difference potentials. *Psychophysiology* 30, 518–524.

Blair, R. C., Karnisky, W., 1994. Distribution-free statistical analyses of surface and volumetric maps. *Functional Neuroimaging: Technical Foundations* (R. W. Thatcher, M. Hallett, T. Zeffiro, E. R. Jony, M. Huerta, eds.), San Diego, California: Academic Press, pp. 19–28.

Braun, C., Kaiser, S., Kinces, W., Elbert, T., 1997. Confidence interval of single dipole locations based on EEG data. *Brain Topography* 10(1), 31–39.

Brookes, M., Gibson, A., Hall, S., Furlong, P., Barnes, G., Hillebrand, A., Singh, K., Holliday, I., Francis, S., Morris, P., 2004. A general linear model for MEG beamformer imaging. *NeuroImage* 23(3), 936–946.

Brooks, M. J., Gibson, A. M., Hall, S. D., Furlong, P. L., Barnes, G. R., Hillebrand, A., Singh, K. D., Holliday, I. E., Francis, S. T., Morris, P. G., 2004. A general linear model for MEG beamformer imaging. *NeuroImage* 23, 936–946.

Brovelli, A., Ding, M., Ledberg, A., Chen, Y., Nakamura, R., Bressler, S., 2004. Beta oscillations in a large-scale sensorimotor cortical network: Directional influences revealed by Granger causality. *Proceedings of the National Academy of Sciences of the United States of America* 101(26), 9849.

Bruns, A., 2004. Fourier-, Hilbert- and wavelet-based signal analysis: Are they really different approaches? *Journal of Neuroscience Methods* 137, 321–332.

Bruns, A., Eckhorn, R., 2004. Task-related coupling from high-to low-frequency signals among visual cortical areas in human subdural recordings. *International Journal of Psychophysiology* 51(2), 97–116.

Canolty, R., Edwards, E., Dalal, S., Soltani, M., Nagarajan, S., Kirsch, H., Berger, M., Barbaro, N., Knight, R., 2006. High gamma power is phase-locked to theta oscillations in human neocortex. *Science* 313(5793), 1626.

Carbonell, F., Galan, L., Valdes, P., Worsley, K., Biscay, R., Diaz-Comas, L., Bobes, M., Parra, M., 2004a. Random field-union intersection tests for EEG/MEG imaging. *NeuroImage* 22(1), 268–276.

Carbonell, F., Galan, L., Valdes, P., Worsley, K., Biscay, R. J., Diaz-Comas, L., Bobes, M. A., Parra, M., 2004b. Random field—Union intersection tests for EEG/MEG imaging. *NeuroImage* 22, 268–276.

Carlson, T., Schrater, P., He, S., 2003. Patterns of activity in the categorical representations of objects. *Journal of Cognitive Neuroscience* 15(5), 704–717.

Chau, W., McIntosh, A. R., Robinson, S. E., Schulz, M., Pantev, C., 2004. Improving permutation test power for group analysis of spatially filtered MEG data. *NeuroImage* 23, 983–996.

Cheyne, D., Bakhtazad, L., Gaetz, W., 2006. Spatiotemporal mapping of cortical activity accompanying voluntary movements using an event-related beamforming approach. *Human Brain Mapping* 27, 213–229.

Christensen, G. E., Johnson, H. J., 2001. Consistent image registration. *IEEE Transactions on Medical Imaging* 20(7), 568–582.

Chung, M. K., 2001. Statistical morphometry in neuroanatomy. Ph.D. thesis, McGill University, Montreal.

Cox, D., Savoy, R., 2003. Functional magnetic resonance imaging (fMRI). *NeuroImage* 19(2), 261–270.

Dalal, S., Sekihara, K., Nagarajan, S., 2006. Modified beamformers for coherent source region suppression. *IEEE Transactions on Biomedical Engineering* 53(7), 1357–1363.

Dale, A. M., Liu, A. K., Fischi, R. B., Buckner, R. L., Belliveau, J. W., Lewine, J. D., Halgren, E., 2000. Dynamic statistical parametric mapping: Combining fMRI and MEG for high-resolution imaging of cortical activity. *Neuron* 26, 55–67.

Darvas, F., Rautiainen, M., Pantazis, D., Baillet, S., Benali, H., Mosher, J. C., Garnero, L., Leahy, R. M., 2005. Investigations of dipole localization accuracy in MEG using the bootstrap. *NeuroImage* 25, 355–368.

De Lange, F., Jensen, O., Bauer, M., Toni, I., 2008. Interactions between posterior gamma and frontal alpha/beta oscillations during imagined actions. *Frontiers in Human Neuroscience* 2, 1–12.

DiNocera, F., Ferlazzo, F., 2000. Resampling approach to statistical inference: Bootstrapping from event-related potentials data. *Behavioral Research Methods, Instruments and Computers* 32(1), 111–119.

Durka, P., Zygierewicz, J., Klekowicz, H., Ginter, J., Blinowska, K., 2004. On the statistical significance of event-related EEG desynchronization and synchronization in the time-frequency plane. *IEEE Transactions on Biomedical Engineering* 51(7), 1167–1175.

Edgington, E. S. (ed.)., 1995. *Randomization Tests*. London, UK: Academic Press.

Edwards, E., Soltani, M., Deouell, L. Y., Berger, M. S., Knight, R. T., 2005. High gamma activity in response to deviant auditory stimuli recorded directly from human cortex. *Journal of Neurophysiology* 94, 4269–4280.

Fischl, B., Serano, M., Tootell, R., Dale, A. M., 1999. High-resolution intersubject averaging and a coordinate system for the cortical surface. *Human Brain Mapping* 8(4), 272–284.

Fisher, R., 1950. *Statistical Methods for Research Workers*, 11th edition. Edinburgh, UK: McGraw-Hill/Appleton and Lange.

Fries, P., 2005. A mechanism for cognitive dynamics: Neuronal communication through neuronal coherence. *Trends in Cognitive Sciences* 9(10), 474–480.

Friston, K., Holmes, A., Price, C., Bqchel, C., Worsley, K., 1999. Multisubject fMRI studies and conjunction analyses. *NeuroImage* 10, 385–396.

Friston, K., Holmes, A., Worsley, K., Poline, J., Frith, C., Frackowiak, R., 1995a. Statistical parametric maps in functional imaging: A general linear approach. *Human Brain Mapping* 2(4), 189–210.

Friston, K. J., Holmes, A. P., Worsley, K. J., Poline, J. B., Frith, C., Frackowiak, R. S. J., 1995b. Statistical parametric maps in functional imaging: A general linear approach. *Human Brain Mapping* 2, 189–210.

Friston, K., Penny, W., Glaser, D., 2005. Conjunction revisited. *NeuroImage* 25, 661–667.

Friston, K. J., Penny, W., Phillips, C., Kiebel, S., Hinton, G., Ashburner, J., 2002. Classical and Bayesian inference in neuroimaging: Theory. *NeuroImage* 16, 465–483.

Friston, K. J., Stephan, K. M., Heather, J. D., Frith, C. D., Ioannides, A. A., Liu, L. C., Rugg, M. D. et al., 1996. A multivariate analysis of evoked responses in EEG and MEG data. *NeuroImage* 3, 167–174.

Fuchs, M., Wagner, M., Kohler, T., Wischmann, H., 1999. Linear and nonlinear current density reconstructions. *Journal of Clinical Neurophysiology* 16, 267–295.

Galan, L., Biscay, R., Rodriguez, J. L., Abalo, M. C. P., Rodriguez, R., 1997. Testing topographic differences between event related brain potentials by using non-parametric combinations of permutation tests. *Electroencephalography and clinical Neurophysiology* 102, 240–247.

Genovese, C., Lazar, N., Nichols, T., 2002. Thresholding of statistical maps in functional neuroimaging using the false discovery rate. *NeuroImage* 15, 870–878.

Gomez-Herrero, G., Atienza, M., Egiazarian, K., Cantero, J., 2008. Measuring directional coupling between EEG sources. *NeuroImage* 43(3), 497–508.

Gross, J., Kujala, J., Hamalainen, M., Timmermann, L., Schnitzler, A., Salmelin, R., 2001. Dynamic imaging of coherent sources: Studying neural interactions in the human brain. *Proceedings of National Academy of Sciences* 98(2), 694–699.

Gross, J., Timmermann, L., Kujala, J., Salmelin, R., Schnitzler, A., 2003. Properties of MEG tomographic maps obtained with spatial filtering. *NeuroImage* 19, 1329–1336.

Hamalainen, M. S., Ilmoniemi, R. J., 1984. Interpreting magnetic fields of the brain: Minimum norm estimates. *Medical and Biological Engineering and Computing* 32(1), 35–42.

Hayasaka, S., Nichols, T. E., 2003. Validating cluster size inference: Random field and permutation methods. *NeuroImage* 20(4), 2343–2356.

Hayasaka, S., Nichols, T. E., 2004. Combining voxel intensity and cluster extent with permutation test framework. *NeuroImage* 23(1), 54–63.

Hayasaka, S., Phan, K. L., Libarzon, I., Worsley, K. J., Nichols, T. E., 2004. Nonstationary cluster-size inference with random field and permutation methods. *NeuroImage* 22, 676–687.

Haynes, J., Rees, G., 2006. Decoding mental states from brain activity in humans. *Nature Reviews Neuroscience* 7(7), 523–534.

Heller, R., Golland, Y., Malach, R., Benjamini, Y., 2007. Conjunction group analysis: An alternative to mixed/random. *NeuroImage* 37, 1178–1185.

Hellier, P., Ashburner, J., Corouge, I., Barillot, C., Friston, K. J., 2002. Inter-subject registration of functional and anatomical data using textSPM. In: *Medical Image Computing and Computer-Assisted Intervention—MICCAI 2002*. Lecture Notes in Computer Science, Vol. 2489, Dohi, T. and Kikinis, R. (Eds). pp. 590–597, Berlin/Heidelberg: Springer.

Hochberg, Y., Tamhane, A. C. (eds.), 1987. *Multiple Comparison Procedures*. Newbury Park, California: Wiley.

Holmes, A., Friston, K. J., 1998. Generalisability, random effects and population inference. *NeuroImage* 7, S754.

Hui, H., Leahy, R., 2006. Linearly constrained MEG beamformers for MVAR modeling of cortical interactions. In: *3rd IEEE International Symposium on Biomedical Imaging: Nano to Macro, 2006*. pp. 237–240, Arlington, Virginia: Institute of Electrical and Electronics Engineers (IEEE).

Hui, H., Pantazis, D., Bressler, S., Leahy, R., 2010. Identifying true cortical interactions in MEG using the nulling beamformer. *NeuroImage* 49(4), 3161–3174.

Hummel, F., Gerloff, C., 2006. Interregional long-range and short-range synchrony: A basis for complex sensorimotor processing. *Event-related Dynamics of Brain Oscillations*, 159(2006), 223–236.

Itier, R. J., Herdman, A. T., George, N., Cheyne, D., Taylor, M. J., 2006. Inversion and contrast-reversal effects on face processing. *Brain Research* 1115, 108–120.

Jacobs, J., Hwang, G., Curran, T., Kahana, M. J., 2006. EEG oscillations and recognition memory: Theta correlates of memory retrieval and decision making. *NeuroImage* 32, 978–987.

Jacques, C., Rossion, B., 2007. Early electrophysiological responses to multiple face orientations correlate with individual discrimination performance in humans. *NeuroImage* 36, 863–876.

Jensen, O., Colgin, L., 2007. Cross-frequency coupling between neuronal oscillations. Trends in cognitive sciences 11(7), 267–269.

Jerbi, K., Bertrand, O., 2009. Cross-frequency coupling in parieto-frontal oscillatory networks during motor imagery revealed by magnetoencephalography. *Frontiers in Neuroscience* 3, 00011.

Jerbi, K., Lachaux, J., N'Diaye, K., Pantazis, D., Leahy, R. M., Garnero, L., and Baillet, S., 2007a. Coherent neural representation of hand speed in humans revealed by MEG imaging. *Proceedings of the National Academy of Sciences* 104(18), 7676.

Jerbi, K., Lachaux, J. P., N'Diaye, K., Pantazis, D., Leahy, R. M., Garnero, L., 2007b. Coherent neural representation of hand speed in humans revealed by MEG imaging. *PNAS* 104(18), 7676–7681.

Joshi, A. A., Shattuck, D. W., Thompson, P. M., Leahy, R. M., April 12–15 2007a. A finite element method for elastic parameterization and alignment of cortical surfaces using sulcal constraints. In: *Biomedical Imaging: From Macro to Nano, 2007. 4th IEEE International Symposium*. pp. 640–643, Arlington, Virginia: Institute of Electrical and Electronics Engineers (IEEE).

Joshi, A. A., Shattuck, D.W., Thompson, P. M., Leahy, R. M., 2007b. Surface constrained volumetric brain registration using harmonic mappings. *IEEE Transactions on Medical Imaging* 26(12), 1657–1669.

Kaiser, J., Lutzenberger, W., Preissl, H., Mosshammer, D., Birbaumer, N., 2000. Statistical probability mapping reveals high-frequency magnetoencephalographic activity in supplementary motor area during self-paced finger movements. *Neuroscience Letters* 283(1), 81–84.

Kaminski, M., Ding, M., Truccolo, W., Bressler, S., 2001. Evaluating causal relations in neural systems: Granger causality, directed transfer function and statistical assessment of significance. *Biological Cybernetics* 85(2), 145–157.

Karnisky, W., Blair, R. C., Snider, A. D., 1994. An exact statistical method for comparing topographic maps with any number of subjects and electrodes. *Brain Topography* 6, 203–210.

Kiebel, S., 2003. The general linear model. In: Frackowiak, R., Friston, K., Frith, C., Dolan, R., Friston, K., Price, C., Zeki, S., Ashburner, J., Penny, W. (eds.), *Human Brain Function*, 2nd Edition. San Diego, California: Academic Press.

Kiebel, S., Tallon-Baudry, C., Friston, K., 2005a. Parametric analysis of oscillatory activity as measured with EEG/MEG. *Human Brain Mapping* 26(3), 170–177.

Kiebel, S. J., Friston, K. J., 2004. Statistical parametric mapping for event-related potentials: I. generic considerations. *NeuroImage* 22, 492–502.

Kiebel, S. J., Tallon-Baudry, C., Friston, K. J., 2005b. Parametric analysis of oscillatory activity as measured with EEG/MEG. *Human Brain Mapping* 26, 170–177.

Kilner, J. M., Kiebel, S. J., Friston, K. J., 2005. Applications of random field theory to electrophysiology. *Neuroscience Letters* 374, 174–178.

Kriegeskorte, N., Goebel, R., Bandettini, P., 2006. Information-based functional brain mapping. *Proceedings of the National Academy of Sciences* 103(10), 3863.

Kucukaltun-Yildirim, E., Pantazis, D., Leahy, R., 2006. Task-based comparison of inverse methods in magnetoencephalography. *IEEE Transactions on Biomedical Engineering* 53(9), 1783–1793.

Kus, R., Kamniski, M., Blinowska, K., 2004. Determination of EEG activity propagation: Pair-wise versus multichannel estimate. *IEEE Transactions on Biomedical Engineering* 51(9), 1501–1510.

Lachaux, J., Rodriguez, E., Martinerie, J., Varela, F., 1999. Measuring phase synchrony in brain signals. *Human Brain Mapping* 8(4), 194–208.

Lakatos, P., Karmos, G., Mehta, A., Ulbert, I., Schroeder, C., 2008. Entrainment of neuronal oscillations as a mechanism of attentional selection. *Science* 320(5872), 110.

Lazar, N., Luna, B., Sweeney, J., Eddy, W., 2002. Combining brains: A survey of methods for statistical pooling of information. *NeuroImage* 16(2), 538–550.

Le Van Quyen, M., Foucher, J., Lachaux, J., Rodriguez, E., Lutz, A., Martinerie, J., Varela, F., 2001. Comparison of Hilbert transform and wavelet methods for the analysis of neuronal synchrony. *Journal of Neuroscience Methods* 111(2), 83–98.

Lin, F., Witzel, T., Hamalainen, M., Dale, A., Belliveau, J., Stufflebeam, S., 2004. Spectral spatiotemporal imaging of cortical oscillations and interactions in the human brain. *NeuroImage* 23(2), 582–595.

Lutzenberger, W., Ripper, B., Busse, L., Birbaumer, N., Kaiser, J., 2002. Dynamics of gamma-band activity during an audiospatial working memory task in humans. *Journal of Neuroscience* 22(13), 5630–5638.

Maris, E., 2004. Randomization tests for ERP topographies and whole spatiotemporal data matrices. *Psychophysiology* 41, 142–151.

Maris, E., Oostenveld, R., 2007. Nonparametric statistical testing of EEG- and MEG-data. *Journal of Neuroscience Methods* 164, 177–190.

Maris, E., Schoffelen, J.-M., Fries, P., 2007. Nonparametric statistical testing of coherence differences. *Journal of Neuroscience Methods* 163, 161–175.

Marzetti, L., Del Gratta, C., Nolte, G., 2008. Understanding brain connectivity from EEG data by identifying systems composed of interacting sources. *NeuroImage* 42(1), 87–98.

McNamee, R., Lazar, N., 2004. Assessing the sensitivity of FMRI group maps. *NeuroImage* 22(2), 920–931.

Monto, S., Palva, S., Voipio, J., Palva, J., 2008. Very slow EEG fluctuations predict the dynamics of stimulus detection and oscillation amplitudes in humans. *Journal of Neuroscience* 28(33), 8268.

Mormann, F., Fell, J., Axmacher, N., Weber, B., Lehnertz, K., Elger, C., Fernandez, G., 2005. Phase/amplitude reset and theta-gamma interaction in the human medial temporal lobe during a continuous word recognition memory task. *Hippocampus* 15(7), 890–900.

Mosher, J. C., Leahy, R. M., 1998. Recursive MUSIC: A framework for EEG and MEG source localization. *IEEE Transactions of Biomedical Engineering* 45(11), 1342–1354.

Mumford, J. A., Nichols, T., 2006. Modeling and inference of multisubject fMRI data. *IEEE Engineering in Medicine and Biology Magazine* 25(2), 42–51.

Nichols, T., Brett, M., Andersson, J., Wager, T., Poline, J.-B., 2005. Valid conjunction inference with the minimum statistic. *NeuroImage* 25, 653–660.

Nichols, T. E., Hayasaka, S., 2003. Controlling the familywise error rate in functional neuroimaging: A comparative review. *Statistical Methods in Medical Research* 12(5), 419–446.

Nichols, T. E., Holmes, A. P., 2001. Nonparametric permutation tests for functional neuroimaging: A primer with examples. *Human Brain Mapping* 15, 1–25.

Nolte, G., Bai, O., Wheaton, L., Mari, Z., Vorbach, S., Hallett, M., 2004. Identifying true brain interaction from EEG data using the imaginary part of coherency. *Clinical Neurophysiology* 115(10), 2292–2307.

Norman, K., Polyn, S., Detre, G., Haxby, J., 2006. Beyond mind-reading: Multivoxel pattern analysis of fMRI data. *Trends in Cognitive Sciences* 10(9), 424–430.

Nunez, P., Srinivasan, R., Westdorp, A., Wijesinghe, R., Tucker, D., Silberstein, R., Cadusch, P., 1997. EEG coherency. I: Statistics, reference electrode, volume conduction, Laplacians, cortical imaging, and interpretation at multiple scales. *Electroencephalography and Clinical Neurophysiology* 103(5), 499–515.

Osipova, D., Hermes, D., Jensen, O., 2008. Gamma power is phase-locked to posterior alpha activity. *PLoS One* 3(12), 1–7.

Palva, J., Palva, S., Kaila, K., 2005. Phase synchrony among neuronal oscillations in the human cortex. *Journal of Neuroscience* 25(15), 3962.

Pantazis, D., Merrifield, W., Darvas, F., Sutherling, W., Leahy, R. M., 2005a. Hemispheric language dominance using MEG cortical imaging and non-parametric statistical analysis. *WSEAS Transactions on Biology and Biomedicine* 2(3), 318325.

Pantazis, D., Nichols, T. E., Baillet, S., Leahy, R. M., 2005b. A comparison of random field theory and permutation methods for the statistical analysis of MEG data. *NeuroImage* 25(2), 383–394.

Pantazis, D., Nichols, T. E., Baillet, S., Leahy, R. M., July 2003. Spatiotemporal localization of significant activation in MEG using permutation tests. In: Taylor, C., Noble, J. A. (eds.), *Proceedings of the 18th Conference on Information Processing in Medical Imaging*. pp. 512–523.

Pantazis, D., Simpson, G., Weber, D., Dale, C., Nichols, T., Leahy, R., April 12–15 2007. Exploring human visual attention in an MEG study of a spatial cueing paradigm using a novel ANCOVA design. In: *2007 IEEE International Symposium on Biomedical Imaging: From Nano to Macro*.

Pantazis, D., Simpson, G., Weber, D., Dale, C., Nichols, T., Leahy, R., 2009. A novel ANCOVA design for analysis of MEG data with application to a visual attention study. *NeuroImage* 44(1), 164–174.

Pantazis, D., Weber, D., Dale, C., Nichols, T., G.V. Simpson, Leahy, R., 2005c. Imaging of oscillatory behavior in event-related MEG studies. In: Bouman, C., Miller, E. (eds.), *Proceedings of SPIE, Computational Imaging III*. Vol. 5674. pp. 55–63.

Park, H., Kwon, J., Youn, T., Pae, J., Kim, J., Kim, M., Ha, K., 2002. Statistical parametric mapping of LORETA using high density EEG and individual MRI: Application to mismatch negativities in schizophrenia. *Human Brain Mapping* 17, 168–178.

Pascual-Marqui, R. D., 2002. Standardized low resolution brain electromagnetic tomography (sLORETA): Technical details. *Methods and Findings in Experimental Clinical Pharmacology* 24D, 5–12.

Pascual-Marqui, R. D., Michel, C. M., Lehmann, D., 1994. Low resolution electromagnetic tomography: A new method for localizing electrical activity in the brain. *International Journal of Psychophysiology* 18, 49–65.

Penny, W., Duzel, E., Miller, K., Ojemann, J., 2008. Testing for nested oscillation. *Journal of Neuroscience Methods* 174(1), 50–61.

Pereira, F., Mitchell, T., Botvinick, M., 2009. Machine learning classifiers and fMRI: A tutorial overview. *NeuroImage* 45(1), S199–S209.

Poline, J.-B., Holmes, A. P.,Worsley, K. J., Friston, K. J., 1997. Statistical inference and the theory of random fields. In: Friston, K., Frith, C. D., Dolan, R. J., Mazziotta, J. C., Frackowiak, R. (eds.), *Human Brain Function*, 1st Edition. San Diego, California: Academic Press.

Rencher, A., 1992. Interpretation of canonical discriminant functions, canonical variates, and principal components. *American Statistician* 46(3), 217–225.

Schack, B., Vath, N., Petsche, H., Geissler, H., Moller, E., 2002. Phase-coupling of theta-gamma EEG rhythms during short-term memory processing. *International Journal of Psychophysiology* 44(2), 143–163.

Schack, B., Weiss, S., 2005. Quantification of phase synchronization phenomena and their importance for verbal memory processes. *Biological Cybernetics* 92(4), 275–287.

Seber, G. A. F., 2004. *Multivariate Observations*. Hoboken, New Jersey: John Wiley & Sons, Inc.

Sekihara, K., Sahani, M., Nagarajan, S. S., 2005. A simple nonparametric statistical thresholding for MEG spatial-filter source reconstruction images. *NeuroImage* 27, 368–376.

Shen, D., Davatzikos, C., 2002. HAMMER: Hierarchical attribute matching mechanism for elastic registration. *IEEE Transactions on Medical Imaging* 21(11), 1421–1439.

Singh, K., Barnes, G. R., Hillebrand, A., 2003. Group imaging of task-related changes in cortical synchronization using nonparametric permutation testing. *NeuroImage* 19, 1589–1601.

Soto, J., Pantazis, D., Jerbi, K., Lachaux, J.-P., Garnero, L., Leahy, R., 2009. Detection of event-related modulations of oscillatory brain activity with multivariate statistical analysis of MEG data. *NeuroImage* 30(6), 1922–1934.

Stouffer, S., Suchman, E., DeVinney, L., Star, S., Williams Jr, R., 1949. *The American Soldier: Adjustment during Army Life. (Studies in Social Psychology in World War II, Vol. 1.).* Princeton, NJ: Princeton University Press.

Tass, P., Rosenblum, M., Weule, J., Kurths, J., Pikovsky, A., Volkmann, J., Schnitzler, A., Freund, H., 1998. Detection of n: m phase locking from noisy data: Application to magnetoencephalography. *Physical Review Letters* 81(15), 3291–3294.

Teolis, A. (ed.), March 1998. *Computational Signal Processing with Wavelets (Applied and Numerical Harmonic Analysis).* Boston: Birkhauser.

Thompson, P., Mega, M., Woods, R. P., Zoumalan, C. I., Lindshield, C. J., Blanton, R. E., Moussai, J., Holmes, C., Cummings, J. L., Toga, A. W., 2001. Cortical change in Alzheimer's disease detected with a disease-specific population-based brain atlas. *Cerebral Cortex* 11(1), 1–16.

Tikhonov, A., Arsenin, V., 1977. *Solutions of Ill-Posed Problems.* Great Falls, Montana: Winston and Sons.

van Veen, B., Drongelen, W. V., Yuchtman, M., Suzuki, A., 1997. Localization of brain electrical activity via linearly constrained minimum variance spatial filtering. *IEEE Transactions of Biomedical Engineering* 44(9), 867–880.

Varela, F., Lachaux, J.-P., Rodriguez, E., Martinerie, J., 2001. The brainweb: Phase synchronization and large-scale integration. *Nature Reviews* 2, 229–239.

Verbeke, G., Molenberghs, G., 2000. *Linear Mixed Models for Longitudinal Data.* New York: Springer-Verlag.

Worsley, K., Friston, K., 2000. A test for a conjunction. *Statistics and Probability Letters* 47(2), 135–140.

Worsley, K. J., Andermann, M., Koulis, T., MacDonald, D., Evans, A. C., 1999. Detecting changes in non-isotropic images. *Human Brain Mapping* 8, 98–101.

Worsley, K. J., Marrett, S., Neelin, P., Vandal, A. C., Friston, K. J., Evans, A. C., 1996. A unified statistical approach for determining significant signals in images of cerebral activation. *Human Brain Mapping* 4, 58–73.

Worsley, K. J., Taylor, J. E., Tomaiuolo, F., Lerch, J., 2004. Unified univariate and multivariate random field theory. *NeuroImage* 23, s189–195.

5

Emergence of Groupwise Registration in MR Brain Study

Guorong Wu*
University of North Carolina

Hongjun Jia
University of North Carolina

Qian Wang
University of North Carolina

Feng Shi
University of North Carolina

Pew-Thian Yap
University of North Carolina

Dinggang Shen
University of North Carolina

5.1 Background

Modern medical imaging technologies such as magnetic resonance imaging (MRI) [1] offer a safe and noninvasive means of performing clinical diagnosis and research, involving human brain development, aging, and disease-induced anomalies. For reliable estimation of disease-related microstructural difference, accurate deformable image registration plays a key fundamental role in dealing with confounding intrasubject variability in longitudinal studies and intersubject variability in cross-sectional studies.

5.1.1 Pairwise Registration

A plethora of pairwise deformable registration algorithms have flourished in the past two decades, comprehensive surveys of which can be found in [2–6]. In general, the goal of image registration is to estimate the deformation field for warping the subject image (or moving image) to the template image (or fixed image) by maximizing a certain similarity measure between the warped subject and the template. Upon successful registration, intra- or intersubject differences are minimized, while at the same time disease-related changes and morphological variations are preserved.

The majority of image registration algorithms fall into three categories: landmark-based [7–9], intensity-based [10–15], and feature-based [16–19]. Landmark-based algorithms take advantage of

* Guorong Wu, Hongjun Jia, and Qian Wang contributed equally to this chapter.

anatomical prior knowledge and are thus computationally fast, since only a few landmarks out of all voxels in an image volume need to be matched. It is, however, a challenging task even for the trained experts to accurately place a sufficient number of anatomical landmarks for achieving accurate registration. Moreover, interrater landmark-placement variability could be large, thus seriously undermining the performance of landmark-based registration algorithms. Intensity-based algorithms take a different approach by aiming to maximize the intensity similarity between a pair of images, which can be fully automated by employing state-of-the-art optimization methods for deformation field estimation. However, intensity similarity does not necessarily imply anatomical correspondence. In light of this, feature-based algorithms formulate image registration as a problem of feature matching for deformation estimation. Anatomical correspondences identified by feature-based registration have been found to be more reliable than those based on intensity alone.

Hierarchical attribute matching mechanism for elastic registration (HAMMER) [17,18]—one of the most popular brain MRI registration algorithms—integrates the advantages of the methods from all three categories, and alleviates their limitations. HAMMER designates an attribute vector to each image point as its morphological signature for efficient determination of anatomical correspondences between an image pair. The attribute vector consists of a variety of image-derived features, including image intensity, edge type, and geometric moment invariants (GMIs) [20] computed for three types of tissues, that is, white matter (WM), gray matter (GM), and cerebrospinal fluid (CSF). The degree of similarity between the GMI-based features of a particular point at the anterior horn of the left ventricle (as indicated by a red cross) and the attribute vector of every other point in the image is color-coded and shown in Figure 5.1, where blue denotes high similarity and red otherwise. To achieve robust registration and to avoid local minima, only a small number of the voxels with the most distinctive attribute vectors—the driving voxels—in both template and subject are selected for guiding the initial registration. As registration progresses, an increasing number of voxels are selected as driving voxels to refine the deformation field. Figure 5.2 illustrates the hierarchical deformation mechanism in HAMMER with points in red, green, and yellow denoting the driving voxels identified in the initial, middle, and final registration stages, respectively. The gradually refined deformation field is shown in the bottom of Figure 5.2.

HAMMER has been evaluated in a number of brain studies and is found to achieve relatively high accuracy, even in the presence of significant morphological differences in cortical regions. In Figure 5.3, some representative registration results of elderly subjects from the Baltimore Longitudinal Study of Aging (BLSA [21]) are shown to demonstrate the performance of HAMMER. The abundance of anatomical details retained in the average image gives a good indication of HAMMER's capability in registering images with significant structural variations.

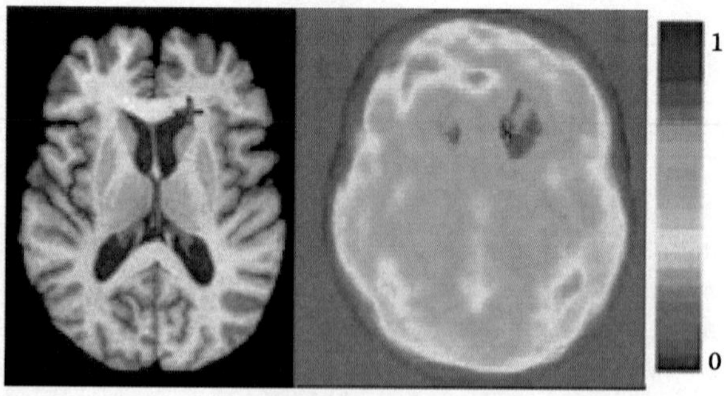

FIGURE 5.1 **(See color insert.)** Color-coded map (right) of the degree of similarity between the attribute vectors of the marked point (the red cross in the left image) and every other point in the brain. Blue denotes for high similarity and red for low similarity. (Adapted from D. Shen and C. Davatzikos, *Medical Imaging, IEEE Transactions on*, 21, 1421–1439, © 2002 IEEE.)

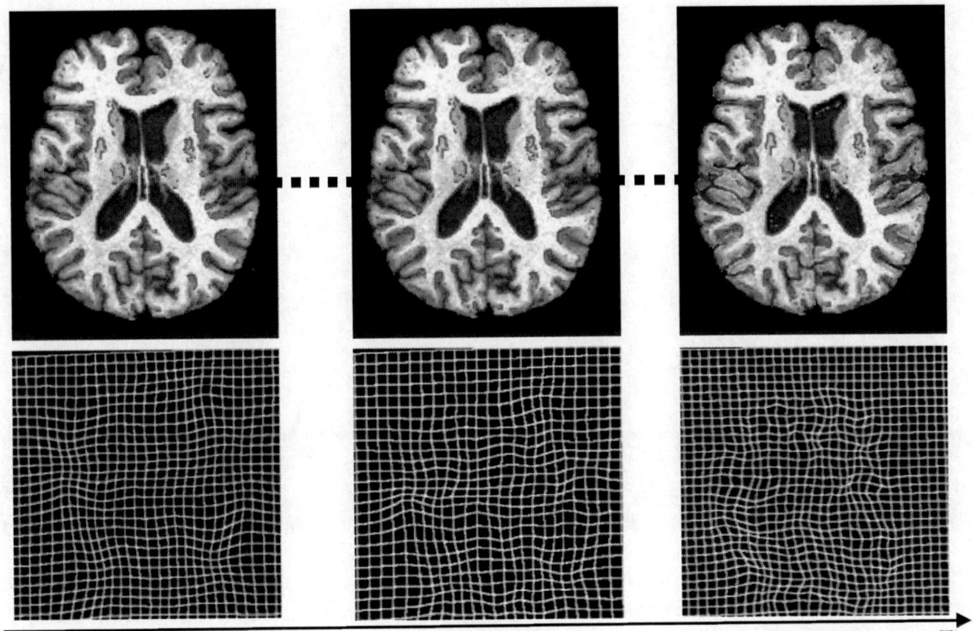

FIGURE 5.2 **(See color insert.)** Hierarchical selection of the driving voxels, and evolution of deformation fields in different registration stages. In the initial stage, only a small number (around approximately 2% of total voxels) of voxels with distinctive attribute vectors (displayed in red), located at sulcal roots, gyral crowns, and ventricular boundaries, are selected to steer the registration of other less distinctive voxels. As registration progresses, more and more voxels are selected as the driving voxels, as shown in green and yellow, respectively. The bottom row shows the corresponding deformation fields estimated at three different stages. It can be observed that, as the number of the driving voxels increases, the deformation field is gradually refined. (Adapted from G. Wu et al., *NeuroImage*, 49, 2225–2233, 2010.)

5.1.2 Limitations of Pairwise Registration

Due to the high anatomic variability among individual human brains, any atlas or clinical diagnostic system based on a single subject's anatomy cannot achieve full success [23]. Although it is applicable to register each subject to the template by pairwise registration for the intra- or interpopulation analysis, registration schemes based on a single reference will introduce systematic bias toward the shape of the selected template. To increase the signal-to-noise ratio (SNR) in subsequent statistical analysis, the registration of a large number of images from different individuals needs to be considered within a unified registration framework, so that the overall registration accuracy for all images in a population can be maximized. Eventually, the anatomical shape differences within and across populations can be better delineated. Thus, groupwise registration algorithms which avoid bias in template selection are recently gaining increasing research interest.

5.1.3 Emergence of Groupwise Registration

To alleviate limitations of pairwise registration, groupwise registration aims to warp all images toward the common space by simultaneously estimating their deformations [24–43]. In other words, given an image population $\boldsymbol{I} = \{I_i \mid i = 1,\ldots,N\}$, the ultimate goal of groupwise registration is to find a set of deformations $\boldsymbol{T} = \{T_i \mid i = 1,\ldots,N\}$ to minimize the variation within the registered subject set $\tilde{\boldsymbol{I}} = \{T_i(I_i) \mid i = 1,\ldots,N\}$. The scheme of groupwise registration is illustrated in the left panel of Figure 5.4.

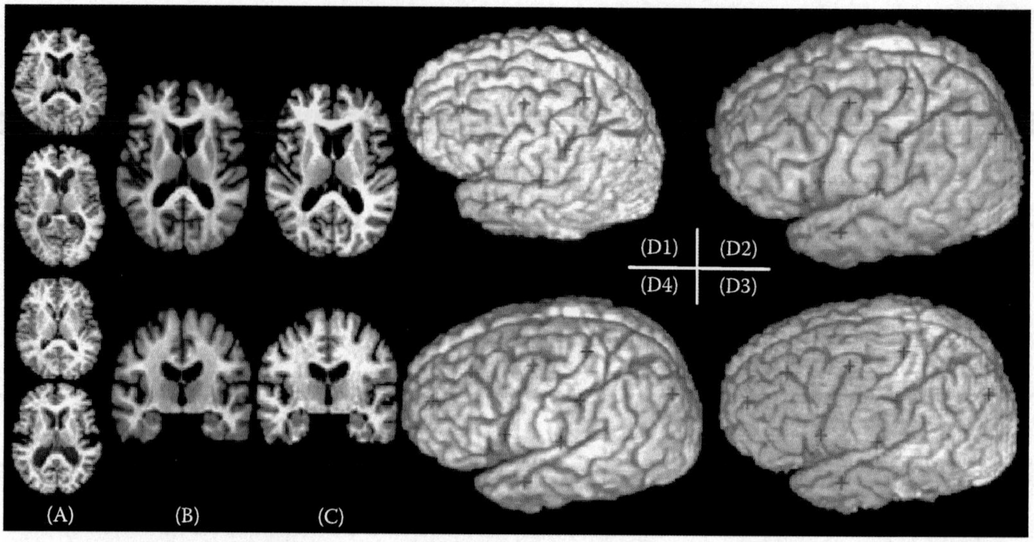

FIGURE 5.3 **(See color insert.)** Results from HAMMER algorithm. (A) Four representative cross sections from BLSA dataset; (B) Representative views from the average of the 18 images after normalization onto the template in (C) by HAMMER; (D1–D4) the 3D rendering of a representative case, its warped configuration using HAMMER, the template and the average of 18 warped brains, respectively. The anatomical details seen in (B) and (D4) are the evidences of the registration accuracy. The red crosses in (D1–D4) are identically placed to allow for visual inspection of point correspondences. (Adapted from Z. Lao et al., *NeuroImage*, 21, 46–57, 2004.)

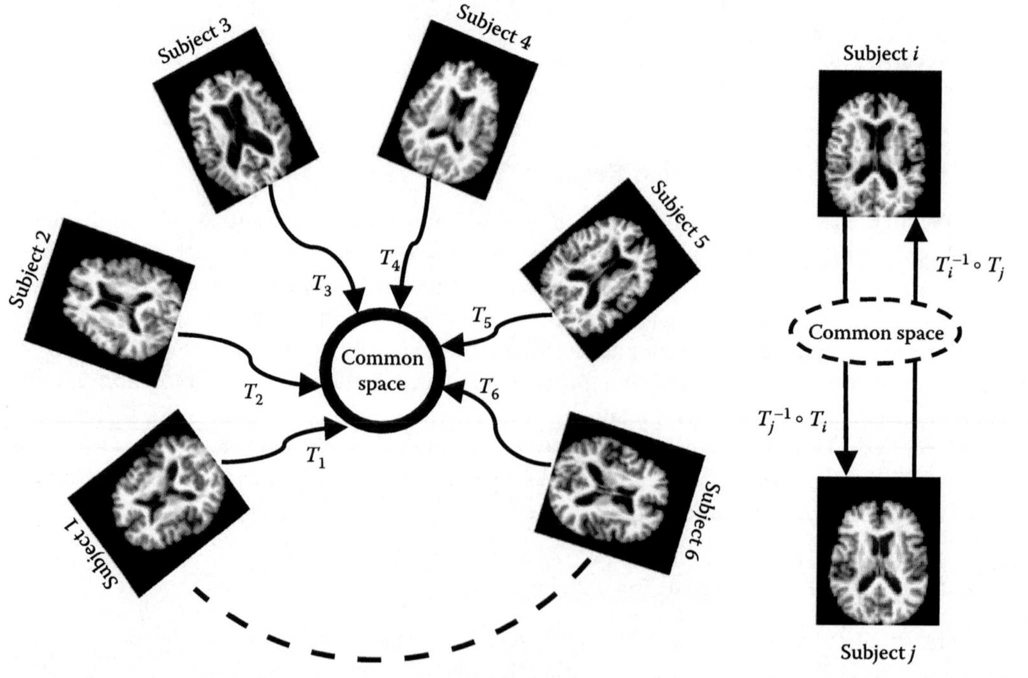

FIGURE 5.4 **(See color insert.)** In groupwise registration, all subjects are warped onto a common space by following their individual deformations (as indicated by red arrows). Also, any subject I_i is connected to another subject I_j via the common space by a composed transformation, that is, $T_j^{-1} \circ T_i$, as shown in the right panel.

Specifically, subject I_i is warped to the common space, following the corresponding deformation T_i. The estimated deformation usually complies with the constraint of invertibility. Then, any two subjects can be connected via the common space. For example, in the right panel of Figure 5.4, subject i can be warped onto the space of subject j by a composed transformation and, that is, $T_j^{-1} \circ T_i$. After all images have been aligned in the common space, any quantitative analysis can be performed.

The majority of the current groupwise registration algorithms can be classified into three classes: (1) pairwise registration derived groupwise registration [24,25]; (2) population center-guided groupwise registration [26,27,32,33,38,40,42]; and (3) hidden common space-based groupwise registration [28–30,36,37,44]. The first class of methods directly applies pairwise registration to achieve the goal of groupwise registration. They attempt to determine an unbiased or least biased atlas by exhaustive pairwise registration of image pairs in a group. We will describe two typical methods of this class in Section 5.2. Recent groupwise registration algorithms take a different approach by simultaneously estimating the deformations in relation to a common space. Specifically, the second class of methods estimates the population center by explicit registration of each subject image to a group mean image. The third class of methods formulates the groupwise registration as an optimization problem with an objective function that drives all subjects toward the hidden common space. We will describe with more details these two classes of groupwise registration algorithms in Sections 5.3, 5.4, respectively. The major difference between the last two classes of methods is that, in the second class, the image in the common space is determined explicitly and is evolved with further registration, while in the third class, the image in the common space is implicit or hidden throughout the optimization. We will provide several typical applications of groupwise registration in Section 5.5, including image parcellation [22], multiple modal image population exploration [31], and infant atlas building [45].

5.2 Pairwise Registration-Derived Groupwise Registration

One of the most straightforward ways of achieving groupwise registration is to apply the pairwise registration directly on the images in the population. In this section, we briefly introduce two such groupwise registration algorithms. Seghers et al. [25] proposed to construct the brain atlas based on the exhaustive pairwise registration, with possible number of registration totaling up to $N(N-1)$. By taking in turn every image I_i in the group as the template, they estimate the deformation fields to all other $N-1$ images with respect to the template, and then warp the template with the average deformation field. Then the final atlas is obtained by the voxelwise averaging of all warped images. However, this method suffers from very heavy computation cost. For example, it takes about 170 days on one 2.6 GHz processor to perform 4032 pairwise registrations for a group of 64 subjects [25].

An alternative method can be found in the work of Park et al. [24]. They perform pairwise registrations among N subjects by taking each subject as a template in turn and registering the rest of the subjects onto this template. Next, instead of averaging all deformed images in [25], they build an $N \times N$ distance matrix with each element denoting a measure of the bending energy of a particular deformation field. Multidimensional scaling (MDS) [46] is performed on the distance matrix to choose the image that is the closest to the population center as the template. Since the distance matrix is assumed to be symmetric, this method is faster since only $N(N-1)/2$ times of pairwise registration need to be performed. Once the least biased template is determined (which is only an approximation to the real population center), all other images can be mapped onto the template space directly using a pairwise registration method. However, the potential bias introduced in the selection of the template, as well as the difficulty in registering images with large deformations to the selected template, limit its application in practice.

In brief, the goal of this kind of method is to construct an unbiased or least-biased atlas. However, the large number of required rounds of pairwise registration limits their application. Possible solution to this is discussed next.

5.3 Population Center-Guided Groupwise Registration

Groupwise registration can be implemented by aligning all images to a population center. In the literature, several groupwise registration methods have been proposed to better estimate and utilize the population center. For example, the group mean method and its extensions [26,40,41] repeatedly estimate the group mean image from the tentatively aligned images and update the deformation of each subject to the newly estimated group mean image. In the tree-based algorithms [27,42], all subjects in the population are connected by a tree structure with the root subject considered as the population center. Thus, all other subjects can be registered to the root by following the path from each individual node to the root node. To better utilize the local and global information of the manifold spanned by all subjects, a method called Atlas Building by Self-Organized Registration and Bundling (ABSORB) [32,33] has been proposed recently. In general, ABSORB warps each subject toward its selected neighbors and assures that all subjects can reach the population center. All these algorithms are detailed next.

To avoid the potential bias in groupwise registration, Joshi et al. [26] proposed to solve the groupwise registration in an iterative manner by estimating the population center via the Fréchet mean of all images. An interim population center is first built by averaging all linearly aligned images. And then all images are warped to this interim population center by a diffeomorphism registration framework. The interim population center is further updated based on all the tentatively warped images, and then the deformations for all images can be refined as well. The two steps of (1) estimating population center and (2) registering images to the population center are interleaved and iteratively performed. As illustrated in Figure 5.5, this method can provide an unbiased population center, and converge fast by a few iterations. However, the registration process of this method could be misled when trying to register individual images (with sharp anatomical structures) to a blurry group mean image (with ambiguous anatomical structures), due to the difficulty in establishing the reliable correspondences between them, especially in the beginning of the registration.

It is worth noting that other registration methods are also applicable to the group mean framework. For example, Marsland et al. [38] introduced a minimum description length (MDL)-based method, which plays as a role similar to the diffeomorphism registration method in [26], for groupwise registration. In MDL, the image population is described by not only a single mean image, but also a set of deformations and a set of residuals, which are encoded according to any given model (e.g., the histogram of the mean image). Based on the information theory, groupwise registration is accomplished when the description length of the population coding is minimized.

Fletcher et al. [40] extended the definition of the geometric median (or the L^1 estimator) to the Riemannian manifold, by adopting geodesic distances between subjects on the manifold and minimizing the distance via gradient-based optimization. The geometric median serves as the population center to guide the subsequent registration. They further proved that the geometric median exists and is unique for any nonpositively curved manifold or under certain conditions for positively curved manifolds.

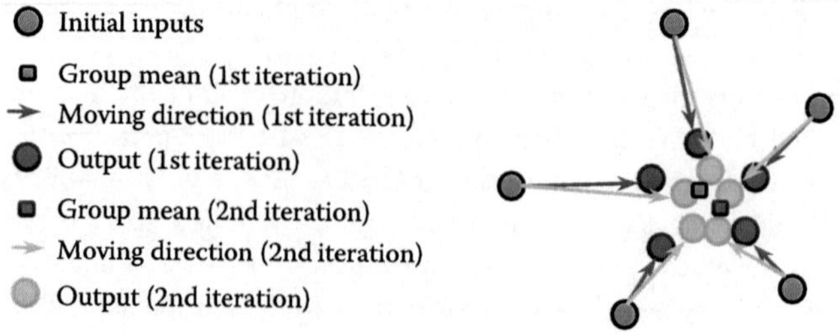

FIGURE 5.5 **(See color insert.)** Illustration of the framework of the group mean method. In each iteration, the subjects are warped toward the tentatively estimated group mean. And the group mean is refined based on newly warped subjects.

In their experiments, this extension was demonstrated to be more robust to outliers than the Fréchet mean used by Joshi et al. [26].

Recently, Wu et al. [41] extended the pairwise HAMMER algorithm [17] to work in a groupwise manner. Instead of simply averaging over the intensities of the cohort of images, they proposed to average images region-by-region according to local anatomical shapes. Starting from an exemplar image which has the minimal distance to all other images, more and more anatomical details are gradually augmented to the mean image as registration progresses. In this way, the mean image can be kept sharp throughout the whole registration process, which is very important to obtain accurate registration results. In their method, each subject is treated differently (according to the alignment of local anatomical structures) in constructing the group mean based on the alignment of local anatomical shape. Two major advantages are demonstrated: (1) the group mean image has minimal anatomical difference to all subjects, and (2) the group mean retains the population information as well as sharp anatomical structures.

It is generally difficult to achieve good registration by directly registering each image to a fixed population center, especially when cross-subject anatomical variation is large. Some algorithms have been proposed to warp the individual images with the help of intermediate template [47–50]. These intermediate templates are produced to pave the path for connecting an individual image to the population center. The final registration result can be obtained by deforming each individual image along its respective path to the population center. This idea is applied to the groupwise registration by building a minimum spanning tree (MST) [51] where each node corresponds to one image and each edge indicates the distance between two connected nodes. The root node of the MST, namely the population center, can be determined by selecting a node that has the minimal edge length to all other nodes or that has the maximal number of children. In Hamm et al. [27], after learning the intrinsic manifold of the whole dataset, the population center is determined as the pseudo-geodesic median image since it minimizes the total path length from each image to the template. The corresponding geodesic paths between individual images and the population center are computed to construct a tree based on the learned manifold. The large deformation between the subject and the population center is thus decomposed into several small ones, and the accuracy of registration is improved. Nevertheless, since the population center is approximated by a fixed image (i.e., the root image) from the dataset, the bias is unavoidable in this scenario.

More recently, a new framework for groupwise registration termed as ABSORB was proposed [32,33]. The basic idea of ABSORB is illustrated in Figure 5.6. This method explores the intrinsic distributions of subjects to guide the registration. The groupwise registration problem is resolved in an iterative manner by warping each image in the population step-by-step on the learned manifold, and, at the same time, maintaining the global distribution of the population. To achieve this goal, two new strategies,

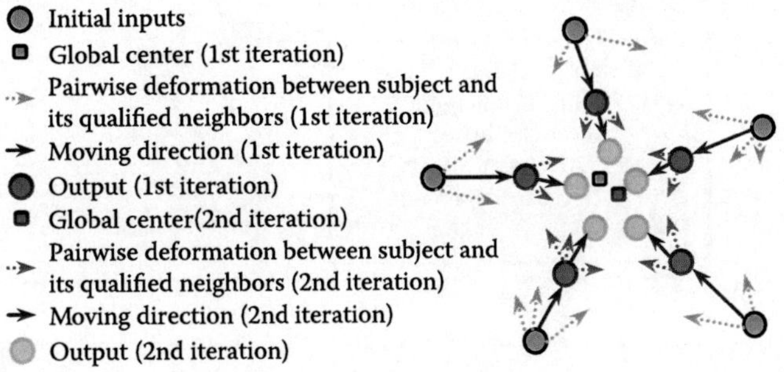

FIGURE 5.6 **(See color insert.)** Illustration of the ABSORB framework. In each iteration, each subject is deformed toward its selected neighbors, which are closer to the population center. The estimated population center is updated iteratively based on the tentatively warped images. (Adapted from H. Jia et al., *NeuroImage*, 51(3), 1057–1070, 2010.)

namely self-organized registration and image bundling are employed. Specifically in the self-organized registration, each image is warped toward a subset of its neighbors that are closer to the population center, in order to condense the global distribution of the population on the manifold. The tentative population center is updated iteratively and used only to guide the selection of qualified neighbors, thereby not directly involved into registration. After several iterations, some nearby subjects become close enough to each other and are, thus, bundled together spontaneously into a subgroup. Then ABSORB jumps to the higher level, where the registration is performed on a much smaller dataset which consists of only the representative images of all subgroups. As the result of this hierarchical registration process, a pyramid of images is built automatically and the population center can be eventually generated once the registration arrives at the upmost level. With ABSORB, the possible registration error can be greatly reduced by only warping each individual subject to its neighbors with similar structures. Also, it can produce a smoother registration path, which traverses each subject image to the final population center, than other groupwise registration methods.

Similar to other approaches that solve the groupwise registration in a "relay" fashion [26,27,42], the complete path from each individual image to the final population center built by ABSORB is composed of a series of small segments. But ABSORB is inherently different from those methods in three ways. First, in ABSORB, no fixed intermediate templates are used for any image in any iteration. Instead, the movement of each individual image on the manifold is driven only by a selected set of its qualified neighboring images, not by a common explicit or implicit template. Second, the number of qualified neighboring images is adaptively determined according to the intrinsic data structure learned online, and the complete path generated from each image to the population center on the manifold is generally smoother and more conservative as ABSORB always warps one image to its nearby location, instead of moving to the population center directly. One example is demonstrated in Figure 5.7. In contrast, in [26,27,42], the direction and the amount of deformation for each image in each iteration are determined by only the selected tentative template, which can often result in a zigzag path if the selected template does not represent the data distribution very well. Finally, the registration path for each image provided by ABSORB is not predetermined before the actual registration starts. In other words, it is a fully

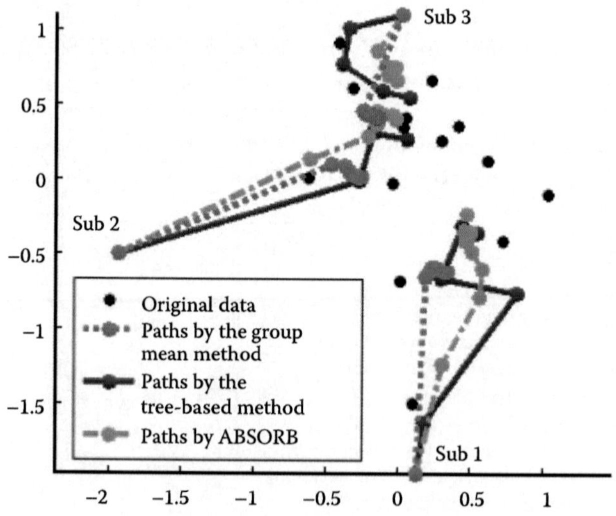

FIGURE 5.7 **(See color insert.)** The registration paths produced by three different methods. The paths generated by ABSORB (with green dashed curves) are much smoother than the tree-based method (with blue solid curves), and the paths given by the group mean method (with red dotted curves) show that there is not much progress after the first iteration of registration. (Adapted from H. Jia et al., *NeuroImage*, 51(3), 1057–1070, 2010.)

data-driven groupwise registration method. On the contrary, a tree in [27,42] is built in the preprocessing step and fixed during the whole registration process.

The information provided by the population center has been demonstrated to be very useful in groupwise registration. But due to the huge gap between the limited number of available subjects and the extremely high dimensions of the data space, it is usually very difficult to estimate the population center robustly, and thus an inaccurate population center might lead the whole registration off the track and degrade the statistical analysis that follows.

5.4 Hidden Common Space-Based Groupwise Registration

For the algorithms illustrated in Section 5.3, groupwise registration is achieved under the guidance by either the selected individual image (such as the root image in the tree-based method) or the group mean image (such as the average of all aligned subjects in [26]). However, both have their limitations. For the former, the difference between the selected individual subject and the real population center cannot be simply ignored even though it might be very close to the real population center. For the latter, since the subjects are far from the good alignment in the initial stage of registration, the tentative mean image by simply averaging all the warped subjects is inevitably fuzzy. Though the mean image guarantees the generation of an unbiased atlas, registration performance might be undermined by the fuzzy mean image due to the lack of structural details for proper correspondence detection.

One common characteristic of the groupwise registration methods described in Section 5.3 is that they all need explicit approximations of the population center. However, explicit estimation of the population center is not a necessity when the goal of groupwise registration is to estimate the deformation fields for warping each subject to a common space. Given a set of images, a unified objective function is developed to help warp all images to a hidden common space in which the variation within the subject images with respect to the deformation fields is minimized. As a result, the estimated deformations for all subjects, which are usually defined in the common space, convey the anatomical diversity across population. The advantage of this kind of groupwise registration algorithm is that it bypasses the estimation of population center by introducing a hidden common space, making the group mean only a by-product of the groupwise registration. In the following, we will summarize several groupwise registration algorithms belonging to this category.

In hidden common space-based groupwise registration, pairwise registration cannot be directly applied since there is no paired relationship between any given image and the specific template. In fact, all images need to be warped to an undetermined destination simultaneously, until they are close enough to each other and converge to a hidden common space. In general, a global objective function is defined to minimize the variation between all to-be-registered images. When the objective function is gradually minimized, the images are progressively pushed to converge to the hidden common space. Therefore, groupwise registration can be regarded as a typical optimization problem, with the optimal solution to the deformations for all images estimated by minimizing the objective function.

The "congealing" method proposed by Miller et al. [28,44] is among the first methods introduced for groupwise registration. In congealing, all images are piled together from top to bottom. Then intensities of the same locations from different images are sampled to form a sequence or a stack, as in the left panel of Figure 5.8. If all input images were identical, the intensity values inside the stack would be the same. The aim of the registration algorithm is then to reduce voxel variation within a stack by minimizing the stack entropy. The local variation measurement, namely stack entropy, is further integrated over the whole image domain to obtain a unified objective function. Given the image set I and the corresponding (tentative) deformations T, the objective function f can be defined as

$$f = \int \mathcal{H}(I(T(x)))\, dx, \tag{5.1}$$

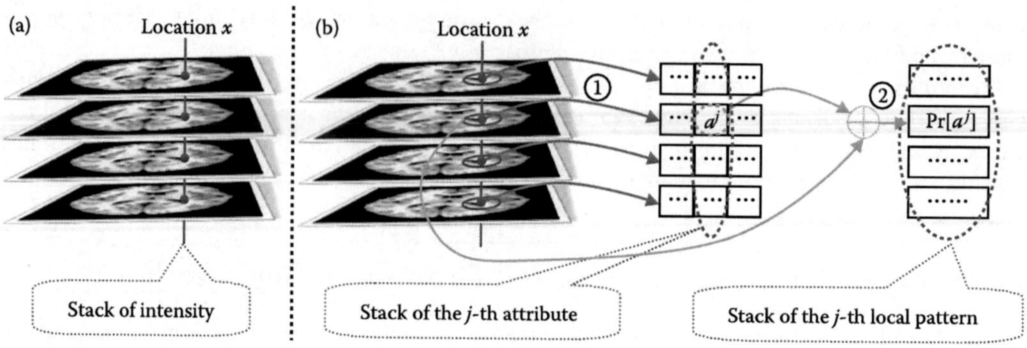

FIGURE 5.8 **(See color insert.)** In (a), a stack of intensities is sampled from the identical locations of different images. (Adapted from Q. Wang et al., *NeuroImage*, 50, 1485–1496, 2010.) In (b), not only the single intensity but also more attributes are sampled to form an attribute vector as a morphological signature of each voxel. Moreover, the neighborhood of each voxel is considered as a local pattern, described by the local probability density function, to construct a robust objective function.

where $\mathcal{H}$ calculates the entropy over the sequence of intensity values sampled from location x of all images. By minimizing f, the optimal estimation of the deformations T can be obtained. Without loss of generality, the notation T will be omitted in the following for convenience, by assuming that the image set I is the tentatively warped results based on the currently estimated deformations T.

An easy way to calculate the entropy of a finite intensity sequence is to adopt the widely used Shannon entropy, although some other measurements, such as the variance in the stack, can also be used. In the case of groupwise registration, the stack sampled at location x consists of the sequence $\{I_1(x), I_2(x), \cdots I_N(x)\}$. However, the number of samples in a stack is very limited, posing great challenge to the accurate estimation of entropy. To alleviate this problem, Parzen window is often used to transfer the discrete sequence into a continuous Gaussian mixture model (GMM). The Gaussians of each GMM, corresponding to individual location x in the image space, center at the sampled pixel values, respectively. Then the cost function can be represented by

$$f = -\int \frac{1}{N}\sum_{i=1}^{N} \log \frac{1}{N}\sum_{j=1}^{N} G_\sigma(I_i(x) - I_j(x))\, dx, \tag{5.2}$$

where G_σ is the Gaussian kernel with variance σ.

The deformation can be parameterized in various ways, the choice of which is often closely related to the optimization. The linear part of the deformation is usually the rigid or affine transformation, while the nonlinear part can be described by a dense deformation field. The congealing method implemented in [29] was based on affine transformations, and was then further extended nonlinearly in [30] by modeling the deformation with B-Splines [52]. For optimization, the common approach is to determine the gradient of the objective function with respect to the deformation parameters, and then search for the optimal solution along the steepest descent direction.

For example, in Wang et al. [34], where a group of point-sets are to be registered, each point-set is modeled as a continuous probability density function using GMM. The Jensen–Shannon (JS) divergence [53] is then used to measure the variation within the group of probability density functions. An objective function is built and further minimized using any gradient-based optimization for estimation of the deformation for each image.

We further note that intensity alone is insufficient for conveying all information needed by registration. It has been proven that attribute vector, consisting of additional information on the top of intensities, can better represent each voxel in an MR image. In HAMMER [17], for example, GMIs are used to determine a set of driving voxels for steering the registration. In fact, many types of features which have been shown to be effective descriptors can be incorporated as attributes for medical image registration.

Wang et al. [36,37] developed a method which integrates the attribute vector into the groupwise registration cost function. Ideally, different attributes in the attribute vector can contribute independent piece of information which is conducive for registration. In Wang et al.'s work [36,37], both intensity and intensity gradient are used as attributes for guiding groupwise registration. Intensity gradient is more sensitive than intensity alone to the subtle mismatch of anatomical boundaries. In the very beginning of registration, the variation within the population of images is high. Therefore, the contribution from intensity gradient is weighted less than that of intensity. As registration progresses, the mismatch between any two images becomes lesser. Then, to increase the accuracy in registration, the weighting for contribution of intensity gradient is increased, with simultaneous decrease in contribution from intensity. It is worth noting that, although only intensity and intensity gradient are used as attributes in Wang et al. [36,37], the framework is flexible enough to accommodate other features for guiding registration.

To further improve the robustness and accuracy of groupwise registration, local pattern is introduced in Wang et al. [36,37]. In particular, given a center voxel in the specific image, its neighborhood is viewed as a local pattern, as in the right panel of Figure 5.8. GMM is estimated to characterize the local pattern. Suppose a^j is the j-th attribute under consideration, then the local pattern centered at location x in image I_i, denoted as $Pr(a^j|i,x)$, is defined as

$$Pr(a^j|i,x) = \frac{1}{K}\sum_{\Delta x} G_\sigma\left(a^j - a^j_{i,x+\Delta x}\right), \tag{5.3}$$

where K is the total number of voxels in the neighborhood and Δx is the allowable offset in the neighborhood.

A single stack now actually connects a set of local patterns. These local patterns are from different images, but centering at the same locations. The variation within the stack of local patterns can be measured with the JS divergence:

$$\text{JS}(x,j) = \mathcal{H}\left(\sum_{i=1}^{N}\pi_i \cdot Pr(a^j|i,x)\right) - \sum_{i=1}^{N}\pi_i \cdot \mathcal{H}(Pr(a^j|i,x)). \tag{5.4}$$

By integrating the JS divergence across the image domain and combining together contributions of different attributes, the final cost function can be formulated. Similarly, gradient-based optimization methods can be used to minimize the cost function.

In general, hidden common space-based groupwise registration can be formulated as an optimization problem with the goal of minimizing variations within the image population. The way of constructing the objective function varies with applications, and should be further explored in the future. By avoiding introducing an explicit image in the common space, results yielded by groupwise registration toward the hidden common space can potentially get rid of bias introduced by impropriate selection of template.

5.5 Applications

Image registration plays a key role in medical image analysis [23,54]. It can be used to concurrently normalize all subjects in a population, and to propagate labels from template to individual subjects. The deformation field generated from registration records the displacement of corresponding voxels between subject and template, which characterizes the global and local morphological differences. In 4D studies

[55,56], the longitudinal changes measured by the registration algorithm can be used to reveal the patterns related to brain development, aging, and neurologic or neuropsychiatric disorders. The use of groupwise registration for morphological measurement has multiple advantages. First, it needs no selection of template, thus avoiding possible bias in data analysis. Second, it is able to generate more representative group mean. Groupwise registration can be easily incorporated into most applications by using it to replace the pairwise registration, for achieving more powerful and unbiased analysis of data. We will present three typical applications of groupwise registration in this section, besides pointing out other possible applications.

5.5.1 Typical Applications

Deformable image registration serves multiple roles in many clinical studies. One of the most popular applications is the evaluation of anatomical variability in human population. By registering each individual subject to a template, a dense deformation field can be obtained, encoding dilation and contraction information of regions of each subject with respect to the template. Therefore, these deformation fields offer ways for pathology detection, identification of gender-specific anatomic patterns, and mapping of dynamic patterns of structural changes in disease-related neuro-developmental and degenerative processes. Taking HAMMER as an example, Figure 5.9 demonstrates several typical clinical

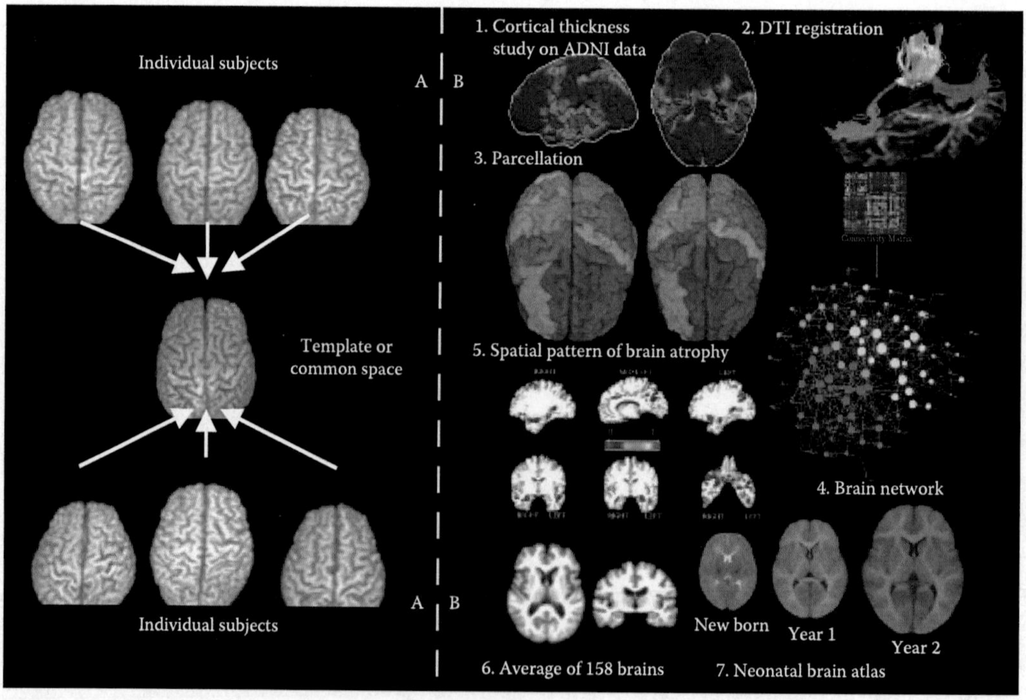

FIGURE 5.9 **(See color insert.)** Illustration of various applications of image registration. Panel (A) shows the procedure of warping individuals subjects (top and bottom rows) to the template (in a pairwise scenario) or common space (in a groupwise scenario). After spatial normalization, numerous clinical applications can be performed, with some typical ones shown in the right panel (B). From (B1) to (B7), we show the illustrative results of (B1) cortical thickness study on ADNI data, (B2) DTI registration, (B3) image parcellation, (B4) brain network discovery on structural images, (B5) spatial pattern of brain atrophy with respect to MCI, (B6) normalization of elderly brains, and (B7) study on infant brain development, respectively.

applications requiring registration of the subject images to the template image (in Figure 5.9 (A)). These applications are further illustrated in Figure 5.9 (B1–B7).

1. After registering all subjects to the template space, subtle changes of cortical thickness [57,58] during pathological or physiological development can be captured, providing a powerful tool for diagnosis and study of a variety of neuro-degenerative and psychiatric disorders [59]. (B1) shows the left and interior views of statistical significance (p-value) of the correlations detected between the thickness and the CDR–SOB scores.
2. Diffusion tensor imaging (DTI) provides unprecedented insight into brain WM structures and is commonly used to delineate subtle abnormalities caused by diseases, including stroke, multiple sclerosis, dyslexia, and schizophrenia. HAMMER has also been extended to DTI image registration [60,61]. (B2) demonstrates the aligned fiber bundles in the genu, splenium, and body of the corpus callosum in green, red, and yellow, respectively.
3. Registration can be used to automatically parcellate and label the brain structures for individual brain images after estimating the deformation field between the subject and the template [22]. (B3) shows 3D renderings of the label map and a representative labeling of an individual's brain after registration to the template. It is worth noting that features extracted from the volumetric measurements of labels can also be used to classify the normal controls and diseased patients.
4. The human brain is considered as a collection of interacting networks with specialized functions to support various cognitive tasks [62]. The connectivity also changes as a consequence of the neuron degeneration, either from natural aging or from diseases such as Alzheimer's disease. After the registration and parcellation on DTI images, the connectivity of two region-of-interests (ROIs) can be identified by the common traversing fibers. This connectivity information is encoded in a connectivity matrix (in the top of (B4)). After properly thresholding the connectivity matrix, a brain network can be obtained, where the spring-embedding visualization is displayed in the bottom of (B4).
5. Computer-based pattern classification of MRI is able to detect patterns of brain structure characterizing subtle anatomical difference between normal and patient subjects after image registration. (B5) shows the representative cross-sections highlighting the brain regions that collectively form a spatial pattern of brain atrophy that is highly indicative of mild cognitive impairment (MCI) [63]. The color coding shows the relative importance of a brain region for classification.
6. HAMMER has been used as the key registration method in one of the most comprehensive longitudinal studies of aging in the world to date (Baltimore Longitudinal Study of Aging—BLSA [21]), in which HAMMER has successfully processed approximately 2100 images. Because of the high accuracy of HAMMER (as the sharp average image of all normalized subjects shown in (B6)), we can now localize longitudinal atrophy and detect abnormal anatomical changes with better spatial specificity and sensitivity.
7. Study of early brain is very challenging because of the insufficient image resolution, low SNR, dynamic myelination of WM, and lack of prior knowledge. (B7) shows the atlases of new born, year 1, and year 2 infants built from the well aligned subjects, which facilitate the infant brain analysis, such as atlas-based tissue segmentation, and brain network construction [42,45,64–66].

5.5.2 Advantages of Groupwise Registration

We demonstrate here the performance gain of groupwise registration over pairwise registration, that is, HAMMER (source code available at http://www.nitrc.org/projects/hammerwml/). Groupwise registration algorithms used in the comparison are the group mean algorithm [26], ABSORB [32,33], and the congealing algorithm [30]. Additionally, we provide the comparison results for the hierarchical groupwise registration algorithm presented in [43], which utilizes the congealing method [30] in the implementation of each level.

We first evaluate these five algorithms on 18 elderly brains from the BLSA dataset [21] by comparing the overlap ratio on WM, GM, and ventricle (VN). Here we use the Jaccard coefficient metric [67] to measure the alignment of two regions with the same tissue. For the two registered regions A and B, the Jaccard coefficient is defined as

$$J(A,B) = \frac{|A \cap B|}{|A \cup B|}, \tag{5.5}$$

where $|\cdot|$ denotes the number of voxels in the underlying region. To evaluate registration accuracy, we employ a majority vote approach by assigning each voxel with a tissue label that is the majority returned by all tissue labels at the same location of all the aligned subjects. Then the Jaccard coefficient between each of the registered label images and the voted label will be calculated. It is worth noting that this is a very strict definition for measurement of ROI overlap, and it emphasizes the importance of groupwise registration in measuring the group performance. In the following experiments, we use the average score of Jaccard coefficients as the overlap ratio for each tissue label.

Figure 5.10 shows a group of 18 elderly brain images. Each image size is of $256 \times 256 \times 124$ and resolution $0.9375 \times 0.9375 \times 1.5$ mm^3. It can be observed that the anatomical structures vary a lot across different subjects, especially for the ventricle and the cortex. To better evaluate the performance of pairwise registration (by HAMMER), we randomly select five individual subjects (shown by red boxes in Figure 5.10) as templates in reporting both the mean and the standard deviation of the overlap ratios over three different tissues (the first row of Table 5.1).

The overlap ratios on WM, GM, and VN, as well as the overall overlap ratio on the whole brain by different groupwise methods are displayed from the second to fifth row in Table 5.1. It can be observed that

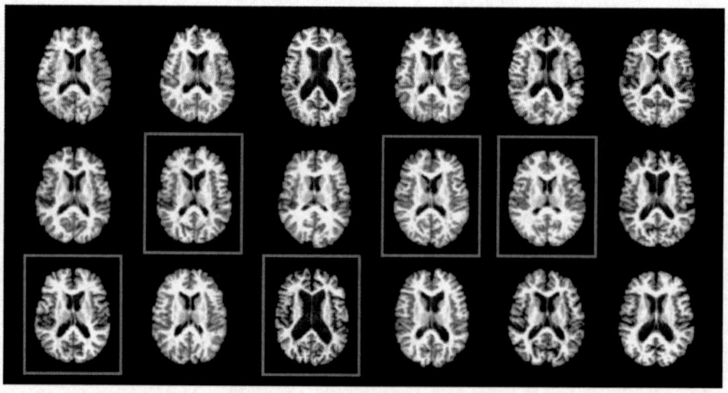

FIGURE 5.10 **(See color insert.)** Eighteen elderly brain images used in evaluation of three registration methods. The five subjects with red rectangles are selected as template images in the pairwise registration algorithm for a fair performance evaluation of the pairwise registration algorithms.

TABLE 5.1 Overall Overlap Ratios of WM, GM, and VN by Five Different Registration Algorithms

	White Matter (%)	Gray Matter (%)	Ventricle (%)	Overall (%)
Pairwise HAMMER	63.86 (±3.87)	57.25 (±2.18)	76.51 (±3.70)	65.64 (±3.15)
Group mean method	73.88	60.51	78.14	70.84
ABSORB	79.01	66.82	82.33	76.05
Congealing method	59.68	51.09	70.61	59.43
Hierarchical congealing	65.64	58.36	78.60	67.54

the second class (i.e., the population center-guided groupwise registration) can achieve much higher overlap ratio than the pairwise algorithm (HAMMER). For example, the overlap ratios of the ABSORB method can reach 79.01% in WM, 66.82% in GM, and 82.33% in VN, which achieves more than 10% improvement in the overall overlap ratio. The congealing method (a hidden common space-based groupwise registration method), however, is not as good as the pairwise counterpart (HAMMER) in terms of overlap ratios at the current stage. One possible reason for this is that much more parameters, compared with those of the pairwise registration method, are involved into the optimization of the objective function (e.g., the stack entropy in the congealing method) in this class of registration methods. In pairwise registration, only the deformation of a single image needs to be estimated, while in groupwise registration the deformations have to be simultaneously refined for all images. Thus, the optimization involved in groupwise registration is more vulnerable to local minima with the same gradient-based optimization method. However, by integrating the congealing method into a hierarchical groupwise registration framework [35,43] which only performs congealing on a set of subjects with similar appearances, the registration performance in terms of the overlap ratio can be improved drastically, as shown in the last row of Table 5.1.

5.5.3 Multiple Modes in Groupwise Registration

The intersubject variation can be so large that a single common space can barely handle the groupwise registration [68]. As discussed previously, an individual subject can be connected to the final population center by a path consisting of segments linking neighboring subjects. In ABSORB, nearby images are automatically bundled together in the self-organized registration progress. A single representative image is selected from each bundle to participate into the further registration in the higher level. In general, images in a population can be better represented by multiple modes. By taking advantage of the multiple mode phenomena, groupwise registration could become more accurate and efficient.

In Wang et al. [35,43], all subjects are hierarchically clustered according to the specific pairwise similarity or distance definition. The top–down hierarchical clustering yields a pyramid, where each leaf node corresponds to an image in the population. In each class, subjects are close to each other. Then registration is always intraclass, as only the images in the identical class are warped to the center of the class in groupwise registration manner. Similar to ABSORB, only a single subject will be produced to represent the whole class when intraclass registration has finished, and contribute to registration in the higher level. From the perspective of the pyramid, the task of intraclass registration happens from the bottom of the pyramid, then climbs up, and finally ends at the top. Meanwhile, all images in the population are warped to the common space, following the path from its corresponding leaf node to the root of the pyramid. In each intraclass registration, subjects involved are much less diverse than the whole population. Therefore, to perform groupwise registration on a class of images is much easier and more accurate than to perform groupwise registration of all images directly. Moreover, the whole computation load is dispatched into several classes where only a small number of subjects are handled, leading to a faster registration algorithm.

An example with only three levels is shown in Figure 5.11, where groupwise registration has been performed on 150 brain MR images. For clarity, only a few subjects are displayed here. In the first level, each class contains a very limited number of subjects, which are quite close to each other. Then intraclass registration yields the representative image for the respective class. And in the second level, intraclass registrations perform again, resulting in fewer modes of the population. The whole process ends in the third level, where a single representative for the whole population is produced. For each image at the leaf node, it can be warped to the common space, following its individual path from the leaf node to the root node of the pyramid.

Groupwise registration can be employed to explore the existence of multiple modes in an image population. Sabuncu et al. [31] incorporated the groupwise registration into a generalized EM framework. Each subject is assigned a label. The assignments are refined, as images of the same label are warped together in a groupwise registration manner. And after the EM process converges, the intrinsic multiple

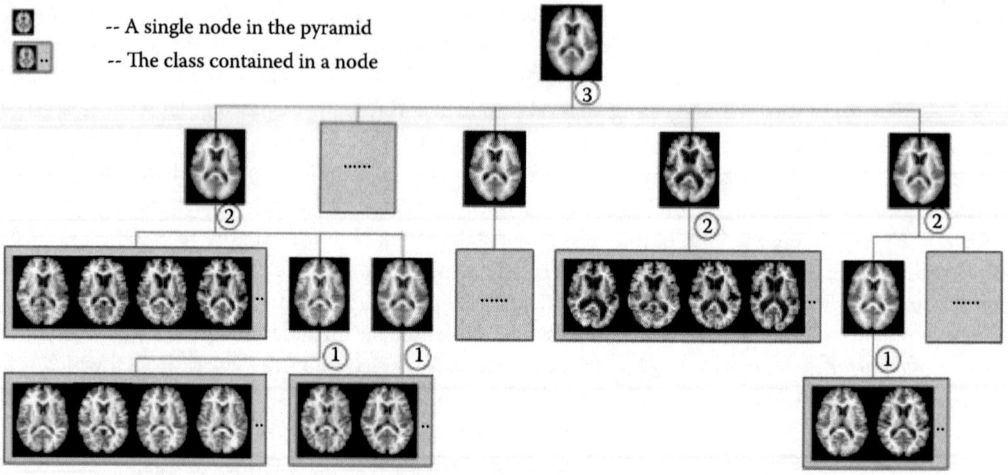

FIGURE 5.11 **(See color insert.)** An image population of 150 brain MR images is hierarchically clustered into a pyramid, based on the similarity definition between any two images. Groupwise registration is performed in each class, producing the representative image for the class (label ϕ). The representative images participate into intraclass registrations in the higher level (label κ). Finally, a single representative is estimated (label λ), as the whole registration process reaches the top of the pyramid. Each input image then can be warped to the common space by following its respective deformation path. (Adapted from Q. Wang et al., *Human Brain Mapping*, 31(8), 1128–1140, 2010.)

modes of the image population are naturally manifested. For example, they can discriminate the subjects from different age groups.

5.5.4 Atlas Building for Infants

Atlas, which refers to a map or spatial record of what we know about a region, is widely used in many disciplines and applications. Brain atlases usually refer to the images incorporated with prior knowledge and take the forms of, for example, an averaged intensity model of the population, as well as the tissue probability maps of WM, GM, and CSF. In many applications, researchers use these atlases as registration templates in spatial normalization, and also as prior knowledge for guiding tissue segmentation. Atlas building is more important and challenging in infant image analysis than in adult because of the poor spatial resolution, low-tissue contrast, and high within-tissue intensity variability of the MR images [55,56,66,73]. An atlas with average-shape can normalize an infant population into the same space, and the prior probability maps can guide the tissue segmentation of infant population, which can be eventually used to disclose the brain development in the infant stage.

To build the infant atlas, we use a longitudinal dataset, in which MR scans were acquired longitudinally in neonates, 1 year old, and 2 years old [45]. We then employ the state-of-the-art longitudinal segmentation and groupwise registration methods to build infant atlases.

This dataset was collected as one of our longitudinal studies, involving 56 infants (27 males and 29 females). Each subject has a set of MR brain images scanned at 3 time points, as neonates (0.9 ± 0.3 months), 1 year old (13.2 ± 0.7 months), and 2 years old (24.9 ± 1.9 months). These healthy subjects were recruited from University of North Carolina at Chapel Hill (UNC–CH) and are free of congenital anomalies, metabolic disease, and focal lesions. Informed consent was obtained from the parents and the experimental protocols were approved by the institutional review board. All subjects were unsedated during MR imaging.

For each subject, T1 and T2 MR brain images were collected using a 3T Siemens scanner. For T1 images, 160 sagittal slices were obtained with parameters: TR = 1900 ms, TE = 4.38 ms, Flip Angle = 7, and resolution = 1 × 1 × 1 mm³. For T2 images, 70 transverse slices were acquired with parameters: TR = 7380 ms, TE = 119 ms, Flip Angle = 150, and resolution = 1.25 × 1.25 × 1.95 mm³.

All images are preprocessed utilizing a standard pipeline. To achieve better tissue contrast, T2 is selected for neonate, and T1 is selected for 1 year old and 2 years old. T2 images are resampled into 1 × 1 × 1 mm³. Nonbrain tissues (such as skull and dura) are stripped with a dedicated learning based algorithm [69], followed by manual editing in ITK–SNAP software [70] to ensure accurate removal. Bias correction is performed in all images with N3 method [71] to reduce the impact of intensity inhomogeneity and thus improve the performance of the subsequent segmentation and registration.

We employ the strategy proposed in [45] to first segment the last time-point image, and then take advantage of the longitudinal follow-up time-point to build a subject-specific tissue probabilistic atlas including WM, GM, and CSF, to guide the earlier time-point segmentation, which has much lower tissue contrast. In particular, the T1 image of 2 years old subjects has shown the early adult pattern, and tissue structures can be well segmented with fuzzy segmentation technique such as adaptive K-means algorithm [72]. Then the tissue probability maps of 2 years old subjects are warped into neonate and 1 year old subjects separately and serve as prior to guide their tissue segmentations. The segmentation results are used to refine the registration to better warp the probability maps of 2 years old subjects to the current time-point. With better prior, the performance of the segmentation can be improved. This joint registration-segmentation iterates until convergence. This technique can substantially improve the tissue segmentation accuracy of infant brain images, especially for neonates. After this procedure, the tissue probability maps for all images are obtained.

Next, we build the average-shape atlas for each age group, including the intensity model and the probability maps for WM, GM, and CSF. The conventional atlas building algorithm selects a subject image from or out of this population to be the template. The atlas constructed is anatomically similar with the selected template and is hence biased. Unbiased registration is more preferable here for determining an atlas which is able to better represent the anatomy of the whole population. We employ the groupwise registration method proposed in [41] for unbiased groupwise atlas building. This groupwise registration algorithm utilizes the attribute vector as the morphological signature to robustly identify the anatomical correspondences. Therefore, more accurate registration results can be achieved compared to the intensity-based algorithms.

We show the constructed average-shape atlases for 0, 1, and 2 years in Figure 5.12. The anatomical proportion of 0–1–2 years is preserved and can be observed from the figure. With these constructed

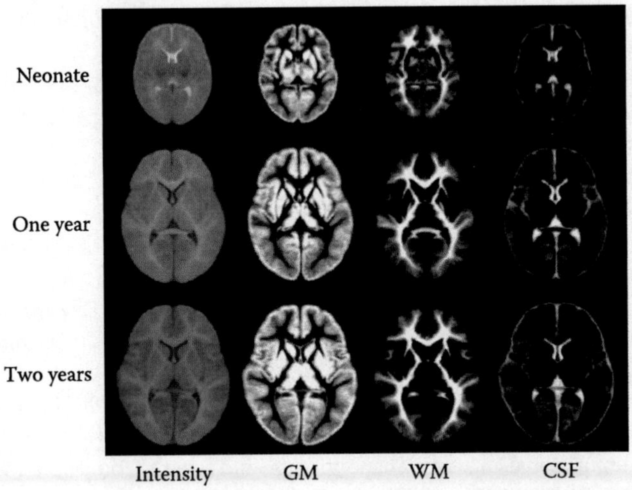

FIGURE 5.12 Illustration of the average-shape atlases of 0–1–2 years. The intensity model and tissue probability maps of WM, GM, and CSF are shown, respectively.

atlases, we now have the tissue probability for the specific age range of infants. We can use these atlases for guiding the segmentation of neonates with missing longitudinal data in the 1 year old or 2 years old, as we did in [65]. The atlases are freely available to the research community at http://bric.unc.edu/idea-group/free-softwares/.

5.6 Summary

In past decades, image registration has been proven to be important for effective medical image analysis. By normalizing an image population to the same space by image registration, qualitative and quantitative analysis on brain anatomies and morphologies can be performed. Plenty of applications have been explored, ranging from brain development study to early disease diagnosis. To meet the booming requirement for the unbiased group analysis, a relatively new family of registration methods, called as groupwise registration has come to the stage. As demonstrated in various applications, groupwise registration algorithms generally demonstrate superior performance over their pairwise counterparts, and thus becomes a hot topic in the field of medical image analysis.

References

1. E. M. Haacke, R. F. Brown, M. Thompson, and R. Venkatesan, *Magnetic Resonance Imaging: Physical Principles and Sequence Design.* New York: J. Wiley & Sons, 1999.
2. J. B. A. Maintz and M. A. Viergever, A survey of medical image registration. *Medical Image Analysis*, 2, 1–36, 1998.
3. B. Zitová and J. Flusser, Image registration methods: A survey. *Image and Vision Computing*, 21, 977–1000, 2003.
4. W. R. Crum, T. Hartkens, and D. L. G. Hill, Non-rigid image registration: Theory and practice. *British Journal of Radiology*, 77, S140–S153, 2004.
5. R. P. Woods, S. T. Grafton, C. J. Holmes, S. R. Cherry, and J. C. Mazziotta, Automated image registration: I. General methods and intrasubject, intramodality validation. *Journal of Computer Assisted Tomography*, 22, 139–152, 1998.
6. R. P. Woods, S. T. Grafton, J. D. G. Watson, N. L. Sicotte, and J. C. Mazziotta, Automated image registration: II. Intersubject validation of linear and nonlinear models. *Journal of Computer Assisted Tomography*, 22, 153–165, 1998.
7. S. Joshi and M. I. Miller, Landmark matching via large deforamtion diffeomorphisms. *IEEE Transactions on Medical Imaging*, 9, 1357–1370, 2000.
8. Z. Xue, D. Shen, and C. Davatzikos, Determining correspondence in 3D MR brain images using attribute vectors as morphological signatures of voxels. *Medical Imaging, IEEE Transactions on*, 23, 1276–1291, 2004.
9. P. J. Besl and H. D. McKay, A method for registration of 3-D shapes. *Pattern Analysis and Machine Intelligence, IEEE Transactions on*, 14, 239–256, 1992.
10. T. Vercauteren, X. Pennec, A. Perchant, and N. Ayache, Diffeomorphic demons: Efficient non-parametric image registration. *NeuroImage*, 45, S61–S72, 2009.
11. D. Rueckert, L. I. Sonoda, C. Hayes, D. L. G. Hill, M. O. Leach, and D. J. Hawkes, Nonrigid registration using free-form deformations: Application to breast MR images. *Medical Imaging, IEEE Transactions on*, 18, 712–721, 1999.
12. J. P. Thirion, Image matching as a diffusion process: An analogy with Maxwell's demons. *Medical Image Analysis*, 2, 243–260, 1998.
13. M. I. Miller, Computational anatomy: Shape, growth, and atrophy comparison via diffeomorphisms. *NeuroImage*, 23, S19–S33, 2004.
14. J. Ashburner, A fast diffeomorphic image registration algorithm. *NeuroImage*, 38, 95–113, 2007.

15. G. E. Christensen and H. J. Johnson, Consistent image registration. *Medical Imaging, IEEE Transactions on*, 20, 568–582, 2001.
16. D. Shen, Image registration by local histogram matching. *Pattern Recognition*, 40, 1161–1172, 2007.
17. D. Shen and C. Davatzikos, HAMMER: Hierarchical attribute matching mechanism for elastic registration. *Medical Imaging, IEEE Transactions on*, 21, 1421–1439, 2002.
18. D. Shen and C. Davatzikos, Very high-resolution morphometry using mass-preserving deformations and HAMMER elastic registration. *NeuroImage*, 18, 28–41, 2003.
19. G. Wu, P.-T. Yap, M. Kim, and D. Shen, TPS-HAMMER: Improving HAMMER registration algorithm by soft correspondence matching and thin-plate splines based deformation interpolation. *NeuroImage*, 49, 2225–2233, 2010.
20. C. H. Lo and H. S. Don, 3-D moment forms: Their construction and application to object identification and positioning. *IEEE Transactions on Pattern Analysis and Machine Intelligence*, 11, 1053–1064, 1989.
21. S. M. Resnick, A. F. Goldszal, C. Davatzikos, S. Golski, M. A. Kraut, E. J. Metter, R. N. Bryan, and A. B. Zonderman, One-year age changes in MRI brain volumes in older adults. *Cerebral Cortex*, 10, 464–472, 2000.
22. Z. Lao, D. Shen, Z. Xue, B. Karacali, S. M. Resnick, and C. Davatzikos, Morphological classification of brains via high-dimensional shape transformations and machine learning methods. *NeuroImage*, 21, 46–57, 2004.
23. A. W. Toga and P. M. Thompson, The role of image registration in brain mapping. *Image and Vision Computing*, 19, 3–24, 2001.
24. H. Park, P. H. Bland, A. O. Hero, and C. R. Meyer, Least biased target selection in probabilistic atlas construction, in *Medical Image Computing and Computer-Assisted Intervention—MICCAI 2005*, Palm Springs, California, pp. 419–426, 2005.
25. D. Seghers, E. D'Agostino, F. Maes, D. Vandermeulen, and P. Suetens, Construction of a brain template from MR images using state-of-the-art registration and segmentation techniques, in *Medical Image Computing and Computer-Assisted Intervention—MICCAI 2004*, Saint-Malo, France, pp. 696–703, 2004.
26. S. Joshi, B. Davis, M. Jomier, and G. Gerig, Unbiased diffeomorphic atlas construction for computational anatomy. *NeuroImage*, 23, S151–S160, 2004.
27. J. Hamm, C. Davatzikos, and R. Verma, *Efficient Large Deformation Registration Via Geodesics on a Learned Manifold of Images—MICCAI 2009*, London, UK, 2009.
28. E. G. Learned-Miller, Data driven image models through continuous joint alignment. *Pattern Analysis and Machine Intelligence, IEEE Transactions on*, 28, 236–250, 2006.
29. L. Zöllei, E. Learned-Miller, E. Grimson, and W. Wells, Efficient population registration of 3D data, in *Computer Vision for Biomedical Image Applications (ICCV)*, Beijing, China, pp. 291–301, 2005.
30. S. K. Balci, P. Golland, M. Shenton, and W. M. Wells, Free-form B-spline deformation model for groupwise registration, in *Medical Image Computing and Computer-Assisted Intervention—MICCAI 2007*, Brisbane, Australia, pp. 23–30, 2007.
31. M. R. Sabuncu, S. K. Balci, M. E. Shenton, and P. Golland, Image-driven population analysis through mixture modeling. *Medical Imaging, IEEE Transactions on*, 28, 1473–1487, 2009.
32. H. Jia, G. Wu, Q. Wang, and D. Shen, ABSORB: Atlas building by self-organized registration and bundling, in *Proceedings of IEEE Conference on Computer Vision and Pattern Recognition*, San Francisco, CA, 2010.
33. H. Jia, G. Wu, Q. Wang, and D. Shen, ABSORB: Atlas building by self-organized registration and bundling, *NeuroImage*, 51(3), 1057–1070, 2010.
34. F. Wang, B. C. Vemuri, A. Rangarajan, and S. J. Eisenschenk, Simultaneous nonrigid registration of multiple point sets and atlas construction. *Pattern Analysis and Machine Intelligence, IEEE Transactions on*, 30, 2011–2022, 2008.

35. Q. Wang, L. Chen, and D. Shen, Group-wise registration of large image dataset by hierarchical clustering and alignment, in *Medical Imaging 2009*. Orlando, Florida, vol. 7259, SPIE, 2009.
36. Q. Wang, P.-T. Yap, G. Wu, and D. Shen, Attribute vector guided groupwise registration, in *Medical Image Computing and Computer-Assisted Intervention—MICCAI 2009*, London, UK, 2009.
37. Q. Wang, G. Wu, P.-T. Yap, and D. Shen, Attribute vector guided groupwise registration. *NeuroImage*, 50, 1485–1496, 2010.
38. S. Marsland, C. J. Twining, and C. J. Taylor, A minimum description length objective function for groupwise non-rigid image registration. *Image and Vision Computing*, 26, 333–346, 2008.
39. S. Marsland and C. J. Twining, Constructing diffeomorphic representations for the groupwise analysis of nonrigid registrations of medical images. *Medical Imaging, IEEE Transactions on*, 23, 1006–1020, 2004.
40. P. T. Fletcher, S. Venkatasubramanian, and S. Joshi, The geometric median on Riemannian manifolds with application to robust atlas estimation. *NeuroImage*, 45, S143–S152, 2009.
41. G. Wu, P.-T. Yap, Q. Wang, and D. Shen, *Groupwise registration from exemplar to group mean: Extending HAMMER to groupwise registration*, in International Symposium of Biomedical Imaging (ISBI), Rotterdam, The Netherlands, 2010.
42. B. C. Munsell, A. Temlyakov, and S. Wang, Fast multiple shape correspondence by pre-organizing shape instances, in *IEEE Conference on CVPR*, Miami, Florida, pp. 840–847, 2009.
43. Q. Wang, L. Chen, P. T. Yap, G. Wu, and D. Shen, Groupwise registration based on hierarchical image clustering and atlas synthesis. *Human Brain Mapping*, 31(8), 1128–1140, 2010.
44. E. G. Miller, N. E. Matsakis, and P. A. Viola, Learning from one example through shared densities on transforms, in *Proceedings of the IEEE Conference on Computer Vision and Pattern Recognition, 2000*. Cambridge, Massachusetts, pp. 464–471, 2000.
45. F. Shi, Y. Fan, S. Tang, J. H. Gilmore, W. Lin, and D. Shen, Neonatal brain image segmentation in longitudinal MRI studies. *NeuroImage*, 49, 391–400, 2010.
46. T. Cox and M. A. A. Cox, *Multidimensional Scaling*, second ed. London: Chapman & Hall, 2000.
47. S. Baloch and C. Davatzikos, Morphological appearance manifolds in computational anatomy: Groupwise registration and morphological analysis. *NeuroImage*, 45, S73–S85, 2009.
48. S. Baloch, R. Verma, and C. Davatzikos, An anatomical equivalence class based joint transformation-residual descriptor for morphological analysis, in *Information Processing in Medical Imaging*, The Netherlands, pp. 594–606, 2007.
49. S. Tang, Y. Fan, and D. Shen, RABBIT: Rapid alignment of brains by building intermediate templates. *NeuroImage*, 47, 1277–1287, 2009.
50. M.-J. Kim, M.-H. Kim, and D. Shen, Learning-based deformation estimation for fast non-rigid registration, in *2008 IEEE Conference on Computer Vision and Pattern Recognition Workshops*, Anchorage, Alaska, pp. 1–6, 2008.
51. J. B. Kruskal, On the shortest spanning subtree of a graph and the traveling salesman problem, *Proceedings of the American Mathematical Society*, 7, 48–50, 1956.
52. K. K. Bhatia, J. V. Hajnal, B. K. Puri, A. D. Edwards, and D.Rueckert, Consistent groupwise non-rigid registration for atlas construction, in *IEEE Int. Symp. Biomed. Imag.: Macro Nano, 2004*. vol. 1, pp. 908–911, 2004.
53. J. Lin, Divergence measures based on the shannon entropy. *Information Theory, IEEE Transactions on*, 37, 145–151, 1991.
54. R. Wolz, P. Aljabar, J. V. Hajnal, A. Hammers, and D. Rueckert, LEAP: Learning embeddings for atlas propagation. *NeuroImage*, 49, 1316–1325, 2010.
55. R. C. Knickmeyer, S. Gouttard, C. Kang, D. Evans, K. Wilber, J. K. Smith, R. M. Hamer, W. Lin, G. Gerig, and J. H. Gilmore, A structural MRI study of human brain development from birth to 2 years. *Journal of Neuroscience*, 28, 12176–12182, 2008.
56. W. Gao, H. Zhu, K. S. Giovanello, J. K. Smith, D. Shen, J. H. Gilmore, and W. Lin, Evidence on the emergence of the brain's default network from 2-week-old to 2-year-old healthy pediatric subjects,

Proceedings of the National Academy of Sciences of the United States of America, 106, 6790–6795, 2009.
57. C. Hutton, E. De Vita, J. Ashburner, R. Deichmann, and R. Turner, Voxel-based cortical thickness measurements in MRI. *NeuroImage*, 40, 1701–1710, 2008.
58. S. R. Das, B. B. Avants, M. Grossman, and J. C. Gee, Registration based cortical thickness measurement. *NeuroImage*, 45867–879, 2009.
59. ADNI, http://www.loni.ucla.edu/ADNI/, 2004.
60. P.-T. Yap, G. Wu, H. Zhu, W. Lin, and D. Shen, Fast tensor image morphing for elastic registration, in *Medical Image Computing and Computer-Assisted Intervention—MICCAI 2009*, London, UK, 2009, pp. 721–729.
61. P.-T. Yap, G. Wu, H. Zhu, W. Lin, and D. Shen, TIMER: Tensor image morphing for elastic registration. *NeuroImage*, 47, 549–563, 2009.
62. P. Hagmann, L. Cammoun, X. Gigandet, R. Meuli, C. J. Honey, V. J. Wedeen, and O. Sporns, Mapping the structural core of human cerebral cortex. *PLoS Biol*, 6, 1479–1493, 2008.
63. C. Davatzikos, Y. Fan, X. Wu, D. Shen, and S. M. Resnick, Detection of prodromal Alzheimer's disease via pattern classification of MRI. *Neurobiology of Aging*, 29, 514–523, 2008.
64. F. Shi, D. Shen, P.-T. Yap, Y. Fan, J. Cheng, H. An, L. L. Wald, G. Gerig, J. H. Gilmore, and W. lin, CENTS: Cortical enhanced neonatal tissue segmentation. *Human Brain Mapping*, 32(3), 382–396, 2011.
65. F. Shi, P.-T. Yap, J. H. Gilmore, W. Lin, and D. Shen, Construction of multi-region-multi-reference atlases for neonatal brain MRI segmentation. *NeuroImage*, 51(3), 1057–1070, 2010.
66. M. Altaye, S. K. Holland, M. Wilke, and C. Gaser, Infant brain probability templates for MRI segmentation and normalization. *NeuroImage*, 43, 721–30, 2008.
67. P. Jaccard, The distribution of the flora in the alpine zone. *New Phytologist*, 11, 37–50, 1912.
68. D. J. Blezek and J. V. Miller, Atlas stratification. *Medical Image Analysis*, 11, 443–457, 2007.
69. F. Shi, L. Wang, Y. Dai, J. H. Gilmore, W. Lin, and D. Shen, LABEL: Pediatric brain extraction using learning-based meta-algorithm, *Neuroimage*, in press, 2012. Available at: http://www.sciencedirect.com/science/article/pii/S1053811912005307?v=s5
70. P. A. Yushkevich, J. Piven, H. C. Hazlett, R. G. Smith, S. Ho, J. C. Gee, and G. Gerig, User-guided 3D active contour segmentation of anatomical structures: Significantly improved efficiency and reliability. *NeuroImage*, 31, 1116–1128, 2006.
71. J. G. Sled, A. P. Zijdenbos, and A. C. Evans, A nonparametric method for automatic correction of intensity nonuniformity in MRI data. *IEEE Trans Med Imaging*, 17, 87–97, 1998.
72. D. L. Pham and J. L. Prince, An adaptive fuzzy C-means algorithm for image segmentation in the presence of intensity inhomogeneities. *Pattern Recognition Letters*, 20, 57–68, 1999.
73. F. Shi, P.-T. Yap, G. Wu, H. Jia, J. H. Gilmore, W. Lin, and D. Shen, Infant brain atlases from neonates to 1- and 2-year-olds, *PLoS ONE*, 6, e18746, 2011.

6

Functional Optical Brain Imaging

Meltem Izzetoglu
Drexel University

6.1 Introduction

Functional imaging is typically conducted in an effort to understand the activity in a given brain region in terms of its relationship to a particular behavioral state, or its interactions with inputs from another region's activity. The advances in noninvasive functional brain monitoring technologies provide opportunities to accurately examine the living brains of large groups of subjects over long periods of time, with little impact on their well-being. Neurophysiological and neuroimaging technologies have contributed much to our understanding of normative brain function, as well as to our understanding of the neural underpinnings of various neurological and psychiatric disorders. Commonly employed techniques such as electroencephalography (EEG), event-related brain potentials (ERPs), magnetoencephalography (MEG), positron emission tomography (PET), single-positron emission computed tomography (SPECT), and functional magnetic resonance imaging (fMRI), have dramatically increased our understanding of a broad range of brain disorders. Nevertheless, there is still much unknown about these syndromes. This is due, in large part, to the inherent complexity of the neurobiological substrates of these disorders and of the mind itself. In addition, each of the research methods used to study brain function and its disorders have methodological strengths as well as their own inherent limitations. These limitations place constraints on our ability to fully explicate the neural basis of neurological and psychiatric disorders both inside and outside of the laboratory setting, and to use the information gleaned from laboratory studies for clinical applications in real-world environments. New techniques that allow data to be gathered under more diverse circumstances than is possible with extant neuroimaging systems should facilitate a more thorough understanding of brain function and its pathologies.

Functional near-infrared spectroscopy (fNIR) has been introduced as a new neuroimaging modality with which to conduct functional brain imaging studies [1–24]. fNIR technology uses specific wavelengths of light, irradiated through the scalp, to enable the noninvasive measurement of changes in the relative ratios of deoxygenated hemoglobin (deoxy-Hb) and oxygenated hemoglobin (oxy-Hb) during brain activity. This technology allows the design of portable, safe, affordable, noninvasive, and minimally intrusive monitoring systems. These qualities make fNIR suitable for the study of hemodynamic changes due to cognitive and emotional brain activity under many working and educational conditions, as well as in the field. Using this technique, several types of brain activity have been assessed, including motor activity, visual activation, auditory stimulation, and the performance of cognitive tasks (e.g., [9]). To date, the outcomes of studies utilizing fNIR compare favorably with previous fMRI and complement EEG findings [21–23].

The purpose of the present chapter is to describe an emerging neuroimaging technology, fNIR, which has several attributes that make it possible to conduct neuroimaging studies of the cortex in clinical offices and under more realistic, ecologically valid parameters. In this chapter, we will first describe general working principles of fNIR and different fNIR instrumentations based on these working principles. Then, we will review algorithms developed for fNIR data processing for artifact removal and used in the extraction of hemodynamic signals from the fNIR intensity measurements. We will discuss the results of various fNIR applications in laboratory settings and in field conditions. Finally, the merits of optical imaging in brain research will be summarized.

6.2 Working Principles

6.2.1 Physiological Principles: How Can Brain Activity Be Measured through Hemodynamic Changes?

Neural activity has a direct relation with hemodynamic changes in the brain [25]. Research on brain-energy metabolism has elucidated the close link between hemodynamic and neural activity [26,27]. Understanding the brain energy metabolism and associated neural activity is of importance for realizing principles of fNIR in assessing brain activity. The brain has small energy reserves and a great majority of the energy used by brain cells is for processes that sustain physiological functioning [28]. Ames III reviewed the studies on brain energy metabolism as related to function and reported that the oxygen (O_2) consumption of the rabbit vagus nerve increased 3.4-fold when it was stimulated at 10 Hz and O_2 consumption in rabbit sympathetic ganglia increased 40% with stimulation at 15 Hz. Furthermore, glucose utilization by various brain regions increased several fold in response to physiological stimulation or in response to pharmacological agents that affect physiological activity [28]. These studies provide clear evidence that large changes occur in brain energy metabolism in response to changes in activity. The levels of compounds involved in energy metabolism and energy metabolites can be outlined as

- Neuronal activity is fueled by glucose metabolism, so increases in neural activity result in increased glucose and oxygen consumption from the local capillary bed. Brain cells consume energy when activated and oxygen is required to metabolize the glucose. The oxygen concentration in the capillaries can support the normal oxygen consumption (about 3.5 $\mu mol\, g^{-1}\, min^{-1}$) for 2 s. [27]. For that reason, a reduction in local glucose and oxygen stimulates the brain to increase local arteriolar vasodilation, which increases local cerebral blood flow (CBF) and cerebral blood volume (CBV), a mechanism known as neurovascular coupling.
- Over a period of several seconds, the increased CBF carries both glucose and oxygen to the neural tissue in the area. Oxygen is transported via oxy-Hb in the blood. The oxygen exchange occurs in the capillary beds. As oxy-Hb gives up oxygen, it is transformed into deoxy-Hb.

- The increased oxygen transported to the area via increased CBF typically exceeds the local neuronal rate of oxygen utilization, the cerebral metabolic rate of oxygen (CMRO2), resulting in an overabundance of cerebral blood oxygenation in active areas [29]. Therefore, local blood is more oxygenated and hence less deoxy-Hb is present [30]. (Although the initial increase in neural activity is thought to result in a focal increase in deoxygenated hemoglobin in the capillary bed as oxygen is withdrawn from the hemoglobin for use in the metabolization of glucose, this feature of the vascular response has been much more difficult to measure, and more controversial, than hyperoxygenation. Please see [31,32], for a more detailed discussion of this topic.)

These changes in the hemodynamic signals occur within a few seconds after the onset of the stimulation and may take 10–20 s to evolve [33,34]. Based on the brain energy metabolism, methods and imaging modalities, such as fNIR and fMRI [35,36] for measurements of slowly changing hemodynamic signals, deoxy-Hb and/or oxy-Hb are implemented to provide correlates of brain activity through oxygen consumption by neurons.

6.2.2 Physical Principles: How Can Hemodynamic Activity Be Measured by Optics?

It is well-known that the functional state of tissue can influence its optical properties, for instance, cyanosis in hypoxia; pallor in anemia. The human brain undergoes a number of physiological changes as it responds to environmental stimuli; these changes in blood levels and electrochemical activity also affect its optical properties. Functional optical imaging capitalizes on the changing optical properties of these tissues by using light in the near-infrared range (700–900 nm) to measure physiological changes. Because oxy-Hb and deoxy-Hb have characteristic optical properties in the visible and near-infrared light range between 700 and 900 nm, the change in concentration of these molecules during neurovascular coupling can be measured using optical methods [9,37]. Most biological tissues are relatively transparent to light in the near-infrared range, largely because major components of most tissues, such as water absorb very little energy at these wavelengths (see Figure 6.1). As such, this spectral band is often referred to as the "optical window" for the noninvasive assessment of brain activation. However,

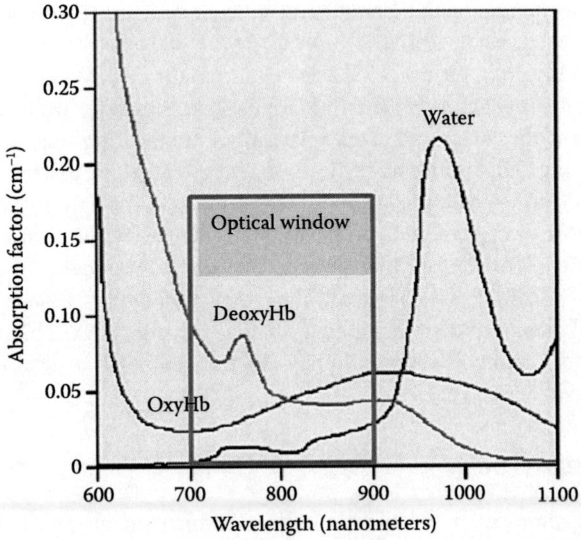

FIGURE 6.1 Absorption spectrum in near-infrared (IR) window.

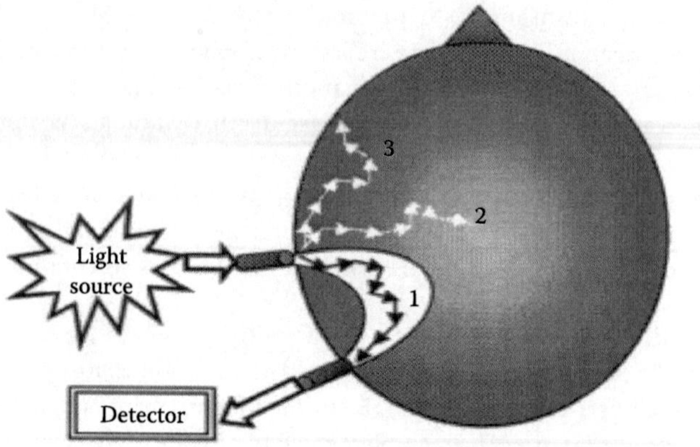

FIGURE 6.2 Photon path inside the human head. Photon 1 undergoes a number of scattering events and leaves the head at the location that the detector is placed and hence will be detected by the system. Photon 2 is absorbed by chromophores after a number of scattering events and cannot continue to travel within the tissue and hence will not be detected by the system. Photon 3 gets scattered in a different direction and leaves the head at a location where no detector is placed and hence will not be detected by the system. Changes in scattering and absorption within the banana-like shaped sampling volume will alter the amount of photons reaching the detector and hence can be monitored and quantified by the system. (From Obrig H et al. 2000. *Int. J. Psychophysiol.*, 35:125–142.)

the chromophores oxy-Hb and deoxy-Hb do absorb a fair amount of energy in this range. Fortunately, in the optical window, the absorption spectra of oxy-Hb and deoxy-Hb remain significantly different than each other as shown in Figure 6.1 allowing spectroscopic separation of these compounds to be possible using only a few sample wavelengths.

Typically, an fNIR apparatus is comprised of a light source that is coupled to the participant's head via either light-emitting diodes (LEDs) or though fiber-optical bundles (the optode), and a light detector that receives the light after it has interacted with the tissue. Photons that enter tissue undergo two different types of interaction, namely absorption and scattering [4,5,19]. When photons get absorbed by the tissue they lose their energy to the medium and hence cannot continue to travel within the tissue. After entering the tissue, photons get diffused and experience multiple scattering events. Hence, a photodetector placed 2–7 cm away from the light source can collect a relatively predictable quantity of photons that are not absorbed and traveled within the tissue along the "banana-shaped path" between the source and detector due to multiple scattering [9,38] as shown in Figure 6.2. When the distance between the source and photodetector is set at 4 cm, the fNIR signal becomes sensitive to hemodynamic changes within the top 2–3 mm of the cortex and extends laterally 1 cm to either side, perpendicular to the axis of source-detector spacing [39]. Studies have shown that at inter-optode distances as short as 2–2.5 cm, grey matter is part of the sample volume [39,40]. If wavelengths of the light sources are chosen to maximize the amount of absorption by oxy-Hb and deoxy-Hb, changes in the chromophore concentrations cause changes in the number of photons that are absorbed and the number of photons that are scattered back to the surface of the scalp. These changes in the attenuation of light measured at the surface of the scalp can be quantified using different techniques, that is, diffusion equation, modified Beer–Lambert law, and so on, and information on changes in oxy-Hb and deoxy-Hb concentrations can be assessed which will be discussed in Section 6.5.

6.3 Instrumentation

A wide variety of both commercial and custom-built fNIR instruments are currently in use [5]. These systems differ with respect to their use and system engineering, with tradeoffs between light sources, detectors, and instrument electronics that result in tradeoffs in the information available for analysis, safety, and cost. Three distinct types of fNIR implementation have been developed: time domain (TD) systems, frequency domain (FD) systems, and continuous wave (CW) spectroscopy systems, each with their own strengths and limitations [3–5]. In TD systems, also referred to as time-resolved spectroscopy (TRS), extremely short (picosecond-order) incident pulses of laser light are applied to the tissue and the temporal distribution of photons that carry the information about tissue scattering and absorption is measured. The emerging intensity is detected as a function of time (the temporal point spread function [TPSF]) with picosecond resolution [7,39,41]. Streak camera systems can provide high-temporal resolution, but they are large, expensive, and have a limited dynamic range. Time-correlated single-photon counting systems can be built with cheaper components and can provide wide dynamic range, however, they have poor temporal resolution. Even though TRS instruments offer absolute measurements of hemodynamic changes since they can be large, expensive, with limited dynamic range or poor temporal resolution, they have originally been developed as laboratory-based devices, and hence are difficult to be implemented in the clinical environment and in the field applications [5]. In FD or phase modulation spectroscopy (PM) systems, the light source is intensity modulated to the frequencies in the order of tens to hundreds of megahertz. The amplitude decay, phase shift, and modulation depth of the detected light intensity with respect to the incident light are measured to characterize the optical properties of tissue [42]. FD methods are low-cost alternatives to time-resolved methods and hence several multichannel FD instruments are now in common use [7,43].

CW systems apply either continuous or a slow-pulsed light to tissue and are limited to measuring the amplitude attenuation of the incident light [45]. These systems utilize less sophisticated detectors than time-resolved and FD systems and they cannot resolve the time-changing component of the light. As such, CW systems provide somewhat less information than time- or FD systems meaning relative measurements as opposed to absolute ones, but this tradeoff results in the capacity to design more compact, portable, easy to engineer, and affordable hardware making it advantageous for various applications [45,46]. They can be laser-based, but LEDs can also be used in CW designs to increase safety (particularly with respect to eye exposure) and comfort, and to again decrease both instrument size and cost, making it possible to deploy these systems in clinical or educational settings [5,7,32]. A detailed list of both commercially available and laboratory prototype fNIR instruments are presented in [43].

6.4 fNIR Measurements

6.4.1 Fast Neuronal Signal

Fast neuronal signal or event-related optical signal (EROS) capitalizes on the changes in the optical properties of the cell membranes themselves that occur as a function of the ionic fluxes during firing [14]. Using invasive techniques, it has been well-established that the optical properties of cell membranes change in the depolarized state relative to the resting state [32,47–49] and that optical methods can be used to detect these changes that occur within the first 200 ms of functional stimulation.

The ability to measure the actual depolarization state of neuronal tissue provides obvious advantages in that it is a direct measure of neural activity, with millisecond-level time resolution as can be measured with EEG and MEG but with the superior spatial resolution lacking in EEG/MEG. However, there are also a number of limitations to the noninvasive use of the EROS signal in humans. A primary disadvantage of the fast optical signal is the low signal- to-noise ratio (SNR) resulting from the need to image through skin, skull, and cerebral-spinal fluid. Basic sensory and motor movements such as tactile stimulation and finger tapping require between 500 and 1000 trials to establish a reliable signal [13]. There have also been failures to replicate the results of experiments reporting the fast optical signal in response to a visual stimulus among normal adult humans [32]. The low SNR may play a role in current difficulties with experimental replication; however, more cross-validation work is warranted. The final constraint is that these methods require a more expensive and cumbersome laser-based light source (vs. an LED-based light source), they are not portable, and the potential risk of inadvertent damage to the eyes is increased relative to the systems available for measuring hemodynamic responses. (LED-based near-infrared sources pose very little, if any, risk upon eye exposure [50]). In spite of these current limitations, the fast optical signal continues to be an important area of investigation because it offers glimpses of the "holy grail" of neuroimaging: the direct measurement of neuronal activity with millisecond time resolution and superior spatial resolution.

6.4.2 Slow Hemodynamic Signal

As explained in Section 6.2.1 through brain-energy metabolism, during brain activity first local oxygen consumption increases to metabolize glucose and provide energy to the activated neurons. Next, blood flow and perfusion increases in the area of activated neurons through neurovascular coupling which in turn changes the hemoglobin concentrations and oxygenation. These slow changes in hemodynamic signal occur within a few seconds after the onset of the stimulation and takes 10–20 min to take its full course to evolve [33,34] and can be measured by fNIR, PET, and fMRI as blood oxygen level dependent (BOLD) signal that is related with the changes in the concentration of deoxy-Hb.

Most fNIR applications are based upon the measurement of the slow hemodynamic responses in terms of deoxy-Hb and oxy-Hb. Typical slow hemodynamic signals together with corresponding fMRI-BOLD signal collected during a finger tapping experiment is shown in Figure 6.3a. Either the full-time course of the hemodynamic signals and/or features that can be extracted from them such as maximum amplitude, time to peak or reaction time, full width half maximum, and so on, as shown in Figure 6.3b are then used for comparison purposes in different task conditions, spatial locations or subject populations which will be discussed in detail in Sections 6.5 and 6.6.

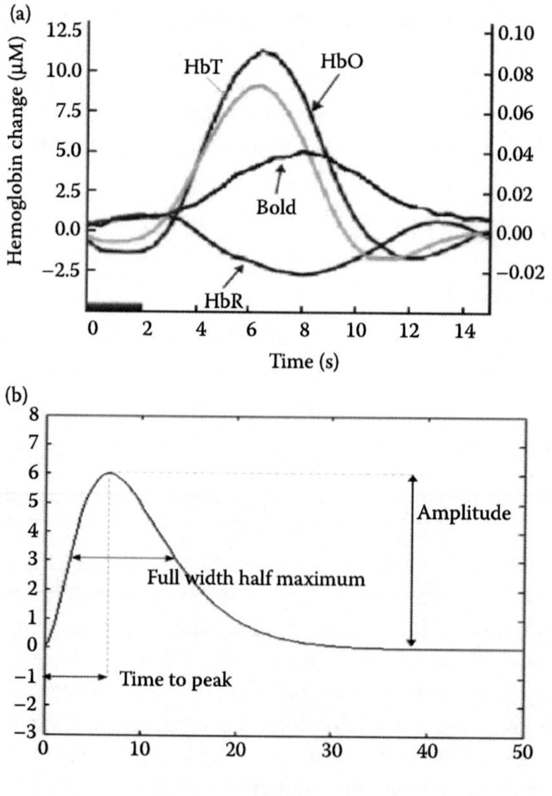

FIGURE 6.3 (a) Example hemodynamic signals. (From Boas DA, Dale AM, Francheschini MA. 2004. *Neuroimage*, 23:S275–S288.) (b) Features that can be extracted from hemodynamic responses.

6.5 fNIR Signal Processing

Analysis of fNIR measurements involves two main steps: (i) artifact and/or noise removal, and (ii) conversion of optical measurements into physiologically relevant signals and/or features. fNIR measurements can get corrupted by different sources of noise that should be suppressed in order to reliably extract information-bearing signals that are related to cognitive activity. Depending on the fNIR system used optical intensity measurements are converted to physiologically relevant signals and features for further processing using different approximations, assumptions, and algorithms. In this section, we will review different sources and characteristics of noise and existing algorithms to suppress them and the algorithms used to extract hemodynamic variables from fNIR intensity measurements.

6.5.1 Signal Separation and Noise Removal

The sources of noise in fNIR measurements can be categorized in two main groups: (i) noise of nonphysiological basis, and (ii) artifacts arise from systemic physiological origins. Noise sources that are not driven by physiological origins can happen as a result of instrumental noise, that is, electrical noise or experimental errors, that is, motion artifact, task-related errors. Since fNIR systems measure changes in hemodynamics, they measure such changes not only related with cognitive activity but also the ones that occur due to heart pulsation, respiration, and so on, resulting in systemic physiological artifacts. A detailed explanation of these noise sources and some algorithms for their suppression is presented in [52]. In this section, we will briefly explain these different sources of noise and summarize currently existing algorithms for their suppression.

Note that, noise in the optical measurements can be removed before and after the conversion of raw intensity measurements to physiological hemoglobin concentrations. The noise of nonphysiological basis such as instrument noise or experimental errors that are not related to underlying physiological changes should be removed prior to conversion of signals into hemodynamic measures. This way, errors across wavelengths will not be propagated causing additional crosstalk in the separation of oxy-Hb and deoxy-Hb. In contrast, noise of physiological origins such as blood pressure changes, heart pulsations, and so on, causes oscillations in hemoglobin concentrations together with changes related to brain activity such biological noise is better removed after the conversion of raw intensity measurements to hemodynamic variables [52].

6.5.1.1 Noise of Nonphysiological Basis

One type of noise that is not related with any physiological changes is electrical/electronic noise from the computer or other hardware in the instrument. Such electrical noise can also be generated by the use of other devices or from the surrounding space that can create interference in the measurements. This type of electrical noise is generally assumed to be white and since hemodynamic response generated by brain activity is generally slow (up to 0.1 Hz), most of the time, high frequency instrument noise are suppressed by simply low-pass filtering the data [52,53] or significantly reduced by adjusting the power of light sources within the safety limits and gain amplification at the detectors.

There can be other types of noise within fNIR measurements whose origins are not directly related with physiological changes within the underlying tissue such as artifacts that may arise as the result of subject motion or noncompliance with the experimental paradigm or the ones that are the direct results of experimental paradigm itself. This type of noise is sometimes called experimental errors [52]. Head movement can cause the fNIR detectors to shift and lose contact with the skin, exposing them to either ambient light or to light emitted directly from the fNIR sources or reflected from the skin, rather than being reflected from tissue in regions of interest. These effects cause sudden increases in the fNIR data. Another consequence of head movement is, it can cause the blood to move toward (or away from) the area that is being monitored, increasing (or decreasing) the amount of oxygen, hence result in an increase (or decrease) in the measured data. Since the dynamics of this type of motion artifact are slow, they can easily be confused with the actual hemodynamic response due to brain activation. Even though it is not as pronounced as in fMRI, motion artifacts in fNIR studies are a serious problem for real-life applications where head immobility is undesirable or untenable such as in studies involving pilots, children, and so on. Hence, cleaning the fNIR data from motion artifacts is an important and necessary task in order to deploy fNIR as a brain monitoring technology in its full potential to many real-life application areas.

The best way to deal with motion artifacts is to avoid them as much as possible which mostly depend on subject compliance, experimental design, and experimenter's expertise in the placement of the fNIR sensor. However, these conditions can be satisfied for experiments involving adults and the ones that can be carried out in the laboratory, in controlled environments or in sitting positions. Different sensor designs and placements are developed to match the requirements of the experiment and reduce dependence on experimenter's expertise for its secure placement [52]. However, such sensor designs may only eliminate motion artifacts that can arise from the shift or pop of sources and/or detectors where motion artifacts of slow nature due to blood movement may still be present if head movement occurs during data acquisition as a result of experimental design or subject incompliance. There are several different algorithms developed for the detection and elimination of motion artifacts. For motion artifacts arising from the physical displacement or movement of the optical probe, detection algorithms such as the one based on outlier detection methods was proposed in [52]. In order to suppress the motion artifact, several methods were proposed such as the ones based on principal component analysis (PCA) [52], wavelet analysis [54] or recently a combined PCA and independent component analysis (ICA) [55]. The novelty in this last method was the use of dark current measurements for the identification of the existence of motion artifacts and their removal by the use of a combined ICA/PCA-based method. This method was applied on a clinical data collected in a highly noisy environment namely operating room and shown to successfully remove motion artifacts. A comparison of algorithms in motion artifact removal based on wavelets, autoregression, adaptive filtering, and ICA are discussed in [56]. For motion artifacts that are the result of the movement of the blood within the tissue that are more slow in nature and have similar frequency spectrum as with the optical signals coming from physiological origins such as hemodynamic response to stimulus, respiration, heart pulsation, and so on, there exists different algorithms based on adaptive, Wiener and Kalman filtering. A detailed analysis of these algorithms in comparison to each other based on their ability to improve SNR on 11 subject data set where slow, medium, and high-speed head movement was tested are given in [57,58]. A sample result is shown in Figure 6.4 where motion free data, adaptive, Wiener and Kalman filtered data are presented on a medium speed head movement case. A separate study for similar type of motion artifact used the observation that motion noise may cause the measured oxy-Hb and deoxy-Hb signals, which are typically strongly negatively correlated, to become more

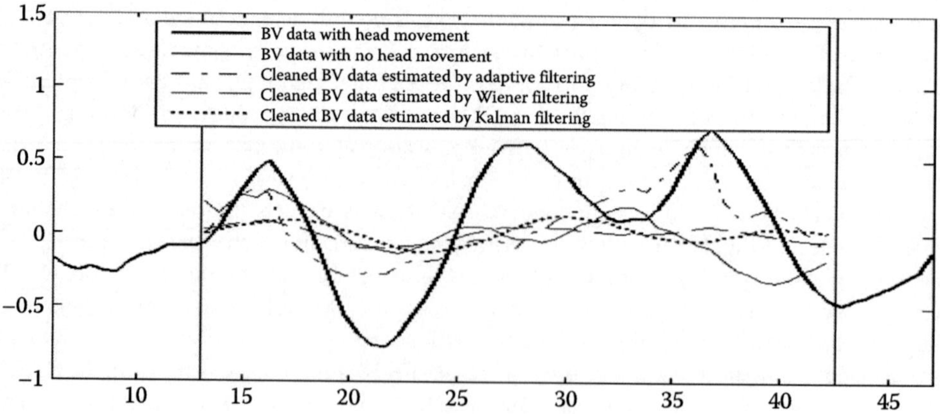

FIGURE 6.4 Comparison of different motion artifact removal algorithms on blood volume (total hemoglobin = oxy-Hb + deoxy-Hb) data.

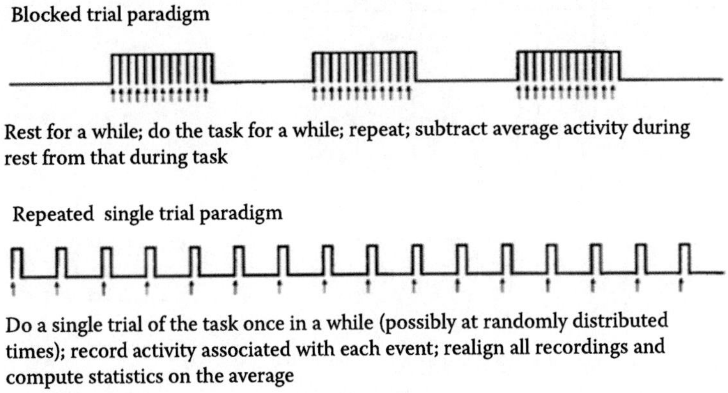

FIGURE 6.5 Schematic diagram of blocked and single-trial paradigms.

positively correlated [59]. A method has been developed to reduce noise-based on the principle that the concentration changes of oxy-Hb and deoxy-Hb should be negatively correlated.

In addition to motion artifacts, experimental errors can also be introduced simply by the design of the functional task or the study itself of it being an event-related or block design or a longitudinal study, and so on. The predominant paradigms used in functional studies are the repeated single trial paradigm and the blocked trial paradigm (Figure 6.5) [60]. Usually in fNIR studies experimental designs are selected similar to the ones used in fMRI or EEG studies. However, additional care must be taken in adjusting the task or selecting data analysis methods while using fNIR. For example, since hemodynamic responses are slow in nature as compared to the fast neuronal signals as measured by EEG, improper design of the timing of an experimental paradigm can introduce errors. In general, this requires that the timing of stimulus presentation in single trial paradigms to be spaced widely apart in time to allow the evoked-hemodynamic signal to evolve completely. If a block design or a rapid event-related design is used, selection of the interstimulus interval is very important for the evoked-hemodynamic responses to still hold the linearity assumption (the assumption that repeated evoked responses will add linearly). For event-related stimulus designs or in block designs where evoked-hemodynamic responses are required to be extracted [61], the total hemodynamic responses measured may be approximated as the linear summation of evoked responses to each single stimulus, provided that the interstimulus interval is longer than around 3–4 s. Another study related error in the measurements can occur during longitudinal studies over a subject group. If the fNIR sensor is not placed on the exact same location at different recording times, the results may not reflect possible changes over time but the optical differences in different tissue area monitored [52].

6.5.1.2 Artifacts That Arise from Systemic Physiological Origins

fNIR technology measures hemodynamic changes which can be as a result of brain activity or simply due to systemic physiological variations such as cardiac pulsations, respiration, and blood pressure. In humans, the cardiac pulsation and respiration typically have a period of 0.7–1.5 s and 3–8 s, respectively. The arterial blood pressure varies on multiple time scales approximately 10 s Mayer waves and slower N50-s variation [51,52,62,63]. Note that, although often times these physiological fluctuations are considered to be artifacts because they may interfere with the evoked-functional responses, if they can be effectively and reliably separated from evoked-hemodynamic responses, it may in fact be a very valuable characteristic of fNIR to be able measure all these physiological signals with just one sensor.

In order to improve the sensitivity and interpretability of fNIR measurements to brain activation, it is necessary to separate systemic physiological signal sources spatially and temporally. There are different techniques developed to suppress or separate the systemic physiological signals from evoked-hemodynamic responses based on either (i) known approximate frequency content of signals, (ii) the spatial covariance of

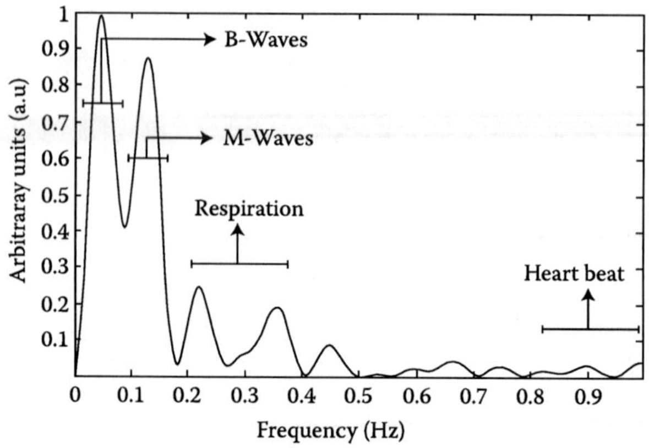

FIGURE 6.6 fNIR signal and artifacts in FD.

physiology, or (iii) the ability to remotely measure physiological signals correlated with the ones appearing in fNIR measurements of interest. Since the frequency bands of the physiological signal sources are known approximately, classical filters, that is, low-pass, band-pass, high-pass filters can effectively and efficiently be used to separate some of those signals. A classic example of the power spectral density (PSD) spectrum of the poststimulus signal segment is shown in Figure 6.6 [60]. The hemodynamic response following neural activation is embedded in the frequencies up to approximately 0.1 Hz. The 0.8 Hz and 0.2 Hz bands correspond to heart rate and respiration, respectively. The B-waves (~0.03 Hz) represent very low frequency oscillations (VLFO) generated by the various brain stem nuclei in the vasomotor tone of cerebral arterioles [64]. The Mayer waves (~0.1 Hz) represent low frequency oscillations reflecting oscillations due to blood pressure. As an example, if a band-pass filter with pass band selected to be between 0.08 and 0.12 Hz is designed, it can remove the high-frequency instrument noise, the fast cardiac oscillations, respiration, and VLFO. Note that, in such application involving band-pass filtering care should be taken to avoid removal of frequencies associated with the evoked-functional hemodynamic response. For example, bandpass filtering can generally not be used to remove Mayer waves, since their frequency band overlaps with the content of the hemodynamic response. Alternatives to conventional bandpass filtering, involve the use of curve fitting [60], adaptive, Wiener and Kalman filtering techniques [60,65,66]. In the Wiener filtering approach, the statistical changes in such physiological artifacts had been taken into account.

Other than classical filters, algorithms that use the spatial persistence nature of systemic physiological signals (specific and repeated spatial pattern across the brain) such as PCA-based physiological filtering methods have been proposed [67] similar to its use for motion correction. There also exist algorithms based on separate measurements providing correlated noise sources with the physiological signals. In these algorithms the cardiac, respiration, and blood pressure signals are separately measured by additional sensors such as with dynamic blood pressure cuff, pneumatic belt, pulse plethysmograph, pulse oximetry, or an electrocardiogram which can provide signals that are correlated with the artifacts that exist within fNIR measurements. Then, algorithm such as least squares regression algorithms [68], adaptive filtering [66], ICA [69] or RETROICOR [70] as developed for fMRI can be used to remove these signals from fNIR measurements to extract evoked-hemodynamic responses. In another technique, correlated measurements of physiological artifacts are measured by using multiple source detector separations. Since penetration depth increases with an increase in source detector separation, by measuring from detectors that are placed close enough to the source, one can guarantee penetration to only superficial tissues and not to brain. On the contrary, detectors placed farther away from the source can measure signals coming from the brain together with all the other superficial layers. Such arrangement is used in different applications to remove physiological signals [66] as well as motion artifacts [71].

6.5.2 Hemodynamic Signal Extraction from fNIR Intensity Measurements

Several different algorithms based on different mathematical models and assumptions have been developed to quantify the fNIR measurements and obtain information about the physiological/optical changes related with brain activity. Depending on the fNIR system and measurement type, appropriate algorithms can be implemented. Here, we will discuss two of the most commonly used methods (i) diffusion theory and (ii) modified Beer–Lambert law both of which are derived from linear transport theory to extract absolute or relative measurements of hemodynamic signals. Within each category, we will describe the mathematical model used, assumptions needed to meet for the algorithm to be applicable, and existing analytical and experimental solutions.

6.5.2.1 Diffusion Theory

Propagation of light in highly diffusive media such as tissue is usually modeled by using linear transport theory (radiative transport or Boltzman transport theory) [7,72–74]. However, analytical solutions to radiative transport equation can only be obtained for very simple geometries. Much simpler approximation can be derived from radiative transport equation based on diffusion theory [7,72–77] under certain assumptions such as (i) scattering coefficient is much greater than the absorption coefficient, (ii) scattering is isotropic, (iii) source detector separations are not too small, and (iv) measurement times are apart from the input times [72,77]. TD diffusion equation is given as [7,72–74]

$$\frac{1}{c}\frac{\partial\Phi(r,t)}{\partial t} - \nabla[D(r)\nabla\Phi(r,t)] + \mu_a(r)\Phi(r,t) = S(r,t), \quad D = [3(\mu_a + (1-g)\mu_s)]^{-1} \tag{6.1}$$

where $\Phi(r,t)$ is the diffuse photon fluence rate at position r and time t, $S(r,t)$ is the photon source, c is the speed of light in the tissue, D is the diffusion coefficient, μ_a is the linear absorption coefficient, μ_s is the linear scattering coefficient, and g is the mean cosine of the scattering angle.

Analytical solutions to diffusion equation as a forward problem (derivation of the resulting measurement given the distribution of light sources and detectors, tissue parameters, and boundaries) can be obtained using Green's function which provides the photon distribution when the source is an impulsive function. Green's function solutions to diffusion approximation have been driven for slab, cylindrical, and spherical geometries. For a semi-infinite half-space geometry one such solution for an impulse input is found as [7,78]

$$R(\rho,t) = \frac{z_o \exp(-\mu_a ct)}{(4\pi Dc)^{3/2} t^{5/2}} \exp\left[-\frac{\rho^2 + z_o^2}{4Dct}\right] \tag{6.2}$$

where $R(\rho,t)$ is the reflected light intensity, $z_o = 1/\mu_s'$ and $\mu_s' = (1-g)\mu_s$ is the reduced scattering coefficient. Solutions to diffusion equation in TD and FD can also be found in [77].

Experimentally, as an inverse problem (derivation of the distribution of tissue optical parameters given the distribution of light sources and measurements [72]), in TD systems the time course of the measured light intensities at different wavelengths are fitted to the solution equation and hence the absolute absorption and scattering parameters of the underlying tissue of interest are estimated [7]. Note that, since information contained in temporal profile of the measured light will also be present in FD, similar approaches to TD techniques can be applied to FD systems to extract optical parameters as an inverse problem.

Optical properties of the tissue such as absorption and scattering coefficients are wavelength dependent. Furthermore, absorption parameter of the tissue changes with the change in the concentrations of underlying tissue chromophores. Since within the optical window (700–900 nm) the dominant tissue chromophores are the oxy-Hb and deoxy-Hb, their absolute concentrations can be calculated using the absorption coefficient estimated at multiple wavelengths [51] using:

$$\mu_a(\lambda) = \varepsilon_{HBO2}(\lambda)C_{HbO2} + \varepsilon_{HB}(\lambda)C_{HB} \tag{6.3}$$

where λ is the photon wavelength, ε is the wavelength and chromophore-dependent extinction coefficients (experimental values are tabulated in [19]) and C_{HBO2} and C_{HB} are the concentrations of oxy-Hb and deoxy-Hb, respectively.

Solutions to diffusion equation cannot be obtained analytically for more complex inhomogeneous geometries. For such cases, numerical solutions are studied based on numerical integral and differential approximation methods such as finite difference methods (FDM), finite element methods (FEM), or perturbative approaches using truncated series approximations such as Born and Rytov approximations and their higher order extensions [72,73]. These numerical solutions suffer from extensive computational cost. Another numerical method used for the solution of the forward problem to study the light propagation in tissue is the Monte Carlo modeling (MCM) [73]. In MCM, photons are assumed to have certain probability of scattering and absorption where many photons are injected into the medium at every source, treated separately and at the end statistical maps of a combination of photons collected at the detectors are obtained.

6.5.2.2 Modified Beer–Lambert Law

Under various simplifying assumptions [79], radiative transport equation can be reduced to the Beer–Lambert Law which states that the attenuation of an absorbing compound dissolved in a nonabsorbent compound is proportional to the concentration of the compound and the optical path length [2,4]. In a purely absorbing medium, the transmitted light I can be expressed in terms of the input light I_o as follows:

$$I = I_o e^{-\mu_a L} \tag{6.4}$$

where μ_a is the absorption coefficient of the homogeneous medium and L is the optical path length. Since absorption coefficient is related to concentration of the absorbing compound C and the extinction coefficient ε as $\mu_a = \varepsilon C$, the absorbance or attenuation (A) in terms of optical density (OD) units can be written as

$$A = \text{OD} = \ln\left(\frac{I_o}{I}\right) = \varepsilon \text{CL} \tag{6.5}$$

If there is more than one absorbing compound within the medium then the attenuation can be given by

$$A = [\varepsilon_1 C_1 + \varepsilon_2 C_2 + \cdots + \varepsilon_N C_N]L \tag{6.6}$$

In a scattering medium where there is no absorption, the light will still be attenuated since the photons will be deflected from their path [80]. Hence similar to absorbing case, in a medium having only one scattering compound with a scattering coefficient μ_s the transmitted light intensity I can be written as

$$I = I_o e^{-\mu_s L} \tag{6.7}$$

Note that when multiple scattering occurs and the light gets diffuse, then isotropic scattering is often assumed and the reduced scattering coefficient $\mu_s' = (1 - g)\mu_s$ is used instead to represent it.

Within the tissue, light attenuation happens due to absorption and scattering together. Both of these effects should be taken into account in order to correctly quantify changes in hemodynamics. Modified Beer–Lambert law (MBLL) accounts for the effects of both the absorption and multiple scattering where the attenuation is expressed as follows:

$$A = \ln\left(\frac{I_o}{I}\right) = \varepsilon \mathrm{CL} + G \tag{6.8}$$

where G represents the light attenuation due to scattering which depends on also on measurement geometry.

MBLL relies on several assumptions such as (i) homogeneous tissue, (ii) constant scattering G, and (iii) known path length L [4,74,80]. Even though these may not be exactly met by the biological tissues, MBLL is by far the most widely used technique in calculating hemodynamic changes especially in CW systems mostly due to its simplicity and no computational cost [74]. It is discussed in [80] that scattering in brain tissue occurs mostly due to cell and subcellular membranes and that scattering due to red blood cells is low. Hence, in functional optical imaging studies, the attenuation due to scattering can be assumed to be constant since even though the concentration of oxy-Hb and deoxy-Hb changes due to brain activity their contribution to scattering can be negligible.

The mean path length (L) that light travels in a highly scattering medium such as tissue is larger than the direct path or geometrical path length (d) between light source and detector. This increase in path length due to tissue scattering is corrected by using a differential path length factor (DPF). Then the mean path length is found as

$$L = \mathrm{DPF} \cdot d \tag{6.9}$$

The DPF for tissues at different anatomical regions such as head (forehead, somatosensory, and occipital regions), calf, fore arm, and so on, for adult and infant populations have been both experimentally (using TD and FD systems) and numerically (using Monte Carlo simulations) studied and the values are tabulated [81–83]. It is noted that DPF is wavelength dependent and there can be subject to subject differences based on gender, age, and so on [83,84].

Even though the DPF can be measured or taken from published values assuming small across subject differences, the absolute quantification of chromophore concentrations cannot be possible since G is unknown. If G is assumed to be constant during the measurement period, then by measuring the A at two or more wavelengths, the relative change in tissue chromophores ΔC such as oxy-Hb and deoxy-Hb versus time can be obtained from relative changes in attenuation ΔA to an arbitrary time as follows:

$$\Delta A = \varepsilon \cdot \Delta C \cdot d \cdot \mathrm{DPF} \tag{6.10}$$

By measuring attenuation change at two distinct wavelengths and using Equation 6.10, changes in oxy-Hb (HbO2) and deoxy-Hb (Hb) can be calculated as follows:

$$\begin{bmatrix} \Delta C_{\mathrm{HbO2}} \\ \Delta C_{\mathrm{Hb}} \end{bmatrix} = \frac{1}{d \cdot \mathrm{DPF}} \begin{bmatrix} \varepsilon_{\lambda 1,\mathrm{HbO2}} & \varepsilon_{\lambda 1,\mathrm{Hb}} \\ \varepsilon_{\lambda 2,\mathrm{HbO2}} & \varepsilon_{\lambda 2,\mathrm{Hb}} \end{bmatrix}^{-1} \begin{bmatrix} \Delta A_{\lambda 1} \\ \Delta A_{\lambda 2} \end{bmatrix} \tag{6.11}$$

The MBLL has been widely used in CW systems for the quantification of hemodynamic changes. However, care should be taken in the selection of the wavelengths of the light sources implemented in order to correctly extract relative changes in tissue chromophores while reducing crosstalk between them [51].

6.6 fNIR Studies

Since the first *in vivo* application of fNIR on cat brain by Jobsis [1], there has been a growing interest in this exciting noninvasive, safe, affordable and portable technology and hence many different applications involving healthy and diseased groups in adult and children populations for laboratory and field conditions had been studied. Here, we will summarize some clinical applications and further give some specific examples of some of the basic research and clinical application studies that have been mainly carried out by the Optical Brain Imaging group at Drexel University within the Cognitive Neuroengineering and Quantitative Experimental Research (CONQUER) Collaborative.

6.6.1 Summary of Basic Research and Clinical Application Studies

In the past decade, brain activation studies employing fNIR have been conducted on the visual system [8], the somatosensory system [10], the auditory system [17,16], and the language system [6], and during motor tasks [5]. fNIR studies have also been used to examine a number of cognitive tasks [6,21–23,53]. In general, these studies have reported localized increases in oxy-Hb in response to functional challenge, and the results have largely been in agreement with corollary fMRI studies.

The first clinical applications of fNIR have been in the investigation of fetal, neonatal, and infant cerebral oxygenation and functional activation. For instance, fNIR studies have revealed developmental alterations in the cerebral hemodynamic response to auditory and visual stimulation [17,85]. Neurological applications have included an evaluation of the hemodynamic response during deep brain stimulation in Parkinson's patients [86], brain activations during induced seizures in patients with intractable epilepsy [87], an exploration of the pathophysiology of seizures in childhood epilepsy [88], and an examination of Alzheimer's patients during verbal fluency and other cognitive tasks [89]. Psychiatric applications have included the comparison of prefrontal brain activations of schizophrenic patients to healthy subjects during a mirror drawing task [90], a self-face recognition test [24], and during a continuous performance task [91]. fNIR was used to predict treatment response in a study of the effects of transcranial magnetic stimulation on depression [92]. A detailed review on clinical application can be found in [93].

6.6.2 Specific Example Studies

6.6.2.1 fNIR Device

In all of the specific example studies that will be discussed in this section a portable CW–fNIR system developed by Drexel University, optical brain imaging team which was originally described by Chance et al. [46] is used. The main components of the system were: (1) the sensor that covers the entire forehead, (2) a control box with integrated power supply for sensor control and data acquisition (current sampling rate is 2 Hz), and (3) a computer for the data analysis software [49,53]. The flexible sensor consisted of four light sources with three built-in LEDs sources having peak wavelengths at 730, 805, 850 nm and 10 photodetectors designed to image cortical areas underlying the forehead (dorsolateral and inferior frontal cortices). With a fixed source-detector separation of 2.5 cm and the implemented data collection scheme, this configuration resulted in a total of 16 signal channels (voxels) as shown in Figure 6.7. Communication between the data analysis computer and the task presentation computer is established via a serial port connection to time-lock fNIR measurement to the task events. The flexible sensor design consists of three parts: (i) a reusable flexible circuit board that carries the necessary infrared sources and detectors, (ii) a replaceable cushioning material, and (iii) a disposable single-use medical-grade adhesive tape that serves to attach the sensor to the participant (see Figure 6.7). The flexible circuit provides a reliable, integrated wiring solution, as well as consistent and reproducible component spacing and alignment. Because the circuit board and cushioning materials are flexible, the components move and adapt to the various contours of the participant's head, allowing the sensor elements to maintain an orthogonal orientation to the skin surface, dramatically improving light coupling efficiency and signal strength.

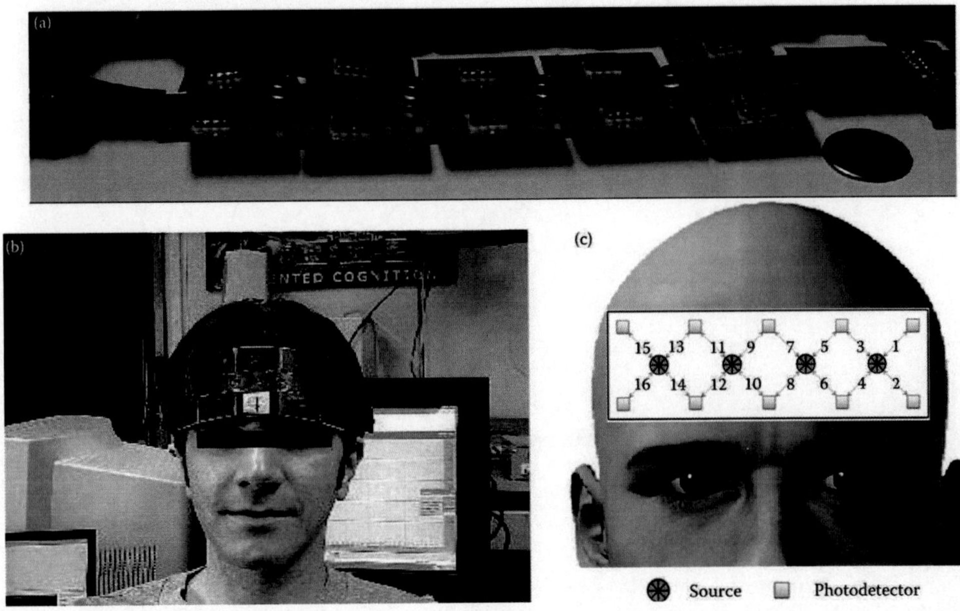

FIGURE 6.7 (a) Flexible fNIR sensor; (b) subject wearing the flexible fNIR sensor; and (c) anatomical location of fNIR measurement channels.

6.6.2.2 Basic Research Studies Targeting Different Cognitive Domains

To date, the fNIR studies of cognition and emotion have focused on functions associated with Brodman's areas BA9, BA10, BA46, BA45, BA47, and BA44. Recent PET and fMRI studies have shown that these areas play a critical role in sustained attention, both the short term storage and the executive process components of working memory, episodic memory, problem solving, response inhibition, and the perception of smell [for a recent review, see 94,95]. In addition, word recognition and the storage of verbal materials activate Broca's area and left hemisphere supplementary and premotor areas [94,96,97]. Some examples of fNIR applications and their results targeting different cognitive domains will be summarized in this section.

6.6.2.2.1 Attention

The protocol used in this study [49,53] to measure attention is a common visual oddball paradigm modified for use with fMRI by McCarthy et al. [98]. The stimuli were two strings of white letters (XXXXX and OOOOO) presented against the center of a dark background. A total of 516 stimuli were presented, 480 context stimuli (OOOOO) and 36 targets (XXXXX). Stimulus duration was 500 ms, with an interstimulus interval of 1500 ms. Target stimuli were presented randomly with respect to context stimuli with a minimum of 12 context stimuli between successive targets to allow the hemodynamic response an opportunity to return to baseline between target presentations. Fifteen right-handed participants (4 females and 11 males with age 20.8 ± 4.2) were required to press one of two buttons on a response pad after each stimulus, while both fNIR and EEG were recorded simultaneously. One button was pressed in response to targets (X's), and another button was pressed in response to context stimuli (O's).

The results for the ERPs were consistent with the literature [99]; targets elicited a pronounced P3 component with an average peak at 365 ms for both electrodes Cz and Pz (see Figure 6.8a for Pz results). The peak amplitude response to target stimuli was larger than the response to context stimuli at both Cz ($t(14) = 7.58$; $p < 0.001$) and Pz ($t(14) = 7.81$; $p < 0.001$). These ERP results confirm that the task parameters and participant responses were comparable to other ERP studies. Repeated-measures ANOVA computed on the fNIR oxygenation data (Oxy = oxy-Hb − deoxy-Hb) revealed that oxygenation values were

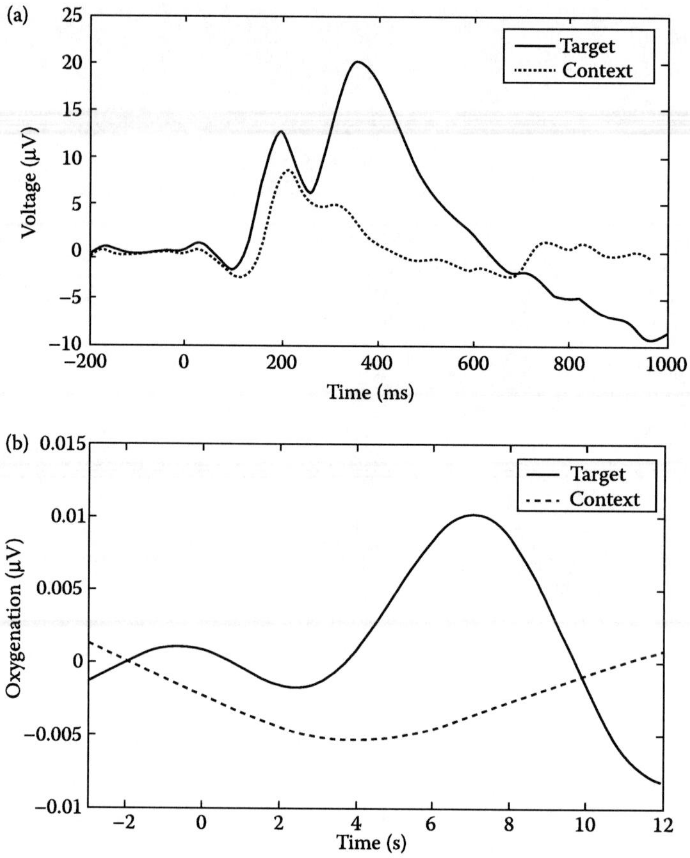

FIGURE 6.8 Averaged (a) ERP from Pz; (b) fNIR data for targets and contexts on voxel 11.

greater in response to targets than to controls in voxel 11, located over middle frontal gyrus of the right. Differentiation occurred between 6 and 9 s poststimulus as shown in Figure 6.8b. These results are consistent with the fMRI literature for visual target categorization with respect to increased oxygenation in response to targets, cortical location, and time course [98,100]. This study also demonstrated the utility of the combined EEG–fNIR system for studies of event-related designs that tap into ubiquitous cognitive functions such as attention [49].

6.6.2.2.2 *Working Memory*

In order to assess the working memory, the n-back task which is a sequential letter task with varied workload conditions that has frequently been used in working memory studies by cognitive psychologists and neuroscientists is used [95,96]. The stimuli are single consonants presented centrally, in pseudorandom sequences, on a computer monitor. Stimulus duration is 500 ms, with a 2500 ms interstimulus interval. Four conditions were used to incrementally vary working memory load from zero to three items. In the 0-back condition, subjects respond to a single prespecified target letter (e.g., "X") with their dominant hand (pressing a button to identify the stimulus). In the 1-back condition, the target is defined as any letter identical to the one immediately preceding it (i.e., one trial back). In the 2-back and 3-back conditions, the targets were defined as any letter that was identical to the one presented two or three trials back, respectively. Subjects pressed one button for targets (approximately 33% of trials) and another for nontargets. This strategy incrementally increased working memory load from the 0-back to the 3-back condition. Each n-back block contained 20 letters whether target

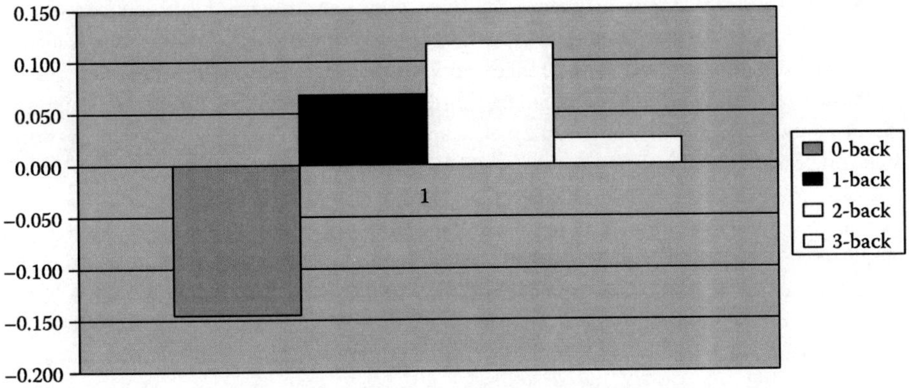

FIGURE 6.9 Averaged mean oxygenation for all subjects for four n-back conditions.

or nontarget and lasted for 60 s with 15 s of rest periods between n-back blocks. Total test included 7 trials of each of the 4 n-back conditions (hence total of 28 n-back blocks) ordered in such a way that within one trial all 4 of the n-back conditions are presented; however, their order is changed randomly from trial to trial.

In the analysis performed on 9 subjects (with age between 18 and 25), statistically significant differences between the n-back conditions in fNIR measurements are obtained on the fourth voxel located on left dorsolateral prefrontal cortex (DLPFC) [53] which is in agreement with the fMRI literature [97]. Statistical analysis revealed that the 0-back condition differed from 1- and 2-back conditions; 1-back > 0-back, $t = 3.21$, $p = .012$; 2-back > 0-back, $t = 2.58$, $p = .032$. After outlier elimination, 1- and 2-back differed from each other; 2-back > 1-back, $t = 2.77$, $p = 0.0275$. No difference was found between 2- and 3-back conditions. A positive relationship between increasing workload and the oxygenation is observed in DLPFC as shown in Figure 6.9, again in agreement with fMRI studies [97]. The drop in the oxygenation values in the most difficult condition (3-back) can be interpreted using a hypothesis similar to the human performance study discussed in Section 6.6.3.1 where subjects get overwhelmed and lost their concentration.

6.6.2.2.3 *Learning and Memory*

This study focused on the physiological effects of repetition on learning and working memory using an adaptation of Luria's Memory Word-Task (LMWT) [101]. The hemodynamic response in DLPFC of 13 healthy subjects (9 female), ranging in age from 23 to 43 while completing LMWT is recorded using fNIR. In LMWT, a list of 10 completely unrelated words is read aloud to the subject for he or she to memorize. This procedure is repeated 10 times. Free word recalls were acquired at the beginning, middle, and end of the task. Behavioral results showed that all subjects could recall the complete word list by the tenth trial, which was considered as successful task accomplishment. In terms of hemoglobin concentrations, it was hypothesized that there will be an increase in oxy-Hb and a decrease in deoxy-Hb in the DLPFC, reflecting activation of this area [102,103], during task learning phase, that is, when the subject is not yet able to recall the complete word list. Conversely, a significant drop in the regional-DLPFC oxy-Hb concentration, along with a significant increase in regional deoxy-Hb, is also expected, reflecting deactivation of the region of interest.

Oxy-Hb and deoxy-Hb results showed significant main effects in periods with ($F[1,12] = 6.31$, $p = 0.027$) and ($F[1,12] = 20.68$, $p < 0.001$), respectively. Post-hoc analyses showed a higher level of oxy-Hb concentration during the first period of LMWT ($M = 0.044$ μM) than during the second ($M = -0.069$ μM). Conversely, a lower level of deoxy-Hb concentration during the first period of the test ($M = -0.037$ μM; corrected $p < 0.01$) than during the second ($M = 0.037$ μM) was found in post-hoc analyses. Significant interactions between channels and period were also detected for oxy-Hb ($F[15,180] = 2.01$; $p = 0.016$) and deoxy-Hb ($F[15,180] = 1.81$; $p = 0.036$). Post-hoc analyses also showed that channels with significant highest differences between the first and second period of the test were left hemisphere channels 2, 3, 4 and right hemisphere channels 13, 14, 15, and 16 (all p's < 0.05) corresponding to BA 45, 46, 9, and 10 bilaterally. These channels also showed a lower deoxy-Hb concentration during the first period of the test (all p's < 0.05).

Correlation analyses showed significant positive correlations between oxy-Hb and memory performance in channels 1–4 and 12–16 for the first period (Spearmann's ρ's ranging from 0.54 to 0.73; p's ranging from 0.03 to 0.005). In these channels, significant negative correlations were found between memory performance and deoxy-Hb (ρ's ranging from −0.59 to −0.78; p's ranging from 0.02 to 0.003). On the contrary, for the second period, significant negative correlations were found between oxy-Hb and memory performance in channels 1–3 and 11–15 (ρ's ranging from −0.51 to −0.66; p's ranging from 0.04 to 0.013). Positive correlations between deoxy-Hb and memory performance were also detected for this period in channels 1–4 and 12–16 (ρ's ranging from 0.54 to 0.61; p's ranging from 0.03 to 0.014).

The comparison of DLPFC hemodynamic activation pattern produced during the first period of word list learning by repetition with that produced during the second period when the list was already learned but the words were still being repeated suggested an attenuation of stimulus-evoked neural activity in prefrontal neurons. These findings indicate that the temporal integration of efficient verbal learning is mediated by a mechanism known as neural repetition suppression (NRS). This mechanism facilitates cortical deactivation in DLPFC once learning is successfully completed. This cortical reorganization is interpreted as a progressive optimization of neural responses to produce a more efficient use of neural circuits. NRS could be considered one of the natural mechanisms involved in the processes of memory learning.

6.6.2.2.4 *Problem Solving*

The protocol used in this study involved presentation of anagram blocks on a computer screen that contains sequences of three letter (3L), four letter (4L), and five letter (5L) anagrams starting from minimal (3L anagrams) proceeding to the maximal level of difficulty (5L anagrams), and then back down again to the starting point of 3L anagrams [61,104]. Between each anagram block session, there is a rest period of 30 s. Each anagram block is displayed for approximately 1 min containing as many anagrams within depending on the number of processed anagrams by the subject. The decision of the subjects on each anagram processed and its timing is recorded on a text file for further analysis.

Since most subjects solve the anagrams within 2–5 s and since hemodynamic response takes 10–20 s period to fully evolve [33] for each anagram stimulus, hemodynamic responses overlap in time which present challenges for data analysis. In order to evaluate the subject's evoked-response times or brain activation for single anagram presentation within a block for graded difficulty analysis, a novel single trial hemodynamic response estimation algorithm was developed [61]. In this algorithm, each event-related hemodynamic response was estimated on the basis of two postulates that: (1) each single-trial hemodynamic response follows a gamma function, $hf_i = A_i t_i^{\alpha_i} e^{\beta_i t_i}$ as given in Figure 6.3b, and (2) the total oxygenation data can be modeled by the summation of individual hemodynamic responses evoked by rapidly presented stimuli, $\text{Oxy} = \sum_{i=1}^{N} hf_i$. Each single trial was estimated by optimizing the error between the total oxygenation data from fNIR measurements and the linear model: $\varepsilon = \min_{A,\alpha,\beta}\left(\text{Oxy} - \sum_{i=1}^{N} hf_i\right)^2$.

All calculations are applied to the data gathered from the left hemisphere of the prefrontal cortex on voxel 5. In block anagram study based on 14 participants (age between 18 and 23), the averaged recorded behavioral response times, the extracted rise times or time to peak (min), and the maximum amplitudes (as given in Figure 6.3b) from the estimated evoked-hemodynamic responses with respect

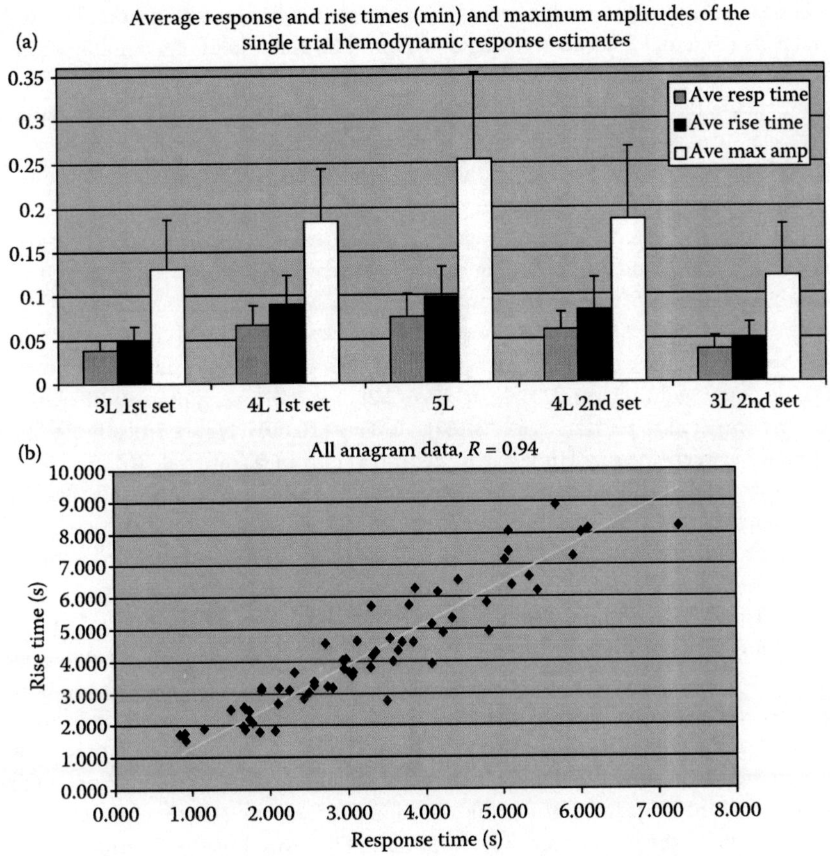

FIGURE 6.10 (a) Subject averages of rise and response times (min) and maximum amplitude; (b) scatter plot of rise time versus response time averages.

to the 3L, 4L, and 5L anagram sets are presented in Figure 6.10a. The estimated rise time which is the time required for the evoked-hemodynamic response to reach its maximum amplitude follows the same pattern as the behavioral (true) response time of the subjects having a correlation of $R = 0.94$ as presented in the scatter plot of the rise time versus response time in Figure 6.10b. Similarly, the estimated maximum amplitudes are correlated with the true response times ($R = 0.73$). The rise times and the maximum amplitude values increase as the difficulty level of the anagram solution increases, meaning that subjects need more time and more oxygen to solve difficult anagrams. Estimation of the event-related signals in a block design allows more precise analysis of the brain's function during a cognitive/problem solving task.

6.6.2.2.5 *Emotion*

Two affective dimensions have been studied extensively in neuroimaging research on emotional stimuli: arousal (exciting or calming) and valence (positive or negative). In this work, a new paradigm in the study of emotional processes through functional neuroimaging is introduced where the influence of the valence and arousal of visual stimuli on the neuroimaging of the evoked-hemodynamic changes are demonstrated [105]. Using fNIR, evoked-cerebral blood oxygenation (CBO) changes in DLPFC during direct exposure to different emotion-eliciting stimuli ("on" period), and during the period directly following stimulus cessation ("off" period) is investigated. It is hypothesized that the evoked-CBO, rather than return to baseline after stimulus cessation, would show either overshoot or undershoot. The study includes 30 healthy subjects (15 female) between the ages of 19 and 51 and a total of 9 stimuli, which consist of video-clips of moderate length (~20 s) with different emotional content (ranging from violence to cartoons) that can ensure that the stimuli will provoke strong lasting responses. The total sample of trials studied (270) is classified according to the valence and arousal ratings given by the subjects.

A significant negative correlation was found between valence and arousal dimensions ($r=-0.58$; $p<0.001$). That is to say, the lower the value in valence dimension, the higher the ratings in arousal. The four-way ANOVA for repeated measures revealed significant main effects for exposure condition ($F[1,234]=27.4$; $p<0.001$) and the grouping factors valence ($F[2,234]=3.93$; $p<0.05$) and arousal ($F[1,234]=6.94$; $p<0.01$). A Student t-test for repeated measures between mean oxy-Hb during "on" and "off" periods revealed a significant mean difference of -0.11 μM ($t[239]=-2.98$; $p<0.01$). Comparisons between valence groups revealed a significant difference in oxygenation of 0.33 μM in unpleasant trials compared to neutral trials ($t[125]=3.28$; $p<0.01$); a significant difference of 0.4 μM was found when compared to pleasant trials ($t[167]=3.84$; $p<0.001$). No statistically significant differences were found between the oxy-Hb levels in neutral versus pleasant trials ($t[182]=0.94$; $p=0.35$). A Student t-test for independent measures between arousing and nonarousing trials revealed a significant mean difference of 0.33 μM ($t(238)=-4.11$; $p<0.001$). There was no main effect for the prefrontal cortex (PFC) region variable ($F[1,234]=1.03$; $p=0.31$) and no significant interactions with this variable. A significant interaction was found between arousal category and exposure condition ($F[1,234]=16.14$; $p<0.001$): in arousing trials, a significant difference of -0.4 μM existed between "on" and "off" conditions ($t[68]=-4.56$; $p<0.001$), while no significant differences were detected in nonarousing trials ($t[170]=0.23$; $p=0.82$).

As a result, one of the main findings of this study is that when the subjective degree of arousal is high, the representation of the stimulus remains in the prefrontal cortex, even when the stimulus is no longer present. The persistence of sources of DLPFC activation during the "off" period is closely related to the degree of arousal that the subject assigns to the stimulus. Furthermore, these results show that valence alone does not determine the persistence of activation in PFC beyond the "on" period, except when the valence is unpleasant. The new and principle finding of this study is that there is an overshoot related to level of arousal in the DLPFC that persists even when the arousing stimulus has disappeared. Data also confirms that valence and arousal have different effects on the course of evoked-CBO response in DLPFC. Significant differences between "on" and "off" periods of DLPFC activation based on valence ratings was not found, but significant poststimulus overshoot related to arousal ratings was observed. These findings provide the first fNIR evidence showing that an increment in subjective arousal leads to activation in DLPFC which persists after stimulus cessation and does not occur with nonarousing stimuli. Note that since arousing stimuli produce longer periods of brain activation than nonarousing stimuli, neuroimaging studies must consider the duration and affective dimensions of the stimulus as well as the duration of the scanning. Not accounting for this difference may contribute to misinterpretation of the data.

6.6.3 Studies Involving Complex Tasks, Field, and Clinical Applications

6.6.3.1 Cognitive Performance Assessment

In this study, the deployment of fNIR for the purpose of cognitive state assessment while the user performs a complex task is presented [21]. This work is based on data collected during the DARPA Augmented Cognition-Technical Integration Experiment session participated by a total of 8 healthy subjects, 3 females and 5 males, ranging in age from 18 to 50. The experimental protocol for this session used a complex task resembling a videogame called the Warship Commander Task (WCT). The WCT was designed and developed by Pacific Science & Engineering Group under the direction of Space and Naval Warfare Systems Center to simulate naval air warfare management [106]. A sample screen shot during WCT is as shown in Figure 6.11a.

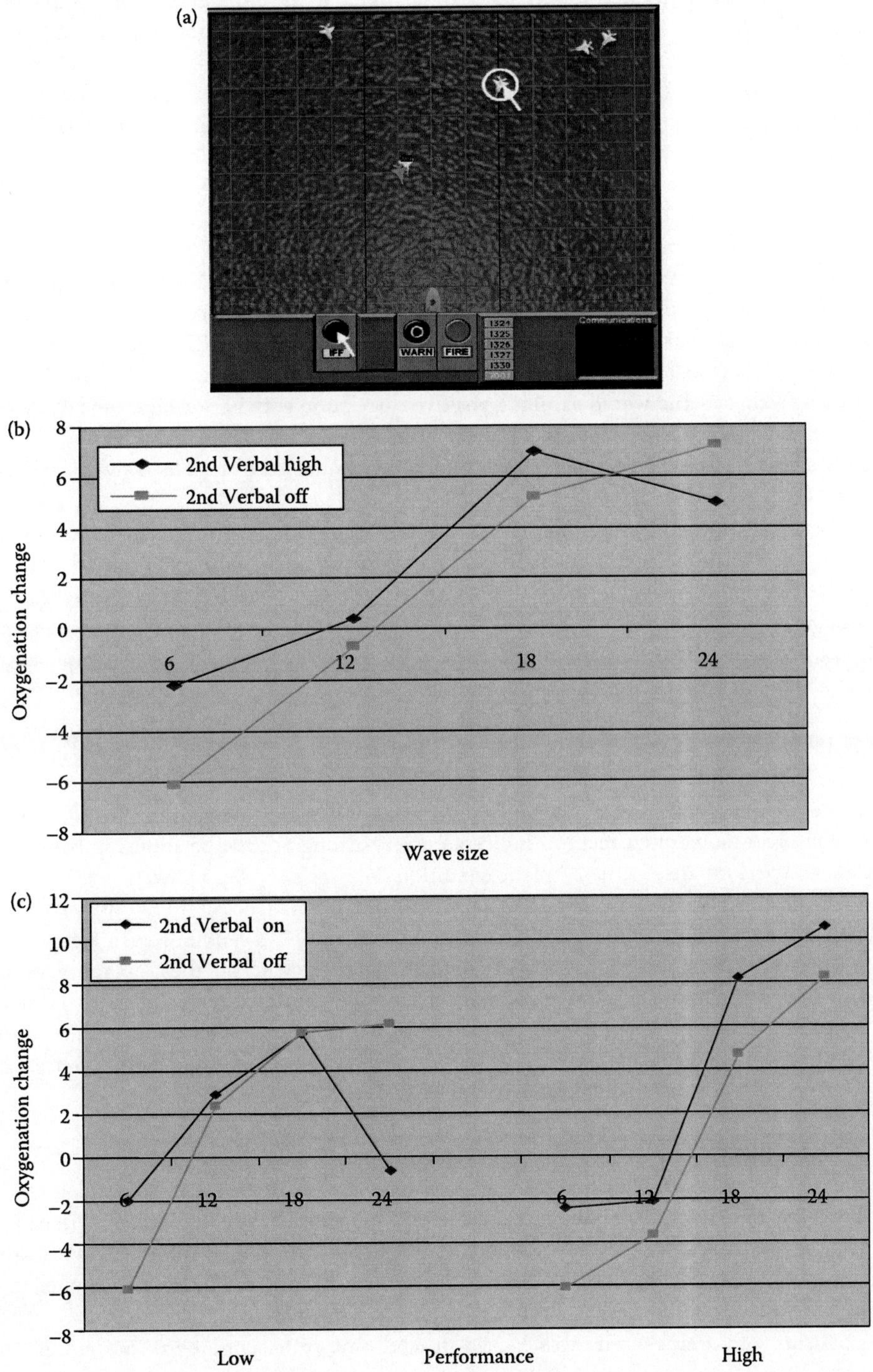

FIGURE 6.11 (a) A snapshot during WCT where air warfare management required the user to monitor "waves" of incoming airplanes, to identify the identity of the unknown ones as friendly or hostile, and to warn and then destroy hostile airplanes using rules of engagement; (b) mean oxygenation change versus wave size ($n = 8$) by secondary verbal task; (c) mean oxygenation change as a function of wave size, secondary verbal task, and average percentage of game score.

Task load and task difficulty were manipulated by changing (i) the number of airplanes that had to be managed at a given time (6, 12, 18, and 24 plane waves), (ii) the number of unknown versus known airplane identities (two levels of difficulty, *low*: 33% of the planes were unknown, and *high*: 67% of the planes were unknown), and (iii) the presence or absence of a verbal memory task (a secondary task causing divided attention). Each participant completed four sets of WCT. Each set was comprised of 3 repetitions of each of the 4 wave sizes (in the order of 6, 18, 12, and 24 planes) where each wave lasted 75 s. The factors of 4 different wave sizes, 2 different task difficulties (*high* vs. *low* percentage of unknown airplanes), and *full* versus *divided* attention (secondary verbal memory task On or Off) were crossed to create a $4 \times 2 \times 2$ repeated-measures design.

The fNIR data analysis explored (1) the relationships among cognitive workload, the participant's performance and changes in blood oxygenation levels of the dorsolateral prefrontal cortex, and (2) the effect of divided attention as elicited by the secondary component of the WCT (the auditory task). The primary hypothesis was that blood oxygenation in the prefrontal cortex, as assessed by fNIR, would rise with increasing task load and would exhibit a positive correlation with performance measures. In support of the primary hypothesis, the results indicated that the rate of change in blood oxygenation was significantly sensitive across both hemispheres ($F = 16.24$, $p < 0.001$) to task load (wave size) changes (see Figure 6.11b when secondary verbal was off).

When attention is divided by the secondary verbal task, the primary effect occurred in the 24-plane wave (the most difficult condition) causing the mean oxygenation for this case to drop below that of the 18-plane wave (see Figure 6.11c). In line with the stated hypothesis, a preliminary interpretation of this finding was that a number of participants had reached their maximal level of performance in this most difficult task level and lost their concentration/effort resulting in a drop in blood oxygenation. The hypothesis also predicts that individuals who were able to stay on task and continue to perform in this difficult condition should demonstrate increased oxygenation relative to both: (1) their own oxygenation levels in the 18-plane wave and (2) individuals who became overwhelmed and disengaged. Because sustained concentration and engagement in the task should result in increased performance, a positive correlation between performance and blood oxygenation would provide support for this interpretation. A Pearson's product-moment correlation indicated a very strong positive relationship between blood oxygenation and performance in the 24-plane condition (Pearson's $r = .89$, $p = .003$).

A median split on the Percentage Game Score provided further evidence of the hypothesized relationship between cognitive effort and the blood oxygenation response. As can be seen in Figure 6.11c, the mean levels of oxygenation were higher for both high and low performers in the 24-plane wave than the 18-plane wave when the secondary verbal task was off. However, when the secondary verbal task was on, the more difficult condition, the individuals who performed well on the 24-plane wave showed a higher mean level of oxygenation for the 24-plane wave than for the 18-plane wave, whereas those who performed poorly showed a decrease in oxygenation relative to the 18-plane wave.

6.6.3.2 Brain–Computer Interface

Brain–computer interface (BCI) is defined as a system that translates neurophysiological signals detected from the brain to supply input to a computer or to control a device. BCI research largely targets to eliminate the need for motor movement and develop mechanisms to relay information directly from the brain to a computer which, in turn, can be used to control or communicate with outside world. Development of alternative communication strategies are a recognized need for clinical applications involving patients with complete paralysis, locked-in syndrome, spinal cord injury, or muscular dystrophy. A technique that bypasses muscles and acquires signals directly from brain would be a notable help. Moreover, this technique should be minimally intrusive, noninvasive, accessible, and safe to be used continuously. In addition to their use in neuroprosthetics, noninvasive BCI systems also have potential applications for healthy individuals especially for enhancing or accelerating the learning process, or in entertainment domains such as in computer games and multimedia applications as a neurofeedback mechanism.

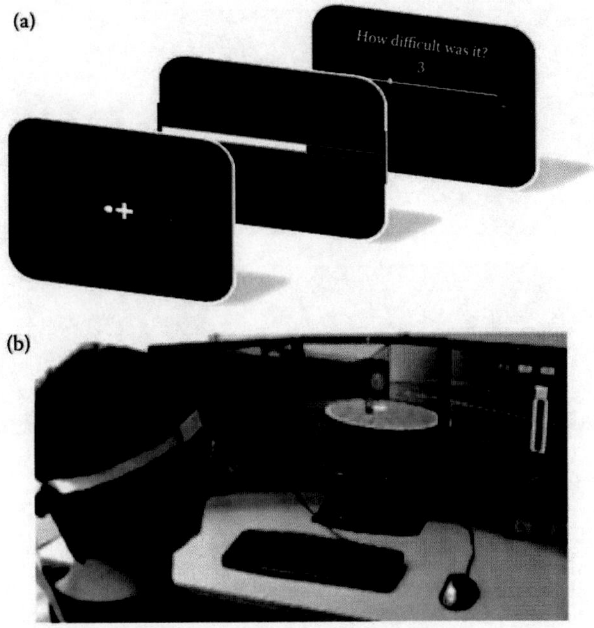

FIGURE 6.12 (a) Bar-size-control task; (b) gaming application.

The purpose of this research is to develop a new fNIR-based BCI to allow communication directly from the brain to a computer. A bar-size-control task based on a closed-loop system was designed and tested with 5 healthy subjects across two days [107]. In a single trial, subjects are first asked to rest for 20 s with a blank screen, after which a vertical or horizontal bar will appear (see Figure 6.12a). Initially, the bar is at 50% size and is mapped to the oxygenation data calculated from fNIR data that is updated at a frequency of 2 Hz. The subject is asked to concentrate on the bar for up to 120 s. Finally, the subject is asked to rate their effort on scale from 0 to 10 with 0 lowest and 10 highest effort/difficulty [108]. The subject has 30 s to complete this effort rating activity. Each trial lasts a maximum of 170 s. Comparisons of the average task and rest period oxygenation changes are significantly different ($p < 0.01$). The average task completion time (reaching + 90%) decreases with practice: day1 (mean 52.3 s) and day2 (mean 39.1 s). These preliminary results suggest that a closed-loop fNIR-based BCI can allow for a human–computer interaction with a mind switch task. Very preliminary studies incorporated fNIR technology into various 3D gaming environments that were built by student teams from Drexel University Digital Media (Figure 6.12b). Use of fNIR in this field is still an ongoing research, however preliminary results suggested that fNIR can allow participants to interact with virtual objects within the 3D environment by their thoughts.

6.6.3.3 Enhancement of Unmanned Aerial Vehicle Operator Training, Evaluation, and Interface Development

As the use of unmanned aerial vehicle (UAV) expand to near-earth applications and force-multiplying scenarios, current methods of operating UAVs and evaluating pilot performance need to expand as well. Research on human factors of UAV flight has identified several reasons underlying mishaps in UAV operations [109]. First, UAV operators have limited situational awareness due to the disembodied nature of UAV flight where operators need to fly UAVs by relying on limited camera angles. Since commands are transmitted over satellite links, UAVs are less responsive to operator input as compared to manned aircraft. In addition to this, typical UAV missions take long durations of time that require transitions

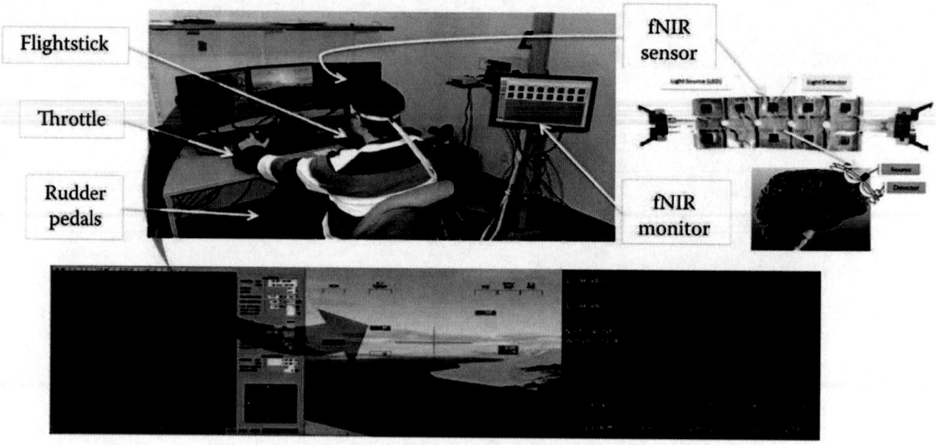

FIGURE 6.13 Computerized flight simulation and data collection environment.

from long periods of dull flight mode to critical moments where operators need to stay alert to engage with a target or to attend to a contingency. Many human factor studies on UAV operations rely on self-reporting surveys to assess the situational awareness and cognitive workload of an operator during a particular task which can make comparisons between operators subjective. In short, physically and cognitively taxing aspects of UAV flight have resulted in a large number of mishaps during military and civilian use. Therefore, devising reliable indices for assessing cognitive load and level of expertise are of critical importance for evaluating training regiments and interface designs, and ultimately for improving the safety and success of UAV operations.

In this project, fNIR is utilized to monitor UAV operator's cognitive workload and situational awareness during simulated missions [110]. The simulation platform is based on Microsoft's Flight Simulator X with the Predator UAV add-on by Firstclass Simulations. Using a complete joystick, throttle, and rudder pedal controller set, this simulation environment approximates an actual MQ-1 Predator user interface (Figure 6.13). After completing a demo session, each subject completes a total of 8 two-hour long training missions within 3 weeks. During each session subjects fly variants of the same mission, where they are asked to successfully take off, locate a submarine in a specified geographical area, pass over it to allow identification photographs to be taken, navigate back to an airfield with given coordinates, fly within 500 ft of the ground en route to the airfield over mountainous terrain, and successfully land after following a contingency maneuver revealed toward the end of the mission. These aspects, as well as other factors such as crosswinds, are added to the simulation to create realistic cognitive and physical demands, similar to those experienced by a real UAV pilot. This simulation environment allows replay of each session. In addition to the flight video, brain activation data is being collected by fNIR, as well as additional parameters such as pitch, roll, yaw, altitude, longitude, latitude, and air speed from within the simulation to aid in the assessment of performance (Figure 6.13).

In this ongoing study, both quantitative and qualitative methods to monitor the progress of each subject will be employed. Critical aspects of the mission that are likely to increase or decrease cognitive load (e.g., actively searching for a target, navigating toward a set of coordinates, and so on), will be identified through video analysis and the flight data. Once critical moments are identified and sampled, fNIR data collected at those moments can be correlated with operator performance to identify cognitive markers indicating expertise development and cognitive workload.

6.6.3.4 Cognitive Workload Assessment of Air Traffic Operators

The Next Generation Air Transportation System, developed by the Joint Planning and Development Office (JPDO), outlines a series of transformations designed to increase the capacity, safety, and security of air traffic operations in the United States [111]. A critical element in achieving this vision for future air-traffic management involves augmenting the current auditory-based communications between air traffic control (ATC) and the flight deck with text-based messaging, or DataComm systems. DataComm systems are expected to allow ATC to manage more air traffic at a lower level of cognitive load, thereby increasing both the capacity of the national airspace system and the safety of passengers. Although self-report measures of workload suggest that DataComm systems require less cognitive effort than voice-based systems to manage the same amount of traffic [112], to date this has not been tested using measures of neural function. The purpose of this research is to provide objective, brain-based measures of neural activity, and to determine the relative cognitive workload of DataComm versus voice-based communications systems (VoiceComm) during realistic simulations using fNIR.

In this study, fNIR has been incorporated into ongoing studies at the federal aviation administration (FAA) William J. Hughes Technical Center's (WJHTC) Research, Development, and Human Factors Laboratory, where 24 certified professional controllers (CPC) between the ages of 24 and 55 who had actively controlled traffic in an Air Route Traffic Control Center between 3 and 30 years were monitored with fNIR while they (i) performed a classic working memory (n-back) task as explained before [95,96] and (ii) managed realistic ATC scenarios under typical and emergent conditions [113]. The primary objective of this study was to use neurophysiological measures to assess cognitive workload during completion of controlled complex cognitive tasks: n-back and ATC.

For the ATC part-task, each CPC controlled traffic on workstations with a high-resolution (2048 × 2048), 29″ radarscope, keyboard, trackball, and direct access keypad for 10 min. To display the air traffic, the DESIREE ATC simulator and the TGF systems that were developed by software engineers at the WJHTC were used. Six simulation pilots were used within scenarios by supporting one sector or two sectors and entering data at their workstations to maneuver aircraft, all based on controller clearances. Two types of communications, either voice (VoiceComm) or data (DataComm) communications were used in separate sessions in a pseudo-random order. For each communication type, task difficulty was varied by the number of aircraft in each sector containing 6, 12, or 18 aircraft.

For the n-back fNIR data, repeated measures ANOVA showed that average oxygenation changes occurred only at voxel 2, that is, close to AF7 in the International 10–20 System, located within the left inferior frontal gyrus in the dorsolateral prefrontal cortex, was significant ($F_{3,69} = 4.37$, $p < 0.05$), see Figure 6.14a. Post-hoc analyses confirmed the differences in oxygenation changes as a function of task difficulty with 3-back is larger than the 0- and 1-back tasks (q0.05/2, 69 = 3.72, $p < 0.05$). For the ATC data, a 2 (Communication: DataComm, VoiceComm) X 2 (Prefrontal Hemisphere: right, left) X 3 (Task Difficulty: 6, 12, 18 aircrafts) ANOVA with repeated measures on all factors was calculated on mean oxygenation. Two subjects (#10, #11) were excluded from the analyses because of high-motion artifact and low signal-to-noise ratios. There were only two significant main effects: (i) task difficulty denoted by number of aircraft [$F_{2,42} = 4.39$, $p < 0.05$] and (ii) communication [$F_{1,21} = 5.09$, $p < 0.05$], which is depicted in Figure 6.14b. Tukey post-hoc tests for task difficulty ($q_{0.05/2,\,42} = 3.44$, $p < 0.05$) showed than the 18 aircrafts condition (M + SD; 0.272 + 0.586 μmol) had significantly higher oxygenation change than the 12 aircrafts condition (−0.015 + 0.409 μmol). There were no other significant differences between aircraft conditions.

As a summary, fNIR results were sensitive to task difficulty specifically at left inferior frontal gyrus in the n-back test. These are in line with the earlier results [21] and with the results of fMRI studies that have used the n-back task [114]. The main hypothesis of this project is that VoiceComm would require more cognitive resources than the DataComm condition. Hence, higher activation for VoiceComm would be expected. The fNIR results from the main effect of communication type ($p < 0.05$) confirms this hypothesis with a small to moderate effect size ($d = 0.36$). These fNIR results are also in line with subjective assessments of operators as reported in earlier studies. This study indicated that operator's cognitive effort for different types of tasks can be objectively assessed by comparing fNIR results. One of the major advantages of using fNIR in this study is that it allowed monitoring brain activity of the ground operators in realistic settings.

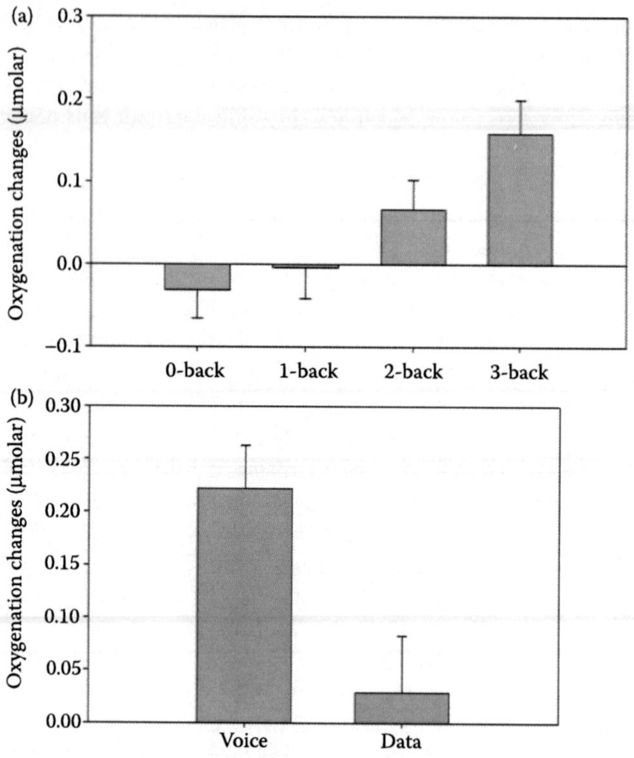

FIGURE 6.14 (a) Average oxygenation changes of all subjects (24 subjects, and 160 trials for each condition) with increasing task difficulty (n-back tasks). (b) Average oxygenation changes for DataComm and VoiceComm ($N = 22$). Error bars are SEM.

6.6.3.5 Cognitive Activity Assessment Following Traumatic Brain Injury on Attention Domain

A commonly observed consequence of traumatic brain injury (TBI) is cognitive impairment, whose assessment represents a considerable challenge. Additionally, the choice of a successful treatment among the many existing neurorehabilitation strategies still relies on behavioral observation, and little information is available about the physiological changes produced at the brain level by the specific intervention. The integration of neuroimaging and electrophysiological measures may be more objective and effective in the evaluation of cognitive impairments. This study evaluates the applicability of fNIR for assessment of TBI-induced impairments of attention [115]. Participants included five male TBI patients between 18 and 37 years old. Brain activation measures were collected during a target categorization (oddball) task as explained before. The pattern of the hemodynamic response elicited by the two classes was in agreement with previous studies that investigated the applicability of fNIR to the study of attention-related tasks. The changes in the concentration of oxy-Hb and deoxy-Hb differ between target-locked and nontarget-locked responses: target stimuli elicited in fact a more marked activation in the areas of the prefrontal cortex monitored by fNIR. This pilot study suggests the potential for fNIR to be applied to the monitoring of attention in the TBI population.

6.6.3.6 Cognitive Activity Assessment Following TBI on Working Memory Domain

Behavioral observation and neuropsychological tests have guided the planning of cognitive rehabilitation and the assessment of its effectiveness. However, the information about the actual changes that rehabilitation interventions induce at the brain level is still limited. The availability of this information would, instead, prove useful for a more objective and individualized approach to the evaluation of a treatment efficacy. To this end, the integration of functional neuroimaging in the evaluation of cognitive impairments could offer a more objective monitoring of rehabilitation outcomes.

The aim of this study is to demonstrate the applicability of fNIR, to the assessment of working memory after TBI [116]. Participants included four TBI and ten healthy controls. Neuropsychological evaluation of attention and working memory was based on the WAIS-III Digit Span and WAIS-III Letter-Number Sequencing. Brain activation measurements were collected through fNIR during a visual n-back task as explained before. Physiologically irrelevant data and noise were eliminated from fNIR measurements and the maximum change in oxy-Hb and deoxy-Hb concentration was obtained for the left and right dorsolateral prefrontal areas.

On the basis of the performance in the neuropsychological tests, the TBI group revealed impaired learning performance as compared to the group of healthy controls. Evaluation of fNIR data revealed a pattern in the hemodynamic activity that was significantly different between the healthy controls and the TBI patients in the DLPFC, known to be involved in the working memory processes. The results obtained in this preliminary study show that fNIR is a promising neuroimaging tool that can prove to be clinically useful to investigate and identify the neurological underpinnings of cognitive functioning after TBI. In particular, fNIR offers to neurorehabilitation some unique advantages over other conventional neuroimaging techniques: fNIR is in fact portable, low-cost, noninvasive, and allows a reasonably flexible task design.

6.6.3.7 Depth of Anesthesia Monitoring

Awareness is an unintended mental state during general anesthesia. An accurate, objective measure of return to consciousness would provide an important safeguard for patients and physicians alike. This exploratory investigation on predicting awareness under general anesthesia examines the hypothesis that the transition from deep to light anesthetic stages is associated with reliable changes in oxygenated, deoxygenated, and total hemoglobin in frontal cortex. Hemodynamic changes during deep and light anesthesia were examined in 26 nonbrain surgery patients [55]. fNIR recordings are collected in the operating room before, during, and after subjects were receiving their scheduled anesthetic and surgical procedures. The results suggest that the rate of deoxygenated hemoglobin change can be used as a descriptive neuromarker to differentiate between deep and light anesthesia stages ($F = 7.61$, $p < 0.01$). This marker is proposed for further development as an index of the depth of anesthesia for the purpose of monitoring awareness under general anesthesia.

In addition to the neuropsychological findings, this research demonstrates engineering and signal processing solutions in the form of customized algorithms and procedures that allow fNIR to measure usable signals under field conditions. ICA and PCA were combined in a novel procedure that employed dark current (i.e., signal from noncortical sources) as a reference measurement. This method provided improved signal-to-noise ratio for the hemodynamic measurements acquired in the operating room, and can be used to increase the signal quality of fNIR for many other applications and field situations.

6.6.4 Future Directions

Since fNIR technology is still relatively new in comparison with other neuroimaging technologies, the research published to date has been relatively conservative—focusing on establishing fNIR as a valid and reliable neuroimaging technology. Furthermore clinical investigations have also been very limited. As a result, the majority of published fNIR studies have not capitalized on the unique capabilities of the technique because of the need to validate the results with known technologies such as fMRI. We believe that the studies explained in the previous section represent examples of how fNIR can be used in research and clinical paradigms that may not be feasible with other neuroimaging technologies and may facilitate research by acquainting clinicians and researchers with the unique merits of fNIR as a brain-imaging technology.

There are several types of clinical applications that could benefit from the unique attributes of fNIR neuroimaging technology in the future:

- Populations that may not be able to readily tolerate the confines of an fMRI magnet, or be able to remain sufficiently still, for example, schizophrenics, autistic children, and neonates
- Populations that require the long-term monitoring of cerebral oxygenation, for example, premature and other high-risk infants
- Studies that require repeated, low-cost neuroimaging, for example, treatment studies that image the cortex for efficacy
- Applications where an fMRI system would be too expensive or cumbersome, for example, for use in a clinical office
- Applications that require ecological validity, for example, working at a computer, or in an educational setting

6.7 Conclusion

fNIR is an emerging technology that uses near-infrared light to measure changes in the concentration of oxygenated and deoxygenated hemoglobin in the cortex. The use of fNIR technology has increased in recent years as a means to measure hemodynamic changes in the cortex in response to cognitive activity. Although fNIR imaging is limited to the outer cortex, it provides neuroimaging that is safe, portable, and very affordable relative to other neuroimaging technologies that can be applied in the laboratory as well as field conditions. Moreover, it is a noninvasive and negligibly intrusive optical imaging modality. It is also relatively robust to movement artifacts, and can readily be integrated with other technologies such as EEG. Current state-of-the-art technologies include portable and wireless fNIR systems, data processing algorithms, and end-user software.

In this chapter, an overview of basis of optical imaging, fNIR instrumentation and signal analysis and cognitive studies carried out in the literature are summarized. In these studies, fNIR has been demonstrated to have adequate validity in the measurement of functional brain activity during a variety of cognitive, emotional, and motor tasks in healthy and diseased subject groups of both adult and children populations, and has the potential to provide a flexible neuroimaging tool for clinicians and researchers alike. The findings are in agreement with the results in current EEG and fMRI literature. The portable and wireless instrumentations, combined with robust analysis algorithms and end-user software, make fNIR a viable option for the study of cognition- and emotion-related hemodynamic changes in both adults and children, under either stationary or ambulant conditions.

Acknowledgments

The author would like to thank Drs. Banu Onaral, Kambiz Pourrezaei, Scott Bunce, Patricia Shewokis, Kurtulus Izzetoglu, Hasan Ayaz, Anna Merzagora, Britton Chance, Shoko Nioka, Jose Leon-Carrion, Murat Cakir, Ajit Devaraj, and Mr. Justin Menda and Mr. Adrian Curtin for their advice and help in the preparation of this chapter and sharing their work and results.

References

1. Jobsis FF. 1977. Noninvasive infrared monitoring of cerebral and myocardial sufficiency and circulatory parameters. *Science,* 198:1264–1267.
2. Cope M, Delpy, D. T. 1988. System for long-term measurement of cerebral blood flow and tissue oxygenation on newborn infants by infra-red transillumination. *Med. Biol. Eng. Comput.,* 26:289–294.

3. Luo Q, Zeng S, Chance B, Nioka S. 2002. Monitoring of brain activation with near infrared spectroscopy. Chapter 8 in *Handbook of Optical Biomedical Diagnostics*, Editor: Valery V. Tuchin, Press Monograph PM107, Bellingham, WA.
4. Rolfe P. 2000. *In vivo* near-infrared spectroscopy. *Annu. Rev. Biomed. Eng.*, 02:715–754.
5. Strangman G, Boas DA, Sutton JP. 2002. Non-invasive neuroimaging using near-infrared light. *Biol. Psychiatry*, 52(7):679–693.
6. Hoshi Y, Tamura M. 1993. Dynamic multichannel near-infrared optical imaging of human brain activity. *J. Appl. Phys.*, 75:1842–1846.
7. Hoshi Y. 2003. Functional near-infrared optical imaging: Utility and limitations in human brain mapping. *Psychophysiology*, 40:511–520.
8. Villringer A, Planck J, Hock C, Schleinkofer L, Dirnagl U. 1993. Near infrared spectroscopy (NIRS): A new tool to study hemodynamic changes during activation of brain function in human adults. *Neurosci. Lett.*, 154:101–104.
9. Villringer A, Chance B. 1997. Non-invasive optical spectroscopy and imaging of human brain function. *Trends Neurosci.*, 20:435–442.
10. Suto T, Ito M, Uehara T, Ida I, Fukuda M, Mikuni M. 2002. Temporal characteristics of cerebral blood volume change in motor and somatosensory cortices revealed by multichannel near infrared spectroscopy. *Int. Congress Series*, 1232:383–388.
11. Maki A, Yamashita Y, Ito Y, Watanabe E, Mayanagi Y, Koizumi H. 1995. Spatial and temporal analysis of human motor activity by using noninvasive NIR topography. *J. Neurosci.*, 11:1458–1469.
12. Gratton E, Toronov V, Wolf U, Wolf M, Webb A. 2005. Measurement of brain activity by near infrared light. *J. Biol. Optics*, 10(1)011008-1-13.
13. Franceschini MA, Boas DA. 2004. Noninvasive measurement of neuronal activity with near-infrared optical imaging. *Neuroimage*, 21:372–386.
14. Gratton G, Corballis PM, Cho E, Fabiani M, Hood DC. 1995. Shades of gray matter: Noninvasive optical images of human brain responses during visual stimulation. *Psychophysiology*, 32:505–509.
15. Heekeren HR, Obrig H, Wenzel R, Eberle K, Ruben J, Villringer K, Kurth R, Villringer A. 1997. Cerebral haemoglobin oxygenation during sustained visual stimulation—A near infrared spectroscopy study. *Physiol. Trans. Biol. Sci.*, 352:743–750.
16. Sato, H, Takeuchi T, Sakai K. 1999. Temporal cortex activation during speech recognition: An optical topography study. *Cognition*, 40:548–560.
17. Zaramella P, Freato F, Amigoni A, Salvadori S, Marangoni P, Suppjei A. 2001. Brain auditory activation measured by near-infrared spectroscopy. *Ped. Res.*, 49:213–219.
18. Son Il-Y, Guhe M, Yazici B. 2005. Human performance assessment using fNIR. *Proc. SPIE*, 5797:158–169.
19. Cope M. 1991. *The Development of a Near-Infrared Spectroscopy System and Its Application for Noninvasive Monitoring of Cerebral Blood and Tissue Oxygenation in the Newborn Infant*. Ph.D. thesis. University College London, London.
20. Bunce SC, Devaraj A, Izzetoglu M, Onaral B, Pourrezaei K. 2005a. Detecting deception in the brain: A functional near-infrared spectroscopy study of neural correlates of intentional deception. *Nondest. Detection Meas. Homeland Security III, Proc. SPIE*, 5769:24–32.
21. Izzetoglu K, Bunce S, Onaral B, Pourrezaei K, Chance B, 2004. Functional optical brain imaging using near-infrared during cognitive tasks. *Int. J. Human-Comp. Int.*, 17(2):211–227.
22. Izzetoglu K, Yurtsever G, Bozkurt A, Yazici B, Bunce S, Pourrezaei K, Onaral B. 2003a. NIR spectroscopy measurements of cognitive load elicited by GKT and target categorization. *Proceedings of 36th Hawaii International Conference on System Sciences*, Philadelphia, PA.
23. Izzetoglu M, Izzetoglu K, Bunce S, Ayaz H, Devaraj A, Onaral B, Pourrezaei K. 2005b. Functional near-infrared neuroimaging. *IEEE Trans. Neural Sys. Rehab. Eng.*, 13(2):153–159.
24. Platek SM, Fonteyn LCM, Izzetoglu M, Myers TE, Ayaz H, Li C, Chance B. 2005. Functional near infrared spectroscopy reveals differences in self-other processing as a function of schizotypal personality traits. *Schizophrenia Res.* 73(1):125–127.

25. Rajapakse JC, Kruggel F, Maisog JM, Von Cramon DY. 1998. Modelin hemodynamic response for analysis of functional MRI time series. *Hum. Brain Mapp.*, 6:283–300.
26. Magistretti PR, Pellerin L. 1999. Cellular mechanisms of brain energy metabolism and their relevance to functional brain imaging. *Phil. Trans. R. Soc. Lond. B*, 354(1387):1155–1163.
27. Magistretti PR. 2000. Cellular bases of functional brain imaging: Insights from neuron-glia metabolic coupling. *Brain Res.*, 886(1–2):108–112.
28. Ames A III. 2000. CNS energy metabolism as related to function. *Brain Res. Brain Res. Rev.* 34:42–68.
29. Fox PT, Raichle ME, Mintun MA, Dence C. 1988. Nonoxidative glucose consumption during focal physiologic neural activity. *Science*, 241:462–464.
30. Buxton RB, Uludag K, Dubowitz DJ, Liu TT. 2004. Modeling the hemodynamic response to brain activation. *Neuroimage*, 23(Suppl. 1):S220–233.
31. Buxton RB. 2001. The elusive initial dip. *Neuroimage*, 13: 953–958.
32. Obrig H, Villringer A. 2003. Beyond the visible—Imaging the human brain with light. *J. Cereb. Blood Flow Metab.*, 23:1–18.
33. Miezin FM, Maccotta L, Ollinger JM, Petersen SE, Buckner RL. 2000. Characterizing the hemodynamic response: Effects of presentation rate, sampling procedure, and the possibility of ordering brain activity based on relative timing. *NeuroImage*, 11:735–759.
34. Haensse D, Szabo P, Brown D, Fauchère JC, Niederer P, Bucher HU, Wolf M. 2005. A new multichannel near infrared spectrophotometry system for functional studies of the brain in adults and neonates. *Optics Exp.*, 13(12):4525–4538.
35. Ogawa S, Lee TM, Nayak AS, Glynn P. 1990. Oxygenation-sensitive contrast in magnetic resonance image of rodent brain at high magnetic fields. *Magn. Reson. Med.*, 14:68–78.
36. Kwong KK, Belliveau JW, Chesler DA, Goldberg IE, Weisskoff RM, Poncelet BP, Kennedy DN. et al. 1992. Dynamic magnetic resonance imaging of human brain activity during primary sensory stimulation. *PNAS*, 89:5951–5955.
37. Chance B, Cope M, Gratton E, Ramanujam N, Tromberg B. 1998. Phase measurement of light absorption and scatter in human tissue. *Rev. Sci. Instrum.*, 69:3457–3482.
38. Gratton G, Maier JS, Fabiani M, Mantulinm WW, Gratton E. 1994. Feasibility of intracranial near-infrared optical scanning. *Psychophysiology*, 31:211–215.
39. Chance B, Leig JS, Miyake H, Smith DS, Nioka S, Greenfeld R, Finander M, Kaufmann K, Levy W. et al. 1988. Comparison of time-resolved and un-resolved measurements of deoxyhemoglobin in brain. *PNAS*, 85:4971–4975.
40. Firbank M, Okada E, Delpy DT. 1998. A theoretical study of the signal contribution of regions of the adult head to near infrared spectroscopy studies of visual evoked responses. *NeuroImage*, 8:69–78.
41. Delpy DT, Cope M, van der Zee P, Arridge S, Wray S, Wyatt J. 1988. Estimation of optical pathlength through tissue from direct time of flight measurement. *Phys. Med. Biol*, 33:1433–1442.
42. Lakowicz, J. R, Berndt, K. 1990. Frequency domain measurement of photon migration in tissues. *Chem. Phys. Lett.*, 166:246–252.
43. Wolf M, Ferrari M, Quaresima V. 2007. Progress of near-infrared spectroscopy and topography for brain and muscle clinical applications. *J. Biomed. Optics*, 12(6):062104–1–14.
44. Obrig H, Wenzel R, Kohl M, Horst S, Wobst P, Steinbrink J, Thomas F, Villringer A. 2000. Near-infrared spectroscopy: Does it function in functional activation studies of the adult brain? *Int. J. Psychophysiol.*, 35:125–142.
45. Boas DA, Franceschini MA, Dunn AK, Strangman G. 2002. *Non-Invasive Imaging of Cerebral Activation with Diffuse Optical Tomography. In-Vivo Optical Imaging of Brain Function.* Boca Raton: CRC Press. pp. 193–221.
46. Chance B, Anday E, Nioka S, Zhou S, Hong L, Worden K, Li C, Murray T, Ovetsky Y, Pidikiti D, Thomas R. 1998. A novel method for fast imaging of brain function, non-invasively, with light. *Optics Exp.*, 2(10):411–423.

47. Rector DM, Poe GR, Kristensen MP, Harper RM. 1997. Light scattering changes follow evoked potentials from hippocampal Schaeffer collateral stimulation. *J. Neurophysiol.*, 78:1707–1713.
48. Stepnoski RA, LaPorta A, Raccuia-Behling F, Blonder GE, Slusher RE, Kleinfeld D. 1991. Noninvasive detection of changes in membrane potential in cultured neurons by light scattering. *PNAS*, 88:9382–9386.
49. Bunce S, Izzetoglu M, Izzetoglu K, Onaral B, Pourrezaei K, 2006. Functional near infrared spectroscopy: An emerging neuroimaging modality. *IEEE Engineering in Medicine and Biology Magazine, Special issue on Clinical Neuroengineering*, 25(4):54–62.
50. Bozkurt A, Onaral B. 2004. Safety assessment of near infrared light emitting diodes for diffuse optical measurements. *Biomed. Eng. Online*, 3(9):1–10.
51. Boas DA, Dale AM, Francheschini MA. 2004. Diffuse optical imaging of brain activation: Approaches to optimizing image sensitivity, resolution, and accuracy. *Neuroimage*, 23:S275–S288.
52. Huppert TJ, Diamond SG, Franceschini MA, Boas DA. 2009. HomER: A review of timeseries analysis methods for near-infrared spectroscopy of the brain. *Appl. Opt.*, 48(10):280–298.
53. Izzetoglu M, Bunce S, Izzetoglu K, Onaral B, Pourrezaei K. 2007. Functional brain imaging using near infrared technology for cognitive activity assessment. *IEEE Engineering in Medicine and Biology Magazine, Special issue on on the Role of Optical Imaging in Augmented Cognition*, 26(4):38–46.
54. Sato H, Tanaka N, Uchida M, Hirabayashi Y, Kanai M, Ashida T, Konishi I, Maki A. 2006. Wavelet analysis for detecting body-movement artifacts in optical topography signals. *Neuroimage*, 33:580–587.
55. Izzetoglu K. 2008. *Neural Correlates of Cognitive Workload and Anesthetic Depth: fNIR Spectroscopy Investigation in Humans*. Ph.D. thesis, Drexel University, Philadelphia, PA.
56. Robertson FC, Douglas TS, Meintjes EM. 2010. Motion artefact removal for functional near infrared spectroscopy: A comparison of methods. *IEEE Trans. Biomed. Eng.*, 57(6):1377–1387.
57. Izzetoglu M, Devaraj A, Bunce S, Onaral B. 2005. Motion artifact cancellation in NIR spectroscopy using Wiener filtering. *IEEE Trans. Biomed. Eng.*, 52(5):934–938.
58. Izzetoglu M, Chitrapu P, Bunce S, Onaral B. 2010. Motion artifact cancellation in NIR spectroscopy using discrete Kalman filtering. *Biomed. Eng. Online*, 9(16):1–10.
59. Cui X, Bray S, Reiss AL. 2010. Functional near infrared spectroscopy (NIRS) signal improvement based on negative correlation between oxygenated and deoxygenated hemoglobin dynamics. *Neuroimage*, 49:3039–3046.
60. Devaraj A. 2005. *Signal Processing for Functional Near Infrared Neuroimaging*. Master's thesis, Drexel University, Philadelphia, PA.
61. Izzetoglu M, Nioka S, Chance B, Onaral B. 2005. Single trial hemodynamic response estimation in a block anagram solution study using fNIR spectroscopy. *Proceedings of ICASSP Conference*, Vol. 5, pp: 633–636.
62. Obrig H, Neufang M, Wenzel R, Kohl M, Steinbrink J, Einhaupl K, Villringer A. 2000. Spontaneous low frequency oscillations of cerebral hemodynamics and metabolism in human adults. *Neuroimage*, 12:623–639.
63. Mayhew J, Askew S, Zheng Y, Porrill J, Westby GWM, Redgrave P, Rector DM, Harper RM. 1996. Cerebral vasomotion: A 0.1 hz oscillation in refleted light imaging of neural acitvity, *Neuroimage*, 4:183–193.
64. Lundberg N. 1960. Continuous recordings and control of ventricular fluid pressure in neurosurgical practice. *Acta Psychiatrica et Neurologica Scandinavica*, 149:1–193.
65. Diamond SG, Huppert TJ, Kolehmainen V, Franceschini MA, Kaipio JP, Arridge SR, Boas DA. 2005. Physiological system identification with the Kalman filter in diffuse optical tomography. *Lecture Notes in Computer Science*, 3750:649–656.
66. Zhang Q, Strangman GE, Ganis G. 2009. Adaptive filtering to reduce global interference in non-invasive NIRS measures of brain activation: How well and when does it work? *Neuroimage*, 45:788–794.
67. Zhang Y, Brooks DH, Francheschini MA, Boas DA. 2005. Eigenvector-based spatial filtering for reduction of physiological interference in diffuse optical imaging. *J. Biomed. Opt.*, 10(1):011014.

68. Gratton G, Corballis PM. 1995. Removing the heart from the brain: Compensation for the pulse artifact in the photon migration signal. *Psychophysiology*, 32:292–299.
69. Morren G, Wolf U, Lemmerling P, Wolf M, Choi JH, Gratton E, De Lathauwer L, Van Huffel S. 2004. Detection of fast neuronal signals in the motor cortex from functional near infrared spectroscopy measurements using independent component analysis. *Med. Biol. Eng. Comput.*, 42(1):92–99.
70. Glover GH, Li TQ, Ress D. 2000. Image-based method for retrospective correction of physiological motion effects in fMRI: RETROICOR. *Magn. Reson. Med.*, 44:162–167.
71. Yamada T, Umeyama S, Matsuda K. 2009. Multidistance probe arrangement to eliminate artifacts in functional near-infrared spectroscopy. *J. Biomed. Opt.*, 14(6):064034.
72. Arridge SR, Schweiger M. 1997. Image reconstruction in optical tomography. *Phil. Trans. R. Soc. Lond. B*, 352:717–726.
73. Boas DA, Brooks DH, Miller EL, DiMarzio CA, Kilmer M, Gaudette RJ, Zhang Q. 2001. Imaging the body with diffuse optical tomography. *IEEE Sign. Proc. Mag.*, 18:57–75.
74. Son IY, Yazici B. 2006. Near infrared imaging and spectroscopy for brain activity monitoring. Advances in Sensing with Security Applications, pp: 341–372, NATO Advanced Study Institute, NATO Security through Science Series-A: Chemistry and Biology, Springer, Edited by J. Byrnes.
75. Ishimaru A. 1997. *Wave Propagation and Scattering in Random Media*. New York: IEEE Press.
76. Tromberg BJ, Svaasand LO, Tsay T, Haskell RC. 1993. Properties of photon density waves in multiple-scattering media. *Appl. Optics*, 32:607–616.
77. Hillman E. 2002. *Experimental and Theoretical Investigations of Near Infrared Tomographic Imaging Methods and Clinical Applications*. Ph.D. thesis, University College London, London.
78. Patterson MS, Chance B, Wilson BC. 1989. Time resolved reflectance and transmittance for the non-invasive measurement of tissue optical properties. *Appl. Optics*, 28(12):2331–2336.
79. Sassaroli A, Fantini S. 2004. Comment on the modified Beer–Lambert law for scattering media. *Phys. Med. Biol.*, 49:N255–N257.
80. Tachtsidis I. 2005. *Experimental Measurements of Cerebral Haemodynamics and Oxygenation and Comparisons with a Computational Model: A Near-Infrared Spectroscopy Investigation*. Ph.D. thesis, University College London, London.
81. Duncan A, Meek JH, Clemence M, Elwell CE, Tyszczuk L, Cope M, Delpy DT. 1995. Optical pathlength measurements on adult head, calf and forearm and the head of the newborn infant using phase resolved optical spectroscopy. *Phys. Med. Biol.*, 40:295–304.
82. Hiraoka M, Firbank M, Essenpreis M, Cope M, Arridge SR, van der Zee P, Delpy DT. 1993. A Monte Carlo investigation of optical pathlength in inhomogeneous tissue and its application to near-infrared spectroscopy. *Phys. Med. Biol.*, 38:1859–1876.
83. Kohl M, Nolte C, Heekeren HR, Horst S, Scholz U, Obrig H, Villringer A. 1998. Determination of the wavelength dependence of the differential pathlength factor from near-infrared pulse signals. *Phys Med Biol.*, 43(6):1771–1782.
84. Duncan A, Meek JH, Clemence M, Elwell CE, Fallon P, Tyszczuk L, Cope M, Delpy DT. 1996. Measurement of cranial optical path length as a function of age using phase resolved near infrared spectroscopy. *Pediatr. Res.*, 39(5):889–894.
85. Meek JH, Firbank M, Elwell CE, Atkinson J, Braddick O, Wyatt JS. 1998. Regional hemodynamic responses to visual stimulation in awake infants. *Pediatr. Res.*, 43:840–843.
86. Sakatani K, Katayama Y, Yamamoto T, Suzuki S. 1999. Changes in cerebral blood oxygenation of the frontal lobe induced by direct electrical stimulation of thalamus and globus pallidus: A near infrared spectroscopy study. *J. Neurol. Neurosurg. Psych.*, 67:769–773.
87. Watanabe E, Maki A, Kawaguchi F, Yamashita Y, Koizumi H, Mayanagi Y. 2000. Noninvasive cerebral blood volume measurement during seizures using multichannel near infrared spectroscopic topography. *J. Biomed. Opt.*, 5:287–290.
88. Haginoya K, Munakata M, Kato R, Yokoyama H, Ishizuka M, Iinuma K. 2002. Ictal cerebral haemodynamics of childhood epilepsy measured with nearinfrared spectrophotometry. *Brain*, 125(9):1960–1971.

89. Hock C, Villringer K, Muller-Spahn F, Hofmann H, Heekeren H, Schuh-Hofer S. 1996. Near infrared spectroscopy in the diagnosis of Alzheimer's disease. *Ann. N.Y. Acad. Sci.*, 777:22–29.
90. Okada F, Tokumitsu Y, Hoshi Y, Tamura M. 1994. Impaired interhemispheric integration in brain oxygenation and hemodynamics in schizophrenia. *Eur. Arch. Psych. Clin. Neurosci.*, 244:17–25.
91. Fallgatter AJ, Strik WK. 2000. Reduced frontal functional asymmetry in schizophrenia during a cued continuous performance test assessed with nearinfrared spectroscopy. *Schizophr. Bull*, 26(4):913–919.
92. Eschweiler GW, Wegerer C, Schlotter W, Spandl C, Stevens A, Bartels M. 2000. Left prefrontal activation predicts therapeutic effects of repetitive transcranial magnetic stimulation (rTMS) in major depression. *Psych. Res.*, 99:161–172.
93. Irani F, Platek SM, Bunce S, Ruocco AC, Chute D. 2007. Functional near infrared spectroscopy (fNIRS): An emerging neuroimaging technology with important applications for the study of brain disorders. *Clin. Neuropsychol.*, 21:9–37.
94. Cabeza R, Nyberg L. 2000. "Imaging Cognition II: An empirical Review of 275 PET and fMRI Studies." *J. Cogn. Neurosci.*, 12:1–47.
95. Smith EE, Jonides J. 1997. "Working Memory: A View from Neuroimaging," *Cogn. Psychol.* 33:5–42.
96. Smith EE, Jonides J. 1999. Storage and executive processes in the frontal lobes. *Science*, 283:1657–1661.
97. Braver TS, Cohen JD, Nystrom LE, Jonides J. Smith EE, Noll DC. 1997. A parametric study of prefrontal cortex involvement in human working memory. *NeuroImage*, 5:49–62.
98. McCarthy G, Luby M, Gore J, Goldman-Rakic P. 1997. Infrequent events transiently activate human prefrontal and parietal cortex as measured by functional MRI. *J. Neurophysiol.*, 77:1630–1634.
99. Polich J, Kok A. 1995. Cognitive and biological determinants of P300: An integrative review. *Biol. Psychol.*, 41:103–146.
100. Ardekani BA, Choi SJ, Hossein-Zadeh G, Porjesz B, Tanabe JL, Lim KO, Bilder R, Helpern JA, Begleiter H. 2002. Functional magnetic resonance imaging of brain activity in the visual oddball task. *Cogn. Brain Res.*, 14:347–356.
101. Leon-Carrion J, Izzetoglu M, Izzetoglu K, Martin-Rodriguez JF, Damas-Lopez J, Martin JM, Dominguez-Morales MR. 2010. Efficient learning produces spontaneous neural repetition suppression in prefrontal cortex. *Behav. Brain Res.*, 208(2):502–508.
102. Strangman G, Franceschini MA, Boas DA. 2003. Factors affecting the accuracy of near-infrared spectroscopy concentration calculations for focal changes in oxygenation parameters. *Neuroimage*, 18:865–879.
103. Huppert TJ, Hoge RD, Diamond SG, Franceschini MA, Boas DA. 2006. A temporal comparison of BOLD, ASL, and NIRS hemodynamic responses to motor stimuli in adult humans. *Neuroimage*, 29:368–382.
104. Chance B., Nioka S., Sadi S., Li C. 2003. Oxygenation and blood concentration changes in human subject prefrontal activation by anagram solutions. *Adv. Exp. Med. Biol.*, 510:397–401.
105. Leon-Carrion J, Martin-Rodriguez JF, Damas-Lopez J, Pourrezai K, Izzetoglu K, Martin JM, Dominguez-Morales MR, 2007. A lasting post-stimulus activation on dorsolateral prefrontal cortex is produced when processing valence and arousal in visual affective stimuli. *Neurosci. Lett.*, 422(3):147–152.
106. John M, Kobus DA, et al. 2002. A multi-tasking environment for manipulating and measuring neural Correlates of cognitive workload". *Proceedings of the IEEE 7th Conference on Human Factors and Power Plants*, 7:10–14.
107. Ayaz H, Shewokis P, Bunce S, Schultheis M, Onaral B. 2009. Assessment of Cognitive Neural Correlates for a Functional Near Infrared-based Brain Computer Interface System. Dylan D. Schmorrow at al. (eds.): Augmented Cognition, HCII 2009, Lecture Notes on Artificial Intelligence, 2009, vol. 5638:699–708, Berlin, Heidelberg: Springer-Verlag (presented at the 13th International Conference on Human-Computer Interaction, July 19–24 2009, San Diego, CA).
108. Paas FGWC, Van Merriënboer JJG. 1993. The efficiency of instructional conditions: An approach to combine mental effort and performance measures. human factors. *J. Hum. Fact. Ergon. Soc.*, 35:737–743.

109. Cooke NJ, Pringle H, Pederson H, Connor O, Salas E. 2006. *Human Factors of Remotely Operated Vehicles.* The Netherlands: Elsevier.
110. Cakir MP, Ayaz H, Menda J, Izzetoglu K, Onaral B. 2010. Connecting brain and learning sciences: An optical brain imaging approach to monitoring development of expertise in UAV piloting. *Proceedings of ICLS2010 Conference,* June 29–July 2 2010, Chicago, IL.
111. JPDO. 2004. Next Generation Air Transportation System Integrated Plan. Retrieved from http://www.jpdo.gov/library/NGATS_v1_1204r.pdf.
112. Hah S, Willems B, Phillips R. 2006. The effect of air traffic increase on controller workload. *Proceedings of the Human Factors and Ergonomics Society Annual Meeting San Francisco,* CA.
113. Ayaz H, Willems B, Bunce S, Shawokis PA, Izzetoglu K, Hah S, Deshmukh AR, Onaral B. 2010. Cognitive workload assessment of air traffic Controllers Using Optical Brain Imaging Sensors. *Proceedings of AHFE2010 Conference,* July 17–20 2010, Miami, FL.
114. Owen AM, McMillan KM, Laird AR, Bullmore E. 2005. N-back working memory paradigm: A meta-analysis of normative functional neuroimaging studies. *Hum. Brain Mapp.,* 25(1):46–59.
115. Merzagora AC., Izzetoglu M., Onaral B., Schultheis M. 2010. "fNIRS as a useful tool for cognitive evaluation following traumatic brian injury", *8th World Congress on Brian Injury,* March 10–14, 2010, Washington, DC.
116. Merzagora A.C, Martin-Rodriguez J.F, Longo Perez A, Leon-Dominguez U, Izzetoglu K, Schultheis M, Onaral B, Leon-Carrion J. 2010. "Applicability of fNIRS to the TBI population: Demonstration on an attention task", *8th World Congress on Brian Injury,* March 10–14, 2010, Washington, DC.

7

Causality Analysis of Multivariate Neural Data

Maciej Kamiński
University of Warsaw

Hualou Liang
Drexel University

7.1 Introduction

With the rapid advances in multielectrode recording and brain-imaging techniques that have occurred in recent years, multichannel data sets have become increasingly obtainable. While standard signal-processing techniques such as crosscorrelations in the time domain and coherence in the frequency domain remain the main statistics for assessing interactions among these multichannel data, it is increasingly felt that these symmetric interdependence measures are no longer sufficient for many intended applications, and further partitioning of relationships among a set of simultaneously recorded signals is needed to parcel out the functional connectivity of complex neural networks. Recent work has begun to explore a class of techniques called Granger causality as a potentially useful addition to the current analytical repertoire in the attempt to add directionality to neural interactions.

In this chapter, we want to give an overview of specific issues concerning multivariate data analysis, present available tools and give a few examples of their applications. The functions will be presented from practical point of view, which means that some technical and mathematical details will not be elaborated here. Instead, for further reading there will be bibliography references. We start with the standard symmetric measures for evaluating the statistical interdependence between two time series. We then discuss practical issues concerning how to estimate such measures from time series data with special emphasis on multivariate autoregressive (MAR) model, from which the Granger causality and its partial measures can be derived. Key technical issues of the causal measures concerning stationarity/nonstationarity, bivariate/multivariate, linearity/nonlinearity, and statistical significance are specifically addressed. Finally, we present several selected applications in the analysis of spike trains, EEG, and fMRI BOLD data, each representing a major recording modality used in neuroscience research, followed by a demonstration of clinical application in seizure localization in epilepsy patients. These applications together demonstrate that causality measures can reveal insights that are not possible with traditional analytical techniques.

7.2 Cross-Estimators, Time, and Frequency Domain

The most important part of multichannel data analysis is estimation of the influence of one signal from the set on the other signal(s). In the case of simultaneous recordings of many quantities, we implicitly record as well relations between these quantities of our multichannel set. To expose these properties we must apply special functions, able to reveal joint properties of multiple signals.

The best-known estimator of that type is covariance or correlation. For two signals $X = \{\ldots, x(0), x(1), x(2),\ldots\} = \{x(t)\}$ and $Y = \{y(t)\}$ covariance R and correlation C are defined as follows (E[·] denotes expectation, μ_x, μ_y are mean values of X and Y, respectively):

$$\begin{aligned} R_{xy}(s) &= \mathrm{E}\left[x(t) - \mathrm{E}[x(t)]\right] \cdot \mathrm{E}\left[y(t+s) - \mathrm{E}[y(t)]\right] = \mathrm{E}\left[x(t) - \mu_x\right] \cdot \mathrm{E}\left[y(t+s) - \mu_y\right] \\ C_{xy}(s) &= \frac{R_{xy}(s)}{R_{xy}(0)} = \frac{R_{xy}(s)}{\sqrt{R_{xx}(0)R_{yy}(0)}} \end{aligned} \tag{7.1}$$

The value of covariance $R_{xy}(s)$ or correlation $C_{xy}(s)$ tells how much the two signals X and Y change together. Correlation may be treated as a normalized version of covariance: its value, unlike covariance, is limited to the [−1, 1] range. Big absolute values of these functions indicate that changes in signal X and changes in signal Y appear in common. Negative values of covariance or correlation indicate that the changes in Y coincide with changes in X, but are in opposite direction. The covariance (correlation) defined above is in fact the covariance (correlation) function. The argument s of these functions, called a time lag, tells us about common changes (of the signals) which are delayed by the value of the time lag (positive or negative). If R is calculated for two different signals it is called cross-covariance function; if $X = Y$ we call R autocovariance function.

The covariance and correlation operate in the time domain; it means that we apply them directly to values of time series and the result is a function over time. In biomedical data analysis area, we are often interested in spectral properties of the recorded signals. A function similar to correlation, but operating in frequency domain is called coherence

$$K_{xy}(f) = \frac{S_{xy}(f)}{\sqrt{S_{xx}(f)S_{yy}(f)}} \tag{7.2}$$

which is constructed from cross-spectrum S_{xy} between signals X and Y normalized by spectra of signals X and Y called here as autospectra (the definition of cross- and autospectra will be given later). This function operates in frequency domain and tells how much common of the signal component of frequency f appear in both signals.

The coherence is a complex number and can be represented in the form

$$K_{ij}(f) = M_{ij}(f)e^{i\Phi_{ij}(f)} \tag{7.3}$$

where

$$M_{ij}(f) = \sqrt{\mathrm{Re}(K_{ij}(f))^2 + \mathrm{Im}(K_{ij}(f))^2} \tag{7.4}$$

is a modulus and

$$\Phi_{ij}(f) = \arctan\frac{\mathrm{Im}(K_{ij}(f))}{\mathrm{Re}(K_{ij}(f))} \tag{7.5}$$

is a phase of the coherence. These quantities are often more handy in presenting the values of analysis and are commonly used to measure similarity of signals in the frequency domain. For two signals in order to be considered coherent their phase difference must be constant which produces high value of coherence modulus and the coherence phase equal to the phase difference of that signals. Sometimes it is said that coherence describes linear phase coupling.

7.3 Practical Realizations of Cross-Measures

7.3.1 Linear Modeling

One successful technique in analysis of biomedical time series is application of linear models, and in particular of autoregressive (AR) model. The linear methods belong to the group of parametric approach in spectral analysis. We assume a model of data generation and then we fit that model to our data. The analysis is then done on the model parameters, not on the data samples. If the model describes our data well, the conclusions from the model can be translated to the properties of the original signals.

Parametric approach in spectral analysis gives us an opportunity to create advanced measures of relations between signals of multichannel set. Most importantly, perhaps, it allows defining causal estimators, which are based on certain models of influence between signals. Nonparametric approach (namely: Fourier analysis) does not give so many possibilities in that area.

In general, signals like EEG or MEG are of stochastic nature—they contain components of specific frequency ranges (rhythms) over a noisy background. This property fits well the theoretical shape of AR model spectrum and that is why the AR model can describe that type of data well and is so popular in the field of biomedical data analysis.

7.3.2 AR Model Introduction

AR model expresses the current value of a process as a linear combination of the previous values of the process. In a multivariate case, the current value $X(t)$ of a process is a vector containing values of all channels of the system.

$$\begin{gathered}\mathbf{X}(t) = (X_1(t), X_2(t), \ldots, X_k(t))^{\mathrm{T}} \\ \mathbf{X}(t) = \sum_{j=1}^{p} \mathbf{A}(j)\mathbf{X}(t-j) + \mathbf{E}(t)\end{gathered} \tag{7.6}$$

or, by assuming $\mathbf{A}(0) = \mathbf{I}$ and changing sign of the rest of $\mathbf{A}(j)$:

$$\mathbf{E}(t) = \sum_{j=0}^{p} \mathbf{A}(j)\mathbf{X}(t-j) \tag{7.7}$$

By applying the Z transform we get

$$\begin{aligned}&\mathbf{E}(Z) = \mathbf{A}(Z)\mathbf{X}(Z), \quad \text{where} \\ &\mathbf{A}(Z) = 1 + \mathbf{A}(1)Z^{-1} + \mathbf{A}(2)Z^{-2} + \cdots + \mathbf{A}(p)Z^{-p} = \sum_{m=0}^{p} \mathbf{A}(m)Z^{-m}\end{aligned} \tag{7.8}$$

Equation 7.8 can be expressed as depending on frequency by substituting $z = \exp(2\pi i f \Delta t)$, where Δt is the inverse of sampling frequency [67,62]:

$$\begin{aligned}
\mathbf{E}(f) &= \mathbf{A}(f)\mathbf{X}(f) \\
\mathbf{X}(f) &= \mathbf{A}^{-1}(f)\mathbf{E}(f) = \mathbf{H}(f)\mathbf{E}(f) \\
\mathbf{H}(f) &= \left(\sum_{m=0}^{p} \mathbf{A}(m)\exp(-2\pi i m f \Delta t)\right)^{-1}
\end{aligned} \tag{7.9}$$

The matrix **H** is called the transfer matrix of the system.

The power spectrum of the signal **X** is defined by the formula:

$$\mathbf{S}(f) = \mathbf{X}(f)\mathbf{X}^*(f) = \mathbf{H}(f)\mathbf{E}(f)\mathbf{E}^*(f)\mathbf{H}^*(f) = \mathbf{H}(f)\mathbf{V}\mathbf{H}^*(f) \tag{7.10}$$

In a multivariate case, the spectrum is a matrix containing autospectra of every channel on the diagonal and cross-spectra off the diagonal. The matrix **V** contains variance of model residual error **E**, which can be interpreted as **X**(t) prediction error. From the spectral matrix elements, we can calculate for instance coherences. The values of $\mathbf{A}(f)$, $\mathbf{H}(f)$, and **V** (Equations 7.9 and 7.10) will be later utilized to construct various measures describing properties of the original dataset.

7.3.3 Model Parameters Estimation

The procedures of fitting of AR model to the data are described in signal analysis handbooks and in our opinion there is no need to present them here. It is rather a technical problem; even a beginner in data analysis using a data processing software package (from wide offer available) can successfully apply that technique, not knowing the implementation particulars. In fact, there are many possible algorithms differing in certain details of their performance on different kind of input data. Probably, the first algorithm was proposed by Yule and Walker. That algorithm is based on solving a set of linear equations constructed from values of correlations between data channels for different time lags.

The other algorithms (like Burg, LWR (Levinson, Wiggins, Robinson), covariance, etc.) are based on slightly different assumptions and are better suited to find sinusoidal components in the stochastic background. On the other hand, Bayesian algorithms estimate specific confidence ranges for the most probable values of the model parameters [14,70]. Application of a particular algorithm in most cases is not a crucial choice; the results obtained by different algorithms can be similar. Discussions about AR model application can be found in the literature [51,52,66,79,82,84,94], and in signal processing textbooks listed at the end of this chapter.

One very important issue concerning the model fitting is the problem of the optimal model order selection. It may seem that the bigger the model order the better the fit, but it is not the case. The number of maxima in the AR model spectrum is related to the model order. For too high orders, the model is likely to create false signal components, typically by splitting the existing "true" spectral maxima. To avoid such situations, certain statistical criteria of model order selection have been developed. Among the most popular ones are Akaike information criterion (AIC), final prediction error (FPE), criterion for AR transfer function (CAT), Bayesian information criterion (BIC) (called also the Schwarz criterion SC) or Hannan–Quinn criterion HQC, and several others. Their descriptions can be found in textbooks and articles [59,62]. Many of the criteria try to balance the variance of the residual error of the model (which gets lower with increasing order) with a penalty term, producing a minimum at certain order value p. Examples of the criteria definitions are given in Equation 7.11: P is the number of parameters, n is the number of data time points, **V** is the residual k-signal model variance matrix of order p ($\mathbf{V}_j$ for order j), and vertical bars denote determinant.

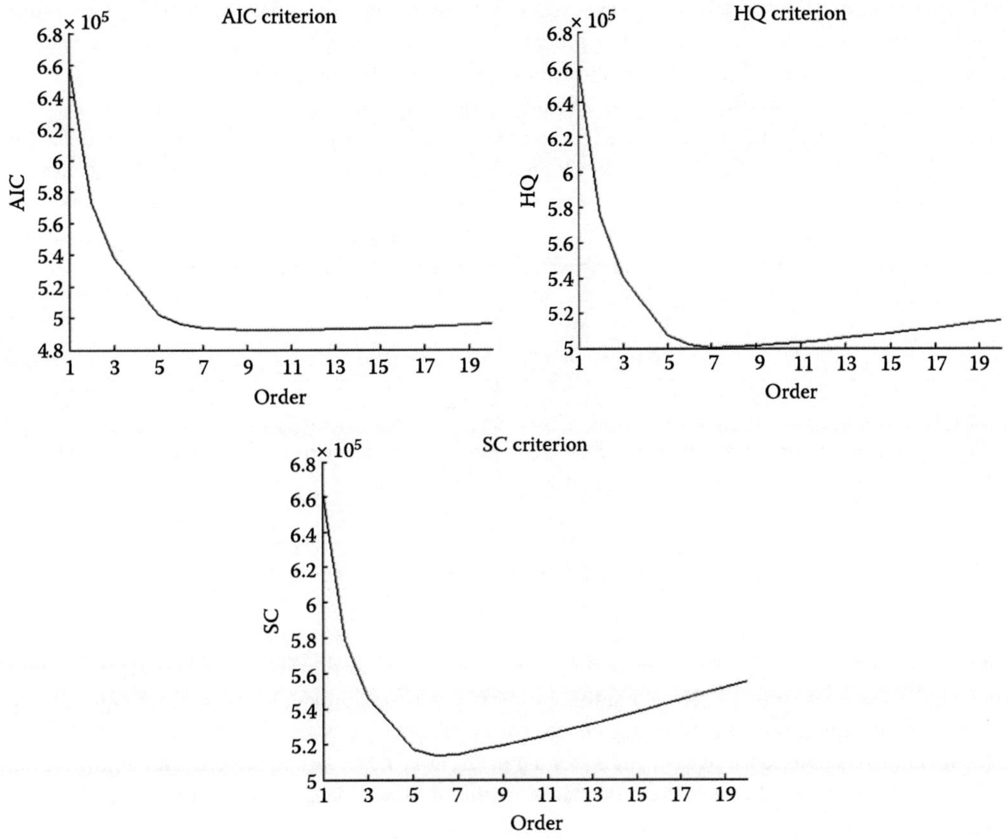

FIGURE 7.1 Example of optimal model order selection criteria. Model orders on horizontal axes, criteria value on vertical axes.

$$
\begin{aligned}
\mathrm{AIC}(p) &= n\log\left|\mathbf{V}\right| + 2P \\
\mathrm{SC}(p) &= n\log\left|\mathbf{V}\right| + 2P\log(n) \\
\mathrm{HQC}(p) &= n\log\left|\mathbf{V}\right| + P\log(\log(n)) \\
\mathrm{FPE}(p) &= \left|\mathbf{V}\right|\left(\frac{n+P}{n-P}\right) \\
\mathrm{CAT}(p) &= \frac{1}{n^2}\sum_{j=1}^{p-1}\frac{n-j}{\left|\mathbf{V}_j\right|} - \frac{n-p}{(n-1)\left|\mathbf{V}\right|}
\end{aligned}
\tag{7.11}
$$

Typically, we calculate criterion values for a range of model orders and look for the first minimum of the obtained function. Although we can encounter slightly different definitions of that criterion in handbooks, the differences in formulas do not change the position of the minimum of those functions. The order at the minimum value is considered the "optimal" one, according to that criterion (Figure 7.1).

7.3.4 Concept of Granger Causality

Very often we are interested in knowing how the elements of the investigated system work together; for instance, we would like to know how the brain areas communicate with each other. That problem can be expressed as the question: which areas are sources of activity or how the signal propagates in our system? Finding sources of activity is sometimes a problem of primary importance and to resolve it; we must define a proper measure utilizing information about relations between signals.

When one area is the source of a signal which propagates and influences another signal, we say that the first signal is *causal* for the second one. For the mathematical purposes, we need a stricter definition of causality. The popular definition, widely adopted in that field, is the definition presented by Granger [34] (derived from a general idea given by Wiener [93]), which is based on predictability of time series.

Let us imagine we have two time series $X = \{x(t)\}$ and $Y = \{y(t)\}$. If we try to predict the current value of time series X using its own previous samples we get a value with certain error ε:

$$X(t) = \sum_{i=1}^{\infty} A_{11}(i)X(t-i) + \varepsilon(t) \tag{7.12}$$

We may add previous values of signal Y to the prediction of the current sample of signal X. In that case the prediction error ε' may be different:

$$X(t) = \sum_{i=1}^{\infty} A'_{11}(i)X(t-i) + \sum_{i=1}^{\infty} A'_{12}(i)Y(t-i) + \varepsilon'(t) \tag{7.13}$$

If the variance of the error ε' is lower than the variance of ε, we say that signal Y is causal for the signal X or signal Y Granger-causes X. Note that this property can be reciprocal, for example, Y can be causal for X and at the same time X may (or may not) be causal for Y.

The formalism presented above is defined for a pair of signals, but can be extended for a multivariate case. First, we try to predict a value of signal X_1 using all available signals except for X_m. We get a prediction error η:

$$X_1(t) = \sum_{\substack{i=1 \\ i \neq m}}^{k} \sum_{j=1}^{p_i} A_{1i}(j)X_i(t-j) + \eta(t) \tag{7.14}$$

Another prediction error η' we get when we use all signals including X_m in the prediction of channel X_1:

$$X_1(t) = \sum_{i=1}^{k} \sum_{j=1}^{p_i} A_{1i}(j)X_i(t-j) + \eta'(t) \tag{7.15}$$

If the variance of η' is smaller than the variance of η, we say that the signal X_m can be called causal for the signal X_1 in the multivariate case. These observations may be used to construct measures of causal influence between signals.

7.3.5 Directional Measures

It may seem straightforward to estimate the direction of influence between signals by analyzing the phase of coherence [33]. However, in practice that approach is possible only for certain simple cases. For biomedical multivariate stochastic data, typically of spectrum rich of components, the coherence phase analysis does not give satisfactory results.

AR model gives us an opportunity to make use of the Granger causality concept directly. We may look at the model equation as it is a prediction of the value $X(t)$. This is what we in fact do during fitting of the model—we try to find the model coefficients in a way which predicts the value of $X(t)$ with the smallest error ε. If we use previous values of many signals in the prediction, we get different set of parameters and different error values. After fitting the multivariate AR model, we get a set of model parameters $\mathbf{A}(i)$ and a matrix of the so-called residual error variance $\mathbf{V}$ which contains estimates of the prediction error variances of every signal from the investigated set. These values may be a basis for the construction of causality estimators based on the Granger causality concept.

7.3.5.1 Measures Derived from Granger Causality

In the literature, there are estimators derived directly from Granger causality definition. In Ref. [31], the measure of linear feedback is defined:

$$F_{y \to x} = \ln\left(\frac{V_x}{V_{xy}}\right) \tag{7.16}$$

where variances of errors are taken from residual variances of the AR models fitted to the data: V_x is the variance of error ε and V_{xy} is the variance of error ε′ (see Equations 7.12 and 7.13). Similar idea was used to define Granger causality index (GCI):

$$\mathrm{GCI}_{y \to x} = 1 - \frac{V_{xy}}{V_y} \tag{7.17}$$

This measure can be extended to a multivariate case:

$$\mathrm{GCI}_{y \to x} = 1 - \frac{V_k}{V_{k-1}} \tag{7.18}$$

Here V_k is the variance of error η′ (in the case when signal Y is included into the set) and V_{k-1} is the variance of error η (cf. Equations 7.14 and 7.15) of the system containing all the signals except for the signal Y.

By its construction the value of GCI is in [0,1] range. When there is no influence on the X_1 signal, no improvement in prediction of the variance should be seen; the variance ratio is equal to 1 and the GCI measures (as well as the linear feedback measure) vanish.

The above-defined measures tell us just if the relation exists, and how strong it may be. We are often interested in frequency relations of causal influence, so we will need another estimator, able to produce results dependent on frequency. In Ref. [16], there is a proposition of Granger causality spectrum estimator, based on ideas from Ref. [31]. It is defined in the form:

$$I_{y \to x}(f) = -\ln\left(1 - \frac{\left(V_{22} - V_{12}^2/V_{11}\right)\left|H_{12}(f)\right|^2}{S_{11}(f)}\right) \tag{7.19}$$

As we see, it utilizes information from power spectrum S, noise variance V, and model transfer function H. More details about these measures can be found in [19,20,32,35,69,81,92].

The Granger causality spectrum is defined for a pair of signals. One of the propositions for a truly multivariate measure (arbitrary number of signals) is the directed transfer function (DTF) introduced in Ref. [43]. Originally that quantity was presented in the normalized form given by the formula:

$$\mathrm{DTF}_{j\to i}(f) = \frac{\left|H_{ij}(f)\right|^2}{\sum_{m=1}^{k}\left|H_{im}(f)\right|^2} \tag{7.20}$$

DTF($j \to i$) describes influence of channel j to channel i at frequency f. More precisely, normalized DTF is a ratio between inflow from channel j to i and inflows from all channels of the set to the channel i at frequency f. This property assures normalization of this quantity in the form:

$$\sum_{j=1}^{k}\mathrm{DTF}_{j\to i}(f) = \frac{\sum_{j=1}^{k}\left|H_{ij}(f)\right|^2}{\sum_{m=1}^{k}\left|H_{im}(f)\right|^2} = 1 \tag{7.21}$$

The values of the normalized DTF are numbers from [0, 1] range; 0 means no transmission.

Often we are interested in absolute transmission value and in that case the nonnormalized version can be helpful. It is defined as

$$\mathrm{NDTF}_{j\to i}(f) = \left|H_{ij}(f)\right|^2 \tag{7.22}$$

The value of the nonnormalized DTF is directly related to the connection strength between signals [44]. This quantity allows for comparison between transmission values and is used for construction of the dynamical extension of DTF, which will be described later.

The value of $\mathrm{DTF}_{j\to i}(f)$ is typically different than $\mathrm{DTF}_{i\to j}(f)$, so we can distinguish the direction of influence by comparing these two values. There may be the case when both values of DTF are big, which means that both signals can be considered causal for each other or the relation is reciprocal. We would not be able to detect such a situation by coherence phase analysis.

7.3.6 Concept of Partial Measures

In systems containing more than two signals, we can observe not only influences between one signal on another, but more complex interactions between signals are possible. To investigate specific properties of such data sets special functions were introduced.

The concept of partialization of relations in a three-channel set can be presented in a following way: we want to measure only the influence of channel 1 on channel 2 with influence of channel 3 removed. In the time domain, we may partialize the covariance $R_{12}(s)$ by subtracting covariations with the third signal:

$$R_{12|3}(s) \sim R_{12}(s) - R_{13}(s)R_{32}(s) \tag{7.23}$$

Precisely, the partial correlation is given by such a formula supplemented by a normalization term:

$$R_{12|3}(s) = \frac{R_{12}(s) - R_{13}(s)R_{32}(s)}{\sqrt{(1 - R_{13}^2(s))(1 - R_{32}^2(s))}} \tag{7.24}$$

In the frequency domain, this concept can be translated to the so-called partial coherence. For a three-channel set, we get a formula for coherence between signals 1 and 2 partialized against signal 3:

$$C_{12|3}(f) = \frac{S_{12}(f) - S_{13}(f)S_{32}(f)}{\sqrt{\left(1-|S_{13}(f)|^2\right)\left(1-|S_{32}(f)|^2\right)}} \tag{7.25}$$

where S_{ij} are elements of the spectral matrix of the process.

In a general (multivariate) case, the partial coherence is defined as

$$C_{ij}(f) = \frac{\mathbf{M}_{ij}(f)}{\sqrt{\mathbf{M}_{ii}(f)\mathbf{M}_{jj}(f)}} \tag{7.26}$$

and describes only "direct" connections between channels i and j, with all linear combinations of influences of other channels removed. In the above formula $\mathbf{M}_{ij}$ is a minor (determinant) of matrix **S** with i-th row and j-th column removed. It can be shown that the Equation 7.26 may be presented using d_{ij}—elements of the inverse of the matrix **S**

$$C_{ij}(f) = (-1)^{i+j}\frac{d_{ji}(f)}{\sqrt{d_{jj}(f)d_{ii}(f)}} \tag{7.27}$$

Values of partial coherence modulus are in [0,1] range.

Another possibility in a three or more channel set is a situation when several channels contain common signal component. To evaluate if a channel is similar to any other channel of the set we use the multiple coherence:

$$G_i(f) = \sqrt{1 - \frac{\det(\mathbf{S}(f))}{S_{ii}(f)\mathbf{M}_{ii}(f)}} \tag{7.28}$$

This quantity tells us if channel i is similar to any other channel from the set. The modulus of multiple coherence takes values from [0,1] range, where zero means that channel i is not coherent with any other channel of the set.

In order to distinguish the different coherence functions, the quantity given by Equation 7.26 is often called the *ordinary* coherence function.

The need to define partial measures in the area of causal influence estimators is expressed by construction of measures able to detect only direct transmissions. DTF detects the fact of signal transmission between channel i and channel j, no matter how that signal was transferred between these locations. The signal could be transferred directly, but in systems of more than two channels, the signal can be transmitted through several other channels before it appears at the destination channel. In order to resolve that problem several functions were proposed in the literature.

Baccalá and Sameshima [7] introduced partial directed coherence (PDC), defined by formula:

$$\gamma_{ij}(f) = \frac{A_{ij}(f)}{\sqrt{\sum_{m=1}^{k}\left|A_{mj}(f)\right|^2}} \tag{7.29}$$

$A(f)$ is the Fourier transformed model coefficient (Equations 7.8 and 7.9). The PDC is a normalized function and takes values from [0,1] range. It presents a ratio between influence of channel i on channel

j and all outflows from channel j. This type of normalization makes the PDC more focused on sinks of activity than on sources. Recently, the modification of PDC called generalized partial directed coherence (GPDC) was proposed [8], according to the formula (for transmission from channel j to i):

$$\pi_{ij}(f) = \frac{A_{ij}(f)\frac{1}{\sigma_i}}{\sqrt{\sum_{m=1}^{k}\left|A_{mj}(f)\frac{1}{\sigma_m}\right|^2}} \tag{7.30}$$

where $\sigma_i^2 = V_{ii}$, the i-th diagonal element of the model noise variance matrix $\mathbf{V}$.

Yet another proposition for a direct causal estimator can be found in Korzeniewska et al. [54]. The direct DTF (dDTF) function presented there is based on a concept of combining DTF with partial coherence. In practical realization it utilizes a modification of the original DTF function, which makes the normalization term independent of frequency.

$$\chi_{ij}^2(f) = F_{ij}^2(f)C_{ij}^2(f) \tag{7.31}$$

dDTF has a nonzero value when both functions simultaneously are nonzero; that situation indicates a presence of transmission while the relation is direct (Figure 7.2).

Various comparisons of performance of different causal estimators can be found in the literature (e.g., [80,94]). Here we present a picture from Ref. [56] where a comparison of selected estimators applied to the real EEG was made. The 21-channels EEG signal was recorded from scalp electrodes (10–20 system [76]) from an adult human subject resting awake with eyes closed. Under such a condition, the alpha rhythm was generated in posterior areas and it was spread toward other derivations to the front of the head. Given the 20-s-long epoch of data (highpass forward and backward filtered above 3 Hz), a MVAR model of order 4 was fitted. DTF, dDTF, and PDC functions were calculated. For presentation purposes integrals of the functions in the range of 7–15 Hz were calculated. Results are plotted in the form of arrows pointing from the source to the destination channels, and the connection of strength (integrated function) is coded in a shade of gray. Only 40 strongest flows are shown.

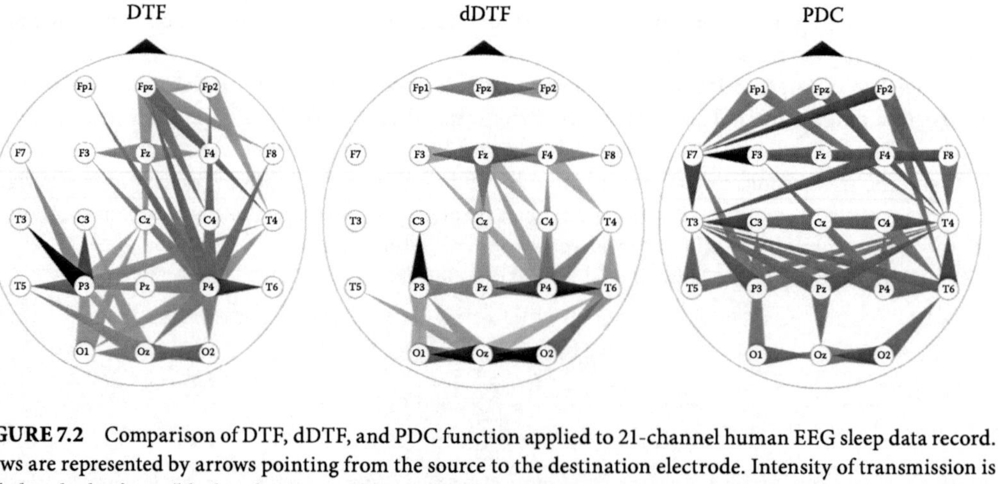

FIGURE 7.2 Comparison of DTF, dDTF, and PDC function applied to 21-channel human EEG sleep data record. Flows are represented by arrows pointing from the source to the destination electrode. Intensity of transmission is coded in shade of gray (black = the strongest). Only 40 strongest flows are shown for each function. (Reprinted from Kuś R, Kamiński M, Blinowska KJ. *IEEE Trans Biomed Eng* 51:1501–1510 © 2004 IEEE.)

In the DTF pattern, we may observe main sources of alpha activity located around P3 and P4 electrodes transmitting their activity in many directions. The dDTF picture lacks most long-distance connections indicating that the direct ones are only the relations between neighbors. The PDC shows quite different pattern. Although the sources at P3 and P4 electrodes are still visible, we see additional sites acting like sources and some sites seem to be sinks of activity.

7.3.7 Dynamical (Nonstationary) Data

When we described the principles of AR model, we said that the model expresses the current value of a process by a linear combination of its previous values with certain constant coefficients $A(i)$. Such a definition implies that we analyze stationary data epochs, where properties of the signals do not vary over time and can be described by the constant model parameters. However, very often we deal with dynamical phenomena with changing patterns of relations. We would like to analyze such processes with AR methodology as well. The solutions present in the literature can be basically divided in two general groups.

The first approach assumes that the model parameters can change over time. This so-called adaptive approach is typically realized by means of Kalman filter methodology, considered to be an optimal linear recursive estimator [83]. During the procedure, we process the nonstationary data and in each step we expand the analyzed epoch of the next sample(s) trying to make corrections to the model in order to improve the fit and minimizing the prediction error. The improvement is done by changing the values of model parameters. In that approach, we need to adjust certain variable controlling the speed of adaptation process; if the speed is too fast the model will follow every fluctuation of the data, if it is too slow the adaptation will not reveal details of changing patterns of relations. The descriptions of practical realizations of the Kalman filter for MVAR modeling can be found in literature [2,9,39,64].

The other possibility is called the short sliding window method [23]. Its application is possible when multiple repetitions (N_T) of an experiment and data recording are available. In that case, we assume that the repetitions of the experiment can be treated as different realizations of the same stochastic process (or, in other words, the process of the same origin and properties). Based on that assumption, we exchange averaging of signal properties over time (as we do in the case of long epochs of stationary data) with averaging over realizations (shorter epochs, multiple trials). This approach makes possible dividing the overall recording epoch into shorter time windows, possibly short enough to treat the data in each window as stationary. During model fitting, we do not average the data; we estimate the correlation matrix for each realization and average these estimates. The averaged correlation matrix is then used to estimate one final MVAR model for that window. Finally, from the model parameters all the interesting quantities: spectrum, coherences and causal estimators can be calculated. The time windows can overlap each other to get smoother results.

The short time window procedure contains certain preprocessing steps and, like in the case of adaptive approach, may need certain adjustments. The most important is the window size (N) selection. A shorter window can better track the dynamics of fast-changing phenomena but choosing the window size too short may compromise the quality of the fit of the model. Although there is no strict rule about the number of data points ($N \cdot N_T \cdot k$) and number of model parameters ($k^2 p$), researchers agree that there should be at least several times more data points than the parameters. It means that having only a few realizations we cannot use too short windows.

If we analyze the signal of evoked response type, where a slower wave appears over ongoing background activity of lower amplitude and higher frequency, it may be advisable to subtract the averaged response (ARP, average over realizations) from each realization. Although it may seem like removing the important information from the signal in fact that step assures better stationarity of the signal, especially for those windows which could contain raising ARP slope, and affects only the lowest part of the signal spectrum.

The results of evaluation of dynamics of spectra, coherences or causal estimators have a form of a matrix of time–frequency maps, so to present them we need to visualize connection between channel i

and channel j over time and frequency. They are called short-time versions of the estimators, like short-time directed transfer function (SDTF) presented in Ref. [58].

7.3.8 Statistical Significance

The coherences and causal estimators, especially in the short-time or adaptive versions, are quantities of distributions rather difficult to describe analytically. The asymptotic distribution for DTF in lack of flow case was recently given by Eichler [26]. However, in most cases the statistical properties can be estimated using methods of resampling statistics and surrogate data, depending on the case. The surrogate data technique is a concept of constructing a dataset based on the original dataset, but modified to lack certain property. For instance, we may think of surrogate data where all interrelations between channels have been cancelled. The practical realizations of such data may adapt random shuffling of each channel samples [44]. The other approach, based on idea given in Ref. [87], involves Fourier transforming the data, randomization of their phases and transforming it back to the time domain. This procedure preserves amplitude spectrum of the data while canceling any phase couplings.

Resampling techniques are used to experimentally estimate the distribution of investigated functions. The functions calculated repeatedly for different datasets produce different values. Multiple generations of surrogate datasets can be used to get the distribution and significance levels for baseline (zero-level) value.

The bootstrap method [24,25,95] is especially useful for multiple repetitions case. In that approach, we randomly draw a pool of realizations (data from repetitions of the experiment) for which we calculate the results obtaining the distribution for the given case. For that empirical distribution, we get the desired significance levels.

7.3.9 Bivariate versus Multivariate

The fact that in a more than two-channel system certain channels can be common sources of signal for several other channels have important consequences in analysis of such data. Let us consider a three-channel system where channel 1 transmits its signal to channel 2 with delay of one sample and to channel 3 with delay of two samples. If we analyze every pair of channels (1–2, 1–3, and 2–3), we will get strong relations in each case. However, the relation found between channels 2 and 3 comes only from the fact that they both have a "common driver" signal, they may be independent in all other aspects. To get the correct pattern of relations, we must include all signals into the analysis and use a truly multivariate method of analysis. That so-called pair-wise approach may lead to results that will be difficult to interpret. Figure 7.3 presents results of DTF analysis of three-channel system constructed in a way described above (simulations are reprinted from Ref. [10]). Signal from channel 1 was transmitted to channels 2 and 3 with different delays. Nevertheless, the DTF analysis reveals true pattern of connections, with no transmission $1 \rightarrow 3$.

In Figure 7.4, we observe that channel 5 becomes a "sink of activity," the surprising effect which is an artifact of the applied method.

In general, the problem arises when we did not include all possible sources of signal in our dataset. Because we cannot detect such a situation my means of any mathematical analysis, the careful experiment planning may be essential to understand the obtained results and the investigated system well.

Many methods for cross-quantities analysis, especially nonlinear ones, are designed for a pair of channels only. One must be aware that the difference between pair-wise and multivariate analysis lies not in flaws of the method itself, but is an inherent property of multivariate systems (Figure 7.5).

7.3.10 Linear versus Nonlinear

All the methods described in this chapter, including MVAR, are considered *linear* which means that they can detect linear relations between signals. What can happen when the signals are connected in a

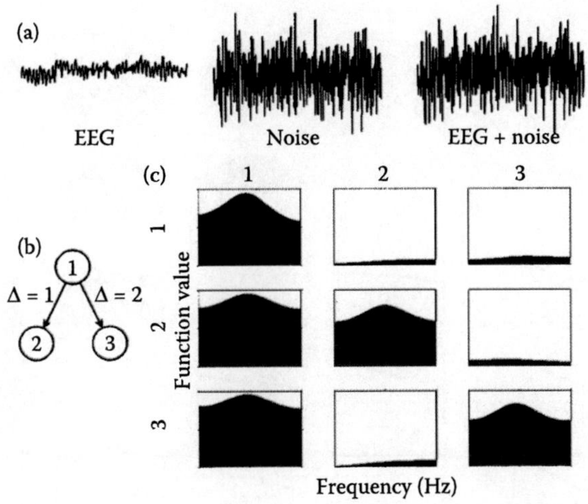

FIGURE 7.3 (a) Simulated signals. (b) Simulation scheme. (c) In each box DTF as functions of frequency (0–25 Hz); the numbers above the columns indicate output channels, the numbers on the left of the rows indicate destination channels. In the next example, we see a five-channel set, where signal from channel 1 appears in the rest of the channels with increasing delays. (Reprinted from Blinowska KJ, Kuś R, Kamiński M. *Phys Rev E* 2004; 70:050902.)

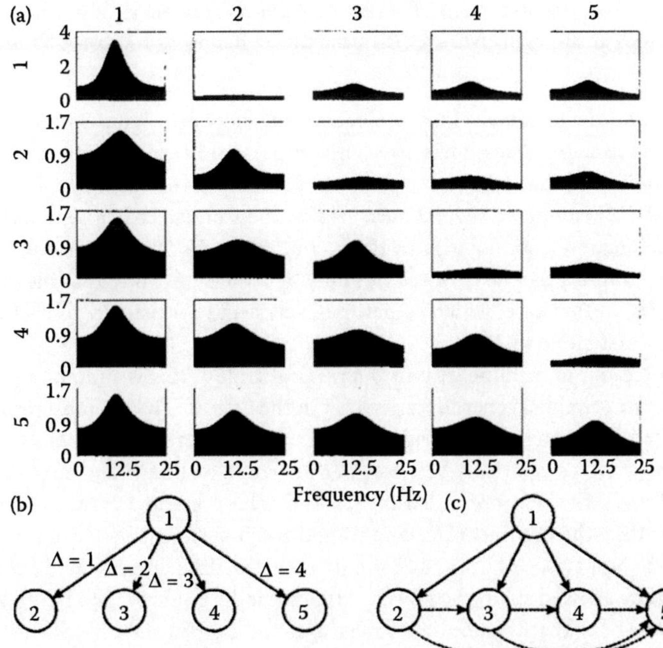

FIGURE 7.4 (a) Granger causality calculated pairwise; each graph represents the function describing transmission from the channel marked above the row to the channel marked on the left of the row. Granger causality in arbitrary units on vertical axes; graphs on the diagonal contain power spectra; frequency on horizontal axes (0–25 Hz range). (b) Simulation scheme. (c) Resulting flow scheme. The black arrows represent true (simulated) flows; the dotted arrows represent false flows found by the applied method. (Reprinted from Blinowska KJ, Kuś R, Kamiński M. *Phys Rev E* 2004; 70:050902.)

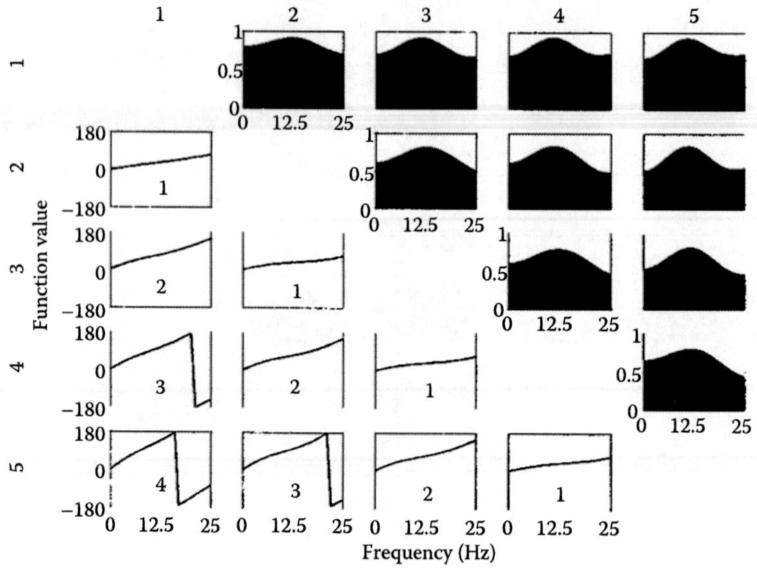

FIGURE 7.5 Pairwise coherences and resulting flows. Top: Coherence amplitude (black graphs above diagonal) and coherence phase (graphs below diagonal); each graph represents the function for the pair of channels marked on the left of the row and above the column; on the horizontal axes frequency (0–25 Hz); on vertical axes coherence amplitudes (0–1 range) or phases (−π–π range); delay values (in samples) estimated from phases, marked by the numbers shown over the phase graphs. Bottom left: Simulation scheme. Bottom right: Resulting flow scheme. The same convention in drawing arrows as in Figure 7.2. (Reprinted from Blinowska KJ, Kuś R, Kamiński M. *Phys Rev E* 2004; 70:050902.)

nonlinear way? Do we need a nonlinear measure of relations between signals? It of course depends on the character of the relation. This question is especially important in the case of brain activity research. Several systematic studies of that type were performed, where linear and nonlinear methods were compared. David et al. [22] compared several measures on the simulated data generated by populations of neurons using different connection patterns, types, and strengths. The conclusion from that work is that in most cases the coupling can be detected not only by a nonlinear but by a linear method too; the sensitivity may be lower in that case, which sometimes may lead to missing a flow. On the other hand, we should not see nonexistent flows.

The problem of detecting of nonlinearity in biomedical time series is present in the literature for many years [29,68,85]. Researchers generally agree that in the case of EEG the most pronounced nonlinear effects can be observed during certain stages of epilepsy. In different conditions there is no definite answer to that question. A comparison between performance of linear and nonlinear approach in forecasting of EEG time series was presented in Ref. [12]. The presented results show that the linear approach is not worse than the nonlinear one and sometimes it performs better in that case.

In Ref. [65], another comparison of linear and nonlinear estimators on simulated examples with noise was presented. The study showed again the power of linear methods in revealing even weak couplings.

Summarizing, we may say that the nonlinear measures should be used only when it is really necessary. Moreover, nonlinear methods are often defined for pairs of signals, which is prone to interpretation difficulties. Considering the fact that nonlinear estimation requires more difficult calculations and the results are often very sensitive to noise, it is advisable to analyze the system with a linear method first to get the overall picture of connections. Such results would be more robust even for noisy signals, which is typical for biomedical data. If some parts of the analysis would require special treatment, the nonlinear analysis can be applied only to that part of the system. Similar conclusions can be found in Ref. [94].

A few examples of nonlinear methods and their applications can be found in Refs. [20,46,72,73,91].

7.4 Examples of Applications in Various Situations

7.4.1 Spike Train Data Analysis

The MVAR methodology cannot be applied directly to analysis of spike train time series. That type of data is characterized by long periods of "silence" (when values of the process do not change or change very little) and fast bursts of activity of high amplitude [15]. The "silent" periods may not have stochastic character at all. However, even spike train data can be adapted to MVAR analysis. The proposition of the procedure can be found in Ref. [50].

In the referred paper, the origin of theta rhythm was investigated in specific structures of the nervous system of rats, namely supramamillary nucleus (SUM), septum (SEP), and hippocampus. It is known that in urethane-anesthetized rats neurons in the SUM fire in synchrony with hippocampal theta rhythm. These neurons project to the septum and hippocampus and it is assumed that they may drive the theta rhythm in the hippocampus. However, the connections between SUM and septohippocampal system are reciprocal and there is evidence that theta rhythm may remain in hippocampus after a lesion of SUM. To investigate connections between these structures, local field potentials (LFP) signals from electrodes implanted in hippocampus and spike trains from SUM neurons were recorded.

To make the MVAR analysis of spike trains possible, a preprocessing procedure was performed. The recording has a form of point process—at the moments of neuron firings the signal has high value and in other time points its value is zero. As the first step, the signal was lowpass filtered. The filter has to preserve the phase of the original signal; it was assured by filtering the data in both directions over time. The cutoff frequency of the filter was at 10% of the Nyquist frequency. Because MVAR model operates on stochastic signals, a small amount (10%) of a noise (uncorrelated with the signal) was added. The signals after the preprocessing steps are presented in Figure 7.6.

To the analysis, 500 samples long (2 s) epochs were selected. Theta oscillations appear around 4 Hz, so the 0–20 Hz frequency range was analyzed. In order to see changes in propagations, the short-time window formalism was used, here applied to the single realization of the experiment; in that study the 2 s long

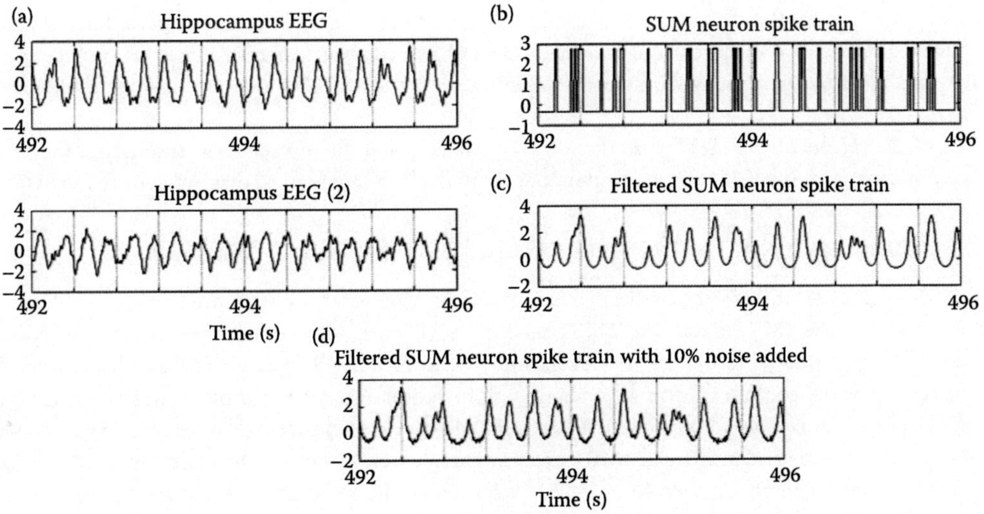

FIGURE 7.6 Preprocessing of signals for DTF. (a) Hippocampal field potentials recorded from hippocampus using two electrodes with a vertical tip separation of 1.5 mm. (b) Standardized spike train from the SUM. (c) Low-pass-filtered spike train. (d) Low-pass-filtered spike train with 10% of noise added. (Reprinted from Kocsis B, Kaminski M. *Hippocampus* 2006; 16(6):531–540.)

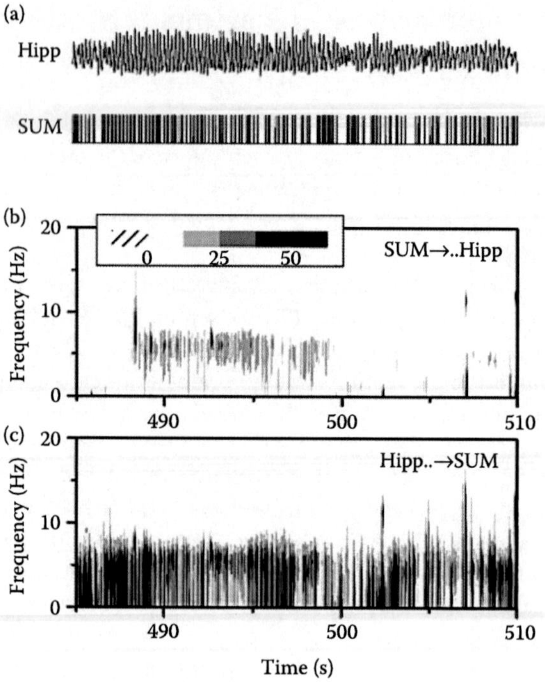

FIGURE 7.7 Activation of the theta drive directed from SUM to hippocampus during sensory stimulation. (a) Traces of rhythmic hippocampal EEG and SUM spike train. Note increase in theta frequency and amplitude during tail pinch between 488 and 499 s. (b) Temporal dynamic of the SUM → Hippocampus DTF. (c) Temporal dynamics of the hippocampus → SUM DTF. (Reprinted from Kocsis B, Kaminski M. *Hippocampus* 2006; 16(6):531–540.)

windows were shifted by 40 ms and in each window the DTF function was calculated. During the experiment the spontaneous theta rhythm was observed. After introducing a stimulus (pinch of the rat's tail), a change in the theta rhythm frequency and amplitude appeared. In Figure 7.7, we see a period of tail pinch and SDTF analysis of that epoch of data. The SUM → hippocampus transmission is low (white color) except for the period of sensory stimulation, when we see higher SDTF values around theta frequency (dark shade).

One of the results of the SDTF study was the conclusion that during sensory stimulation the theta rhythm originates in the SUM while spontaneous theta rhythm seems to be driving neurons in SUM.

7.4.2 Connectivity of Active Areas Found by fMRI Data Analysis

The work of Sato et al. [77] shows that linear modeling can be as well adapted to estimate causal connectivity for the fMRI data. The fMRI technique became popular because of its noninvasive character and high-spatial resolution; however, time resolution of fMRI scans is of the order of seconds. The images typically contain information about concentration of oxygenated blood in brain areas (the quantity called BOLD—blood oxygenated level dependent). Certain methods proposed to assess connectivity between areas identified in fMRI experiments can be found in literature [18,30,37,63]. The problem is that these methods need some *a priori* knowledge about the investigated system and its connections. MVAR modeling is free of such limitations (see also Ref. [61]). In the presented paper, fMRI images were collected during a language-related task. Incomplete sentences were presented on screen for 2.5 s followed by a blank screen. After 700 ms the missing word appeared and subject had to respond if that word completed the sentence or not. Eighty sentences were presented to the subjects. During the experiment, gradient echo-planar images were acquired at the Maudsley Hospital, Institute of Psychiatry,

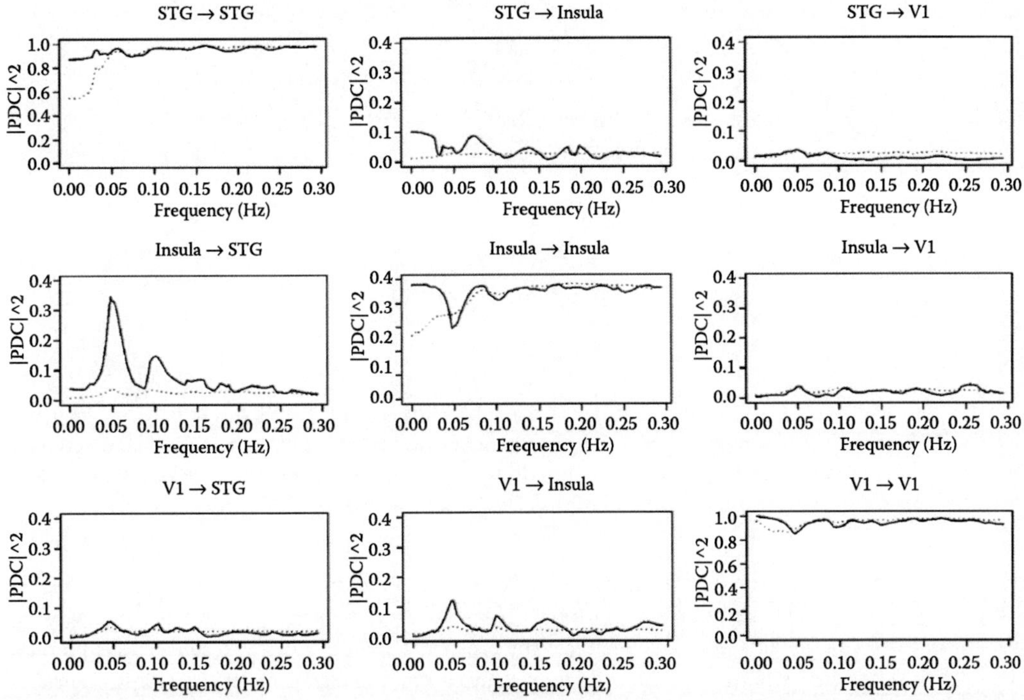

FIGURE 7.8 ROIs' multisubject median PDC. The dotted line shows the 95% confidence upper bound under the hypothesis of no connectivity between the nodes. (Reprinted from Sato JR et al. *Hum Brain Mapp* 2009; 30:452–461.)

King's College, London. The fMRI data was preprocessed by using head motion realignment, slice time correction, spatial smoothing, and normalization to Talaraich and Tournoux space [86]. Brain group activation maps were calculated and based on them primary visual cortex (V1), superior temporal gyrus (STG), and Insula were selected as regions of interest (ROI). For the connectivity analysis the GPDC function was used. The time series were constructed from averaged BOLD data from selected ROIs, normalized to zero mean, and unit variance. Spectral analysis of the ROI time series shows significant power at 0.049 Hz frequency and its harmonic, which is equal to the stimulation frequency. During GPDC analysis data from multiple subjects were incorporated. The authors proposed a complete algorithm for assessing statistical significance of the results in that case, based on the bootstrap method.

Significant connectivity was found around the maximum power frequencies, as it is shown on the graph (Figure 7.8). One can notice strong information flow from the Insula to STG and also from V1 to the Insula. The conclusion is that the information is first transmitted from visual cortex (V1) to the Insula and to the STG. These results were compared with coherence analysis which agrees with the GPDC results but was unable to show the detailed pattern of transmissions. Although fMRI experiments do not provide information about what, where, and how the information is processed during a task, the method introduced in the presented paper was able to show existence of connectivity networks based on the collected data (see also [90]) (Figure 7.9).

7.4.3 Dynamics of Transmissions during a Cognitive Task: Scalp EEG Data Analysis

Another example of MVAR model application is estimation of general dynamical pattern of connectivity from scalp EEG. In the paper [11], the continuous attention test (CAT [89]) was investigated.

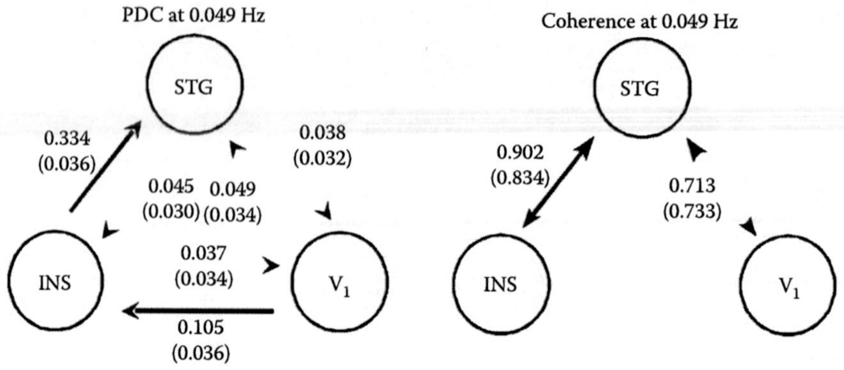

FIGURE 7.9 Multisubject median PDC at 0.049 Hz, simple coherence at 0.049 Hz (using the same bootstrap algorithm). The frequency of stimulation in the language paradigm was 0.049 Hz. The thick solid lines describe the links with relevant intensity of information flow. The critical regions at 5% of significance are values greater than the shown in parentheses. (Reprinted from Sato JR et al. *Hum Brain Mapp* 2009; 30:452–461.)

The experiment was performed at Department of Biomedical Physics, University of Warsaw, Poland. Visual stimuli (small checkerboards type) were presented on screen in random time intervals for human subjects. The subjects were asked to react (by pressing a switch) when two consecutive pictures were identical ("target" situation). Each of 16 young human male subjects observed 720 patterns, 120 of them were identical to preceding ones. EEG was collected during the experiment from 23 scalp electrodes with locations conforming to 10–20 standard [76]. After artifact-removal procedure, nine subjects were left for analysis. The data were filtered in the range of 15–45 Hz. Epochs from 0.5 s before to 1 s after the stimulus presentation were selected. The analysis was done by means of the SDTF function. Because the experiment was performed many times, multiple repetitions of the datasets were available. This allowed using the short-time methodology with windows short enough to capture changes in the relations between signals. A set of 12 selected channels was used in calculations. The sliding window of 20 samples (160 ms) was used, shifted each time by 2 samples (8 ms, overlapped windows). Trials were synchronized according to the motor reaction. The first 0.5 s at the beginning of the considered record was used as a reference to assess significant changes of transmissions during the test.

For statistical testing of the differences between the flows during the CAT test performance and the reference period, the methodology presented in Ref. [53] was used. It assumes that the nonstationary SDTF consists of a smooth trend and a noise component. The smooth trend was estimated and its values are considered different for a certain time value if they are different for every value of the reference period at a given frequency. The details can be found in Ref. [53].

The statistically significant changes of flow were analyzed for "target" (the switch was pressed when it should be) and "nontarget" (the switch was not pressed when it should not be) situations. For better visualization purposes, the SDTF values were integrated over frequency values of interest: beta (15–25 Hz) and gamma (25–45 Hz). The integrated values were presented in forms of arrows on an image of the head. The value of flow change was coded in color and transparence of an arrow (Figure 7.10).

Certain consistent patterns of transmissions were observed for multiple subjects. During the first stage, connected with the mental comparison of displayed pattern and decision making, the propagation from prefrontal electrodes was visible. The next stage was "silent" for target condition while for the nontarget condition propagation from electrode F8 to electrode C3 was observed, interpreted as active inhibition from right inferior cortex to hand motor area. In the third stage in target condition propagation from C3 appeared, connected with performing the hand movement (pressing the switch).

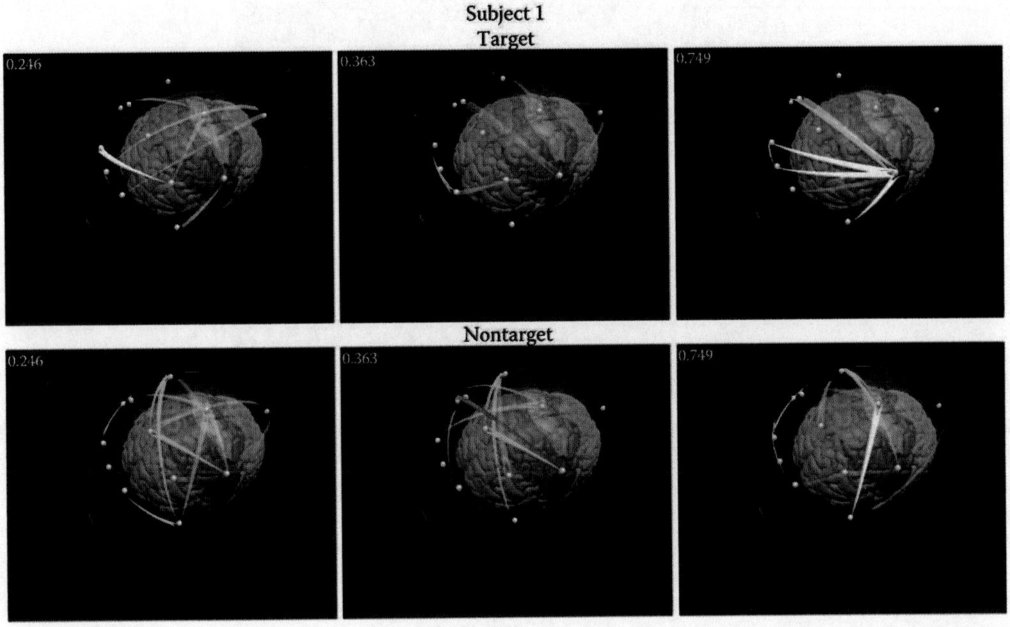

FIGURE 7.10 **(See color insert.)** Snapshots from the movie presenting significant changes in transmissions in one subject, for target (upper) and nontarget (lower part). Intensity of flow changes for increase: from pale yellow to red, for decrease: from light to dark blue. In the right upper corner the time after cue presentation (in seconds). (Reprinted from Blinowska K et al. *Brain Topogr* 2010; 23:205–213.)

Another version of data analysis in that experiment, with trials aligned according to the stimulus presentation time, can be found in Ref. [55].

The method of estimation of EEG signal propagation based on SDTF gives information on processes acting in the scale of milliseconds and allows for understanding the dynamical interactions between brain structures, even during tasks involving complex brain functions.

This section showed straightforward analysis of scalp EEG recordings. An interesting extension of scalp EEG research is presented in Refs. [3–5] or [6]. The authors record scalp EEG data and but before the analysis they perform regularized linear inverse source evaluation of cortical current density which estimates currents at the chosen ROIs from the values at the recording electrodes. The further analysis of functional cortical connectivity is done by computing the DTF or PDC on the estimated cortical current density waveforms in the ROIs. That way the results concern the precisely chosen locations. Together with the EEG analysis other types of data (fMRI, MEG) are simultaneously processed showing validity of the estimates.

7.4.4 Localization of Epileptic Foci: LFP Data Analysis

An important ability of multivariate causal estimators is locating sources of activity. This property can be used, for instance, to trace a localization of an epileptogenic focus. It is known that certain types of epilepsy are originated from an area of pathologically functioning tissue called a focus. In cases of seizures refractory to medical therapy, a possible treatment is to find and resect such a focus. Before that, electrodes are implanted in selected structures of the nervous system in order to provide recordings which are visually inspected by neurologists. In the presented paper ([28], see also [27]) cases of three patients were reanalyzed (after the actual surgery) using the DTF method. The data from patients were recorded at University of Maryland at Baltimore, USA. 32-contact subdural grid array was placed over the lateral temporal lobe and one or two 8-contact depth electrode arrays were placed in mesial temporal

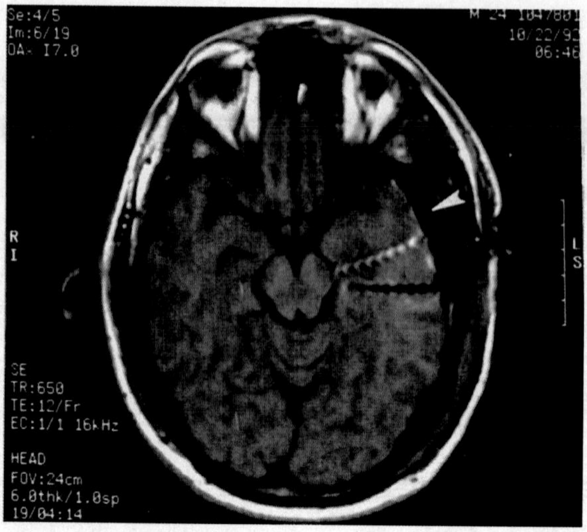

FIGURE 7.11 T1-weighted axial MRI image revealing two depth electrode arrays passing through 32-contact subdural grid array (arrow). The subdural grid array overlies the lateral temporal surface. The deepest contacts of the depth electrode array are in the amygdala and hippocampus, respectively. (Reprinted from Franaszczuk PJ, Bergey GK, Kamiński M. *Electroenceph Clin Neurophys* 1994; 91:413–427.)

structures as it was shown in the MRI image (Figure 7.11). Total of 64 channels of data during several seizures were collected with sapling frequency of 200 Hz.

To the analysis 16-channel segments of 200 samples (1 s) were selected. In the case of highly nonstationary signals longer epochs with more channels were analyzed. The results were calculated in 1–25 Hz frequency range; above 25 Hz the spectral power was low. Because both surface and depth electrodes were implanted, it was possible to see activity spreading from deeper structures to the cortex surface. For the first patient the epileptic activity was identified around 18 Hz. The DTF and autospectra graphs for the selected set of depth electrodes are shown in Figure 7.12. We see spectral peak at 18 Hz and at the same frequency high values of H2 → H1 and H2 → H3 transmissions and transmissions from H1 electrode to several others, suggesting the location of the source around H2 depth electrode. In that case epileptogenic focus was indeed located in deep mesial structures.

In the paper all three cases are discussed. We present only the analysis of the first patient case. As the conclusion, we see that MVAR formalism can be applied even for seizure recordings, when the nonlinear character of signal generation is probably most prominent for all EEG recordings. Selecting stationary fragment of such data from different parts of a seizure allows determining the patterns of seizure onset and propagation. In addition, the DTF method can provide evidence regarding patterns of flow of seizure activity that are not readily apparent from visual inspection. Moreover, we can determine if the initial focus continues to be the source of a given frequency or whether other areas become secondary generators.

7.5 Summary

Simultaneous recording from many different neurons and/or neural assemblies offers a window into how neurons work in concert to generate specific brain functions. Yet, it also presents important signal processing challenges that must be resolved to answer questions about how the brain works. Multivariate time series analysis provides the basic framework for analyzing the patterns of neural interactions in these data. Without substantial methodological development, our ability to understand the brain functions will be significantly hampered because the traditional methods fall short of what ultimately required for the analysis of multivariate neural data.

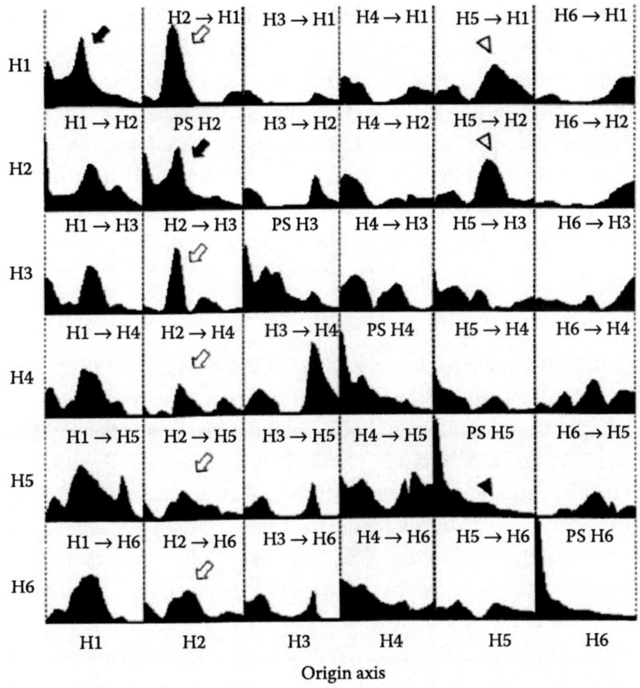

FIGURE 7.12 DTF for the seizure activity recorded from the hippocampal depth electrode during the third second of the seizure. The power spectra for each depth electrode contact are on the diagonal. The peak on the power spectra at 18 Hz is best seen in the deepest contact (H1, H2: solid arrows) but is also seen in the intermediate contacts (H3, H4). The open arrows identify prominent peaks in the DTF graphs corresponding to this peak in the power spectra (column H2). The most important peaks in the DTF graphs are those that have corresponding peaks in the power spectra. Peaks can be identified in the H5 column (open arrowheads) but there is no prominent peak at this frequency in the power spectrum for H5: only a small peak is seen (closed arrowhead). Each individual DTF is labeled to reflect the pattern of flow shown (e.g., H1 → H2). The model order was 5. The horizontal scale for each box is 0.5–50 Hz. The vertical scale for the DTF is 0–1 (full scale). The power spectra are normalized to unit power. (Reprinted from Franaszczuk PJ, Bergey GK, Kamiński M. *Electroenceph Clin Neurophys* 1994; 91:413–427.)

Therefore, in this chapter we have reviewed recent advances of causal influence measures for analyzing multivariate neural data under the framework of MAR modeling. Practical technical issues including stationarity/nonstationarity, bivariate/multivariate, linearity/nonlinearity, and statistical significance are specifically discussed. A variety of applications ranging from basic neuroscience research to clinical relevance are presented. For basic applications, we have stressed the typical applications in the analysis of spike trains, EEG, and fMRI BOLD data, each representing a major recording modality used in neuroscience research. For clinical applications, we have selected the epileptogenic seizure localization as a direct demonstration. We believe that Granger causality analysis offers a new outlook for examining patterns of neural interactions in complex brain networks, and should be a useful addition to the current analytical repertoire in revealing causal influences and directions of driving among multiple neural signals.

We should stress here that by analyzing biomedical data, especially EEG, MEG, or others (fMRI) in order to find interrelations between nervous system structures, we estimate the so-called *functional connectivity* [17]. That term refers to fact, that we observe and record acts of influence between measured regions, as it is realized in the moment of recordings. On the other hand, we may want to know *anatomical connectivity* between these regions. That knowledge comes from anatomical and histological research rather than data analysis. We may note that revealed paths of functional connectivity should be realized over existing paths of possible anatomical connections. However, as we have seen in this chapter, some connections may not be direct and signal may travel from its source to the destination (where it was recorded) by a more complex path. The actual transmission may be realized only over some paths, not every potentially possible. Some paths may be reciprocal and the direction of influence is what we want to reveal, and that is the place for multivariate data analysis methods.

We did not cover all possible approaches in biomedical data analysis, like graph theory or mutual information analysis, but the issues discussed in this chapter should be helpful in all typical problems possible to encounter in research practice. For further reading, there are many signal analysis handbooks [1, 13,21,36,38,42,47,49,60,62,71,74, 75,81] and overview articles available [40,41,45,48,51,52,78,79,84,88].

References

1. Anderson TW. *An Introduction to Multivariate Statistical Analysis*. New York: John Wiley & Sons, 1984.
2. Arnold M, Miltner WHR, Bauer R, Braun C. Multivariate autoregressive modeling of nonstationary time series by means of Kalman filtering. *IEEE Trans Biomed Eng* 1998; 45:553–62.
3. Astolfi L, Cincotti F, Mattia D, Babiloni C, Carducci F, Basiliasco A, Rossini PM, Salinari S, Ding L, Ni Y. Assessing cortical functional connectivity by linear inverse estimation and directed transfer function: Simulations and application to real data. *Clin Neurophysiol* 2005; 116(4):920–932.
4. Astolfi L, Cincotti F, Mattia D, Marciani MG, Baccala LA, de Vico Fallani F, Salinari S, Ursino M, Zavaglia M, Babiloni F. Assessing cortical functional connectivity by partial directed coherence: Simulations and application to real data. *IEEE Trans Biomed Eng* 2006; 53(9):1802–1812.
5. Babiloni F, Cincotti F, Babiloni C, Carducci F, Mattia D, Astolfi L, Basiliasco A et al. Estimation of the cortical functional connectivity with the multimodal integration of high-resolution EEG and fMRI data by directed transfer function. *Neuroimage* 2005; 24(1):118–131.
6. Babiloni F, Mattia D, Babiloni C, Astolfi L, Salinari S, Basilisco A, Rossini PM, Marciani MG, Cincotti F. Multimodal integration of EEG, MEG and fMRI data for the solution of the neuroimage puzzle (Proceedings of the International school on magnetic resonance and brain function—Frontiers of brain functional MRI and electrophysiological methods). *Magn Reson Imaging* 2004; 22(10):1471–1476.
7. Baccalá LA, Sameshima K. Partial directed coherence: A new concept in neural structure determination. *Biol Cybern* 2001; 84:463–474.
8. Baccala LA, Takahashi, YD, Sameshima K. Generalized partial directed coherence. *Proc. of the 2007, 15th International Conference on Digital Signal Processing. IEEE*, 2006; 1:162–166.
9. Benveniste A, Metivier M, Priouret P. *Adaptive Algorithms and Stochastic Approximations*. Berlin: Springer-Verlag, 1990.
10. Blinowska KJ, Kuś R, Kamiński M. Granger causality and information flow in multivariate processes. *Phys Rev E* 2004; 70:050902.
11. Blinowska K, Kus R, Kaminski M, Janiszewska J. Transmission of brain activity during cognitive task. *Brain Topogr* 2010; 23:205–213.
12. Blinowska KJ, Malinowski M. Non-linear and linear forecasting of the EEG time series. *Biol Cybern* 1991; 66:159–165.
13. Box G, Jenkins GM, Reinsel G. *Time Series Analysis: Forecasting and Control*. Englewood Cliffs, NJ: Prentice-Hall, 1994.
14. Box GEP, Tiao GC. *Bayesian Inference in Statistical Analysis*. New York: John Wiley, 1992.
15. Brillinger DR. Comparative aspects of the study of ordinary time series and point processes. *Dev Stat* 1978; 5:33–133.
16. Brovelli A, Ding M, Ledberg A, Chen Y, Nakamura R, Bressler SL. Beta oscillations in a large-scale sensorimotor cortical network: Directional influences revealed by Granger causality. *Proc Natl Acad Sci* 2004; 101(26):9849–9854.
17. Büchel C, Friston K. Characterizing functional integration. In: Frackowiak RSJ, Friston KJ, Frith CD, Dolan RJ, Mazziotta JC, (eds.). *Human Brain Function*. New York: Academic Press, 1997; pp. 127–140.

18. Büchel C, Friston K. Modulation of connectivity in visual pathways by attention: Cortical interactions evaluated with structural equation modeling and fMRI. *Cereb Cortex* 1997; 7:768–778.
19. Chen Y, Bressler SL, Ding M. Frequency decomposition of conditional Granger causality and application to multivariate neural field potential data. *J Neurosci Meth* 2006; 150:228–237.
20. Chen Y, Rangarajan G, Feng J, Ding M. Analyzing multiple nonlinear time series with extended Granger causality. *Phys Lett A* 2004; 324:26–35.
21. Dahlhaus R, Kurths J, Maass P, Timmer J (eds.). *Mathematical Methods in Time Series Analysis and Digital Image Processing (Understanding Complex Systems)*, Berlin: Springer, 2008.
22. David O, Cosmelli D, Friston KJ. Evaluation of different measures of functional connectivity using a neural mass model. *NeuroImage* 2004; 21:659–673.
23. Ding M, Bressler SL, Yang W, Liang H. Short-window spectral analysis of cortical event-related potentials by adaptive multivariate autoregressive modeling: Data preprocessing, model validation, and variability assessment. *Biol Cybern* 2000; 83:35–45.
24. Efron B. Bootstrap methods: Another look at the jackknife. *Ann Stat* 1979; 7:1–26.
25. Efron B, Tibshirani RJ. *An Introduction to the Bootstrap*. London: Chapman & Hall, 1993.
26. Eichler M. On the evaluation of information flow in multivariate systems by the directed transfer function. *Biol Cybern* 2006; 94(6):469–482.
27. Franaszczuk PJ, Bergey GK. Application of the directed transfer function method to mesial and lateral onset temporal lobe seizures. *Brain Topogr* 1998; 11:13–21.
28. Franaszczuk PJ, Bergey GK, Kamiński M. Analysis of mesial temporal seizure onset and propagation using the directed transfer function method. *Electroenceph Clin Neurophys* 1994; 91:413–427.
29. Freiwald WA, Valdes P, Bosch J, Biscay R, Jimenez JC, Rodriguez LM, Rodriguez V, Kreiter AK, Singer W. Testing non-linearity and directedness of interactions between neural groups in the macaque inferotemporal cortex. *J Neurosci Meth* 1999; 94:105–119.
30. Friston KJ, Harrison L, Penny W. Dynamic causal modeling. *Neuroimage* 2003; 19:1273–1302.
31. Geweke J. Measurement of linear dependence and feedback between multiple time series. *J Am Stat Assoc* 1982; 77:304–324.
32. Geweke J. Measures of conditional linear dependence and feedback between time series. *J Am Stat Assoc* 1984; 79:907–915.
33. Govindan RB, Raethjen J, Kopper F, Claussen JC, Deuschl G. Estimation of time delay by coherence analysis. *Physica A* 2005; 350:277–295.
34. Granger CWJ. Investigating causal relations in by econometric models and cross-spectral methods. *Econometrica* 1969; 37:424–438.
35. Guo S, Seth AK, Kendrick KM, Zhou C, Feng J. Partial Granger causality—Eliminating exogenous inputs and latent variables. *J Neurosci Meth* 2008;172:79–93.
36. Hamilton JD. *Time Series Analysis*. Princeton, NJ: Princeton University Press.
37. Harrison L, Penny WD, Friston K. Multivariate autoregressive modeling of fMRI time series. *NeuroImage* 2003; 19:1477–1491.
38. Hayes MH. *Statistical Digital Signal Processing and Modeling*. New York: Wiley & Sons, 1996.
39. Hesse W, Möller E, Arnold M, Schack B. The use of time-variant EEG Granger causality for inspecting directed interdependencies of neural assemblies. *J Neurosci Meth* 2003; 124:27–44.
40. Isaksson A, Wennberg A, Zetterberg LH. Computer analysis of EEG signals with parametric models. *Proc IEEE* 1981; 69:451–61.
41. Jansen BH. Analysis of biomedical signals by means of linear modeling. *CRC Crit Rev Biomed Eng* 1985; 12(4):343–392.
42. Jenkins GM, Watts DG. *Spectral Analysis and its Applications*. SF: Holden-Day, 1968.
43. Kamiński M, Blinowska KJ. A new method of the description of the information flow in brain structures. *Biol Cybern* 1991; 65:203–210.

44. Kamiński M, Ding M, Truccolo W, Bressler S. Evaluating causal relations in neural systems: Granger causality, directed transfer function and statistical assessment of significance. *Biol Cybern* 2001; 85:145–157.
45. Kaminski M., Liang H. Causal influence: Advances in neurosignal analysis. *Crit Rev Biomed Eng* 2005; 33(4):347–430.
46. Kantz H, Schreiber T. *Nonlinear Time Series Analysis*. Cambridge: Cambridge University Press, 2004.
47. Kay SM. *Modern Spectral Estimation*. Englewood Cliffs, NJ: Prentice-Hall, 1988.
48. Kelly EF, Lenz JE, Franaszczuk PJ, Truong YK. A general statistical framework for frequency-domain analysis of EEG topographic structure. *Comput Biomed Res* 1997; 30:129–164.
49. Kemp B, Lopes da Silva FH. Model-based analysis of neurophysiological signals. In: Weitkunat R, (ed.). *Digital Biosignal Processing*. Amsterdam: Elsevier, 1991; pp. 129–155.
50. Kocsis B, Kaminski M. Dynamic changes in the direction of the theta rhythmic drive between supramammillary nucleus and the septohippocampal system. *Hippocampus* 2006; 16(6):531–540.
51. Korhonen I, Mainardi L, Baselli G, Bianchi A, Loula P, Carrault G. Linear multivariate models for physiological signal analysis: Applications. *Comput Meth Prog Biomedic* 1996; 51:121–30.
52. Korhonen I, Mainardi L, Loula P, Carrault G, Baselli G, Bianchi A. Linear multivariate models for physiological signal analysis: Theory. *Comput Meth Prog Biomedic* 1996; 51:85–94.
53. Korzeniewska A, Crainiceanu C, Kus R, Franaszczuk PJ, Crone NE. Dynamics of event-related causality (ERC) in brain electrical activity. *Hum Brain Mapp* 2008; 29:1170–1192.
54. Korzeniewska A, Mańczak M, Kamiński M, Blinowska KJ, Kasicki S. Determination of information flow direction between brain structures by a modified Directed Transfer Function method (dDTF). *J Neurosci Meth* 2003; 125:195–207.
55. Kus R, Blinowska KJ, Kaminski M, Basinska-Starzycka A. Transmission of information during Continuous Attention Test. *Acta Neurobiol Exp* 2008; 68:103–112.
56. Kuś R, Kamiński M, Blinowska KJ. Determination of EEG activity propagation: Pair-wise versus multichannel estimate. *IEEE Trans Biomed Eng* 2004; 51:1501–1510.
57. Liang H, Bressler SL, Ding M, Desimone R, Fries P. Temporal dynamics of attention-modulated neuronal synchronization in macaque V4. *Neurocomputing* 2003; 52–54:481–487.
58. Liang H, Ding M, Nakamura R, Bressler SL. Causal influences in primate cerebral cortex during visual pattern discrimination. *Neuroreport* 2000; 11:2875–2880.
59. Lutkepohl H. Comparison of criteria for estimating the order of a vector autoregressive process. *J Time Ser Anal* 1985; 6(1):35–52.
60. Lutkepohl H. *Introduction to Multiple Time Series Analysis*. New York: Springer, 1993.
61. Mader W, Feess D, Lange R, Saur D, Glauche V, Weiller C, Timmer J, Schelter B. On the detection of direct directed information flow in fMRI. *IEEE J Sel Top Sig Proc* 2008; 2(6):965–974.
62. Marple SL. *Digital Spectral Analysis with Applications Prentice-Hall Signal Processing Series*. New Jersey: Simon & Schuster, 1987.
63. McIntosh AR, Gonzalez-Lima F. Structural equation modeling and its application to network analysis of functional brain imaging. *Hum Brain Map* 1994; 2:2–22.
64. Möller E, Schack B, Arnold M, Witte H. Instantaneous multivariate EEG coherence analysis by means of adaptive high-dimensional autoregressive models. *J Neurosci Meth* 2001; 105:143–158.
65. Netoff TI, Caroll L, Pecora LM, Schiff SJ. Detecting coupling in the presence of noise and nonlinearity. In: Scheleter B, Winterhalder M, Timmer J. (eds.). *Handbook of Time Series Analysis*. Weinheim: Wiley VCH, 2006.
66. Neumaier A, Schneider T. Estimation of parameters and eigenmodes of multivariate autoregressive models. *ACM Trans Math Software* 2001; 27(1):27–57.
67. Oppenheim AV, Schafer RW. *Discrete-time Signal Processing*. Englewood Cliffs, NJ: Prentice-Hall, 1989.
68. Paluš M. Detecting nonlinearity in multivariate time series. *Phys Lett A* 1996; 213:138.

69. Pascual-Marqui RD. Instantaneous and lagged measurements of linear and nonlinear dependence between groups of multivariate time series: Frequency decomposition. arXiv:0711.1455 [stat.ME], 2007; http://arxiv.org/abs/0711.1455.
70. Penny WD, Roberts SJ. Bayesian multivariate autoregressive models with structured priors. *IEE Proc Vision Image Sig Proc* 2002; 149:33–41.
71. Percival DB, Walden AT. *Spectral Analysis for Physical Applications*. Cambridge, UK: Cambridge University Press, 1993.
72. Pereda E, Quiroga RQ, Bhattacharya J. Nonlinear multivariate analysis of neurophysiological signals. *Prog Neurobiol* 2005; 77:1–37.
73. Pereda E, Rial R, Gamundi A, Gonzalez J. Assessment of changing interdependences between human electroencephalograms using nonlinear methods. *Physica D* 2001; 148:147–158.
74. Priestley MB. *Spectral Analysis and Time Series*. London: Academic Press, 1981.
75. Proakis JG, Manolakis DG. *Digital Signal Processing: Principles, Algorithms and Applications*. Englewood Cliffs, NJ: Prentice-Hall, 1996.
76. Rechtschaffen A, Kales A. A manual: Standardized terminology, techniques and scoring system for sleep stages of human subjects. *Brain Information Service. Brain Research Institute, UCLA*, 1968.
77. Sato JR, Takahashi DY, Arcuri SM, Sameshima K, Morettin PA, Baccala LA. Frequency domain connectivity identification: An application of partial directed coherence in fMRI. *Hum Brain Mapp* 2009; 30:452–461.
78. Seth AK. Causal networks in simulated neural systems. *Cogn Neurodyn* 2008; 2:49–64.
79. Schneider T, Neumaier A. Estimation of parameters and eigenmodes of multivariate autoregressive models. *ACM Trans Math Soft* 2001; 27:27–57, 58–65.
80. Schelter B, Winterhalder M, Eichler M, Peifer M, Hellwig B, Guschlbauer B, Lücking HC, Dahlhaus R, Timmer J. Testing for directed influences among neural signals using partial directed coherence. *J Neurosci Meth* 2005; 152:210–219.
81. Schelter B, Winterhalder M, Timmer J (eds.). *Handbook of Time Series Analysis*. Berlin: Wiley-VCH, 2006.
82. Schlögl A. A comparison of multivariate autoregressive estimators. *Signal Processing* 2006; 86:2426–2429.
83. Simon D. *Optimal State Estimation: Kalman, H Infinity, and Nonlinear Approaches*. Hoboken, NJ: Wiley-Interscience, 2006.
84. Spyers-Ashby JM, Bain PG, Roberts SJ. A comparison of fast Fourier transform (FFT) and autoregressive (AR) spectral estimation techniques for the analysis of tremor data. *J Neurosci Meth* 1998; 83:35–43.
85. Stam C, Pijn JPM, Suffczyński P, Lopes da Silva FH. Dynamics of the human alpha rhythm: Evidence for non-linearity? *Clin Neurophys* 1999; 110:1801–1813.
86. Talairach J, Tournoux P. *Co-planar Stereotaxic Atlas of the Human Brain*. New York: Thieme, 1988.
87. Theiler J, Eubank S, Longtin A, Galdrikian B, Farmer D. Testing for nonlinearity in time series: The method of surrogate data. *Physica D* 1992; 58:77–94.
88. Thomson DJ. Spectrum estimation and harmonic analysis. *Proc IEEE* 1982; 70:1055–1096.
89. Tiplady B. Continuous attention: Rationale and discriminant validation of a test designed for the use in psychopharmacology. *Behav Res Methods Instrum Compt* 1992; 24:16–21.
90. Valdés-Sosa PA, Sánchez-Bornot JM, Lage-Castellanos A, Vega-Hernández M, Bosch-Bayard J, Melie-García L, Canales-Rodríguez E. Estimating brain functional connectivity with sparse multivariate autoregression. *Phil Trans R Soc B* 2005; 360:969–981.
91. Veeramani B, Narayanan K, Prasad A, Iasemidis LD, Spanias AS, Tsakalis K. Measuring the direction and the strength of coupling in nonlinear systems—A modeling approach in the state space. *IEEE Sig Proc Lett* 2004; 11:617–620.
92. Verdes PF. Assessing causality from multivariate time series. *Phys Rev E* 2005; 72:026222.
93. Wiener N. The theory of prediction. In: Beckenbach EF, (ed.). *Modern Mathematics for Engineers*. New York: McGraw-Hill, 1956.

94. Winterhalder M, Schelter B, Hesse W, Schwab K, Leistritz L, Klan D, Bauer R, Timmer J, Witte H. Comparison of linear signal processing techniques to infer directed interactions in multivariate neural systems. *Signal Process* 2005; 85:2137–2160.
95. Zoubir AM, Boashash B. The bootstrap and its application in signal processing. *IEEE Sig Proc Mag* 1998; 15:56–76.

Index

C

D

H

I

J

K

L

Q

R

S

U

V

W

Z